D1642768

Test	Reference range	Notes
cholesterol (HDL)	Male 0.9–2.0 mmol/l Female 1.0–2.3 mmol/l	cardiovascular sequelae, hypercholesterolaemia can be caused by diabetes, nephrotic syndrome and biliary obstruction; hypertriglyceridaemia can accompany diabetes, nephritic syndrome pancreatitis, alcohol and oral contraceptives Low levels of HDL are associated with a high risk of myocardial infarction
triglycerides (fasting)	<2.0 mmol/l	Triglyceride values increase with ageing
Osmolality serum	285–295 mOsm/kg	↑ Fluid depletion ↑ Fluid excess
Thyroxine (total)	60–140 mmol/l	↑ Hyperthyroidism (Graves' disease) can be confirmed with TRH chal[...] ↓ Hypothyroidism should be confirmed with TSH measurement and challenge. Thyroxine levels may be decreased by salicylates and p[...] binding displacement
Free T_4	10–25 pmol/l	
Free T_3	5–10.2 pmol/l	
Urate (serum)	Male 0.24–0.48 mmol/l Female 0.16–0.36 mmol/l	↑ May lead to gout. May be due to increased production, e.g. from metabolic defect and carcinoma, or from diminished excretion, e.[...] failure, acidosis and with diuretics
Vitamin B_{12} (serum)	160–900 ng/l	↑ Leads to macrocytic anaemia and peripheral neuropathy. May be c[...] deficiency, pernicious anaemia, ileitis or short-bowel syndrome. St[...] for 2–4 years. Cause can be verified by the Schilling test

*Large variation between labs.
CSF = cerebrospinal fluid; HDL = high-density lipoprotein; IBC = iron-binding capacity; RBC = red blood cells; T_3 = triiod[...]
T_4 = thyroxine; TIBC = total iron-binding capacity; TRH = thyrotrophin-releasing hormone; TSH = thyroid-stimulating ho[...]

Clinical Pharmacy

Commissioning Editors: Ellen Green; Timothy Horne
Development Editor: Ailsa Laing
Project Manager: Gail Wright
Senior Designer: Sarah Russell
Illustrations Buyer: Merlyn Harvey
Illustrator: David Gardner

Clinical Pharmacy

Edited by

Nick Barber BPharm PhD MRPharmS FRSM
Professor of the Practice of Pharmacy,
The School of Pharmacy, University of London,
London, UK

Alan Willson BPharm MSc PhD MRPharmS
Director of Service Development,
National Leadership and Innovation Agency for
Healthcare, Llanharan, Glamorgan, UK

SECOND EDITION

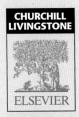

CHURCHILL
LIVINGSTONE

ELSEVIER

EDINBURGH LONDON NEW YORK OXFORD
PHILADELPHIA ST LOUIS SYDNEY TORONTO 2007

An imprint of Elsevier Limited

© Elsevier Limited 1999
© 2007, Elsevier Limited. All rights reserved.

First edition 1999
Second edition 2007

ISBN-13: 978-0-443-07443-1
ISBN-10: 0-443-07443-7

British Library Cataloguing in Publication Data
A catalogue record for this book is available from the British Library

Library of Congress Cataloging in Publication Data
A catalog record for this book is available from the Library of Congress

Note
Knowledge and best practice in this field are constantly changing. As new research and experience broaden our knowledge, changes in practice, treatment and drug therapy may become necessary or appropriate. Readers are advised to check the most current information provided (i) on procedures featured or (ii) by the manufacturer of each product to be administered, to verify the recommended dose or formula, the method and duration of administration, and contraindications. It is the responsibility of the practitioner, relying on their own experience and knowledge of the patient, to make diagnoses, to determine dosages and the best treatment for each individual patient, and to take all appropriate safety precautions. To the fullest extent of the law, neither the Publisher nor the Editors assume any liability for any injury and/or damage to persons or property arising out or related to any use of the material contained in this book.

The Publisher

Printed in China

CONTENTS

CONTRIBUTORS

Caroline Ashley BPharm MSc MRPharmS
Principal Pharmacist Renal Services, Royal Free Hampstead NHS Trust, London, UK

Nick Barber BPharm PhD MRPharmS FRSM
Professor of the Practice of Pharmacy, The School of Pharmacy, University of London, London, UK

Stephanie Barnes BSc MSc MRPharmS
Prinicipal Pharmacist, Clinical Governance (Medicines), Guy's and St Thomas' NHS Foundation Trust, London, UK

Ros Batty BPharm MSc MRPharmS
Principal Pharmacist, North Thames Pharmacy Service, Clinical Pharmacy Unit, Northwick Park and St Mark's NHS Trust, Harrow

Dianne C Berry DPhil CPsychol ACSS
Pro-Vice-Chancellor (Research) and Professor of Psychology, School of Psychology, Reading, UK

Kim Brackley DipPharm(Dist) MSc MRPharmS
Principal Pharmacist, North Thames Pharmacy Services, Chelsea and Westminster Health Care Trust, London

Judy Cantrill BSc MSc FRPharmS
Professor of Medicines Usage, Evaluation and Policy, School of Pharmacy and Pharmaceutical Sciences, University of Manchester, Manchester, UK

Sarah Clifford BA(Hons) MSc PhD
Lecturer in Medicines in Health, Department of Practice & Policy, The School of Pharmacy, University of London, London, UK

J. Graham Davies BPharm MSc PhD MRPharmS
Professor of Clinical Pharmacy and Therapeutics, School of Pharmacy and Biomolecular Sciences, University of Brighton, Brighton, UK

Soraya Dhillon BPharm PhD MRPharmS
Foundation Professor and Head of School, The School of Pharmacy, University of Hertford, Hatfield, UK

Rachel Elliott BPharm PhD MRPharmS
Clinical Senior Lecturer, School of Pharmacy and Pharmaceutical Sciences, University of Manchester, Manchester, UK

David Erskine BPharm MSc FCPP Hon MRPharmS
Acting Director, London and South East Medicines Information Service, Guy's and St Thomas' NHS Foundation Trust, London, UK

Bryony Dean Franklin BPharm MSc PhD MRPharmS
Principal Pharmacist, Clinical Services and Director, Academic Pharmacy Unit, Hammersmith Hospitals NHS Trust/ The School of Pharmacy, University of London, London, UK

Mark Gilchrist MPharm DipClinPharm MRPharmS
Pharmacist Specialist, Clinical and Infectious Diseases, Hammersmith Hospitals NHS Trust, Charing Cross Hospital Pharmacy Department, London, UK

Jatinder Harchowal BPharm MSc MRPharmS
Chief Pharmacist, Ealing Hospital NHS Trust, London, UK

Jamie Hayes MRPharmS
Director, Welsh Medicines Resource Centre (WeMeReC), Penarth, UK

Ann Jacklin BPharm CHSM MRPharmS
Chief Pharmacist, Hammersmith Hospital NHS Trust, London, UK

Nicola John DFPH BPharm MPhil DMS MRPharmS
Director of Public Health, Merthyr Tydfil Local Health Board, National Public Health Service for Wales, UK

Andrzej Kostrzewski BSc MSc MmedEd MRPharmS
Principal Pharmacist, Guy's and St. Thomas' School of Medicine, and Clinical Lecturer, The School of Pharmacy, University of London, London, UK

Peter Knapp PhD BA RGN
Senior Lecturer, Pharmacy Practice & Medicines Management Group, University of Leeds, Leeds, UK

Beryl Langfield BPharm MRPharmS
Principal Pharmacist, Computer Services, Pharmacy Department, Hammersmith Hospitals NHS Trust, London, UK

Wendy Lawson BSc(Hons) GradDipPharm(Hosp) MRPharmS
Pharmacist Advanced, Infectious Diseases, Hammersmith Hospitals NHS Trust, London, UK

Adele Mackeller
Outpatient Dispensary, Wythenshaw Hospital, South Manchester University Hospitals NHS Trust, Wythenshaw, UK

Andrew McCoig BPharm MRPharmS
Community Pharmacist, McCoig Pharmacy, Croydon, UK

D. K. (Theo) Raynor PhD BPharm MRPharmS
Professor of Pharmacy Practice, School of Healthcare, University of Leeds, Leeds, UK

Kay Roberts MPhil FRPharmS
Independent Pharmacy Consultant and Chairman, Pharmacy Misuse Advisory Group, UK

Janie Sheridan PhD MRPharmS MPS(NZ) BPharm(Hons) BA(Hons) Registered Pharmacist New Zealand Pharmacy Council
Associate Professor of Pharmacy Practice, School of Pharmacy, The University of Auckland, Auckland, New Zealand

Ian Smith BSc
Boots Teacher/Practitioner, Drug Usage and Pharmacy Practice, School of Pharmacy and Pharmaceutical Sciences, University of Manchester, Manchester, UK

Norman J Vetter MD FFCM
Department of Epidemiology, Cardiff University, Cardiff, UK

Judith Vincent BScPharm MRPharmS
Deputy Director for Clinical Development, Swansea Local Health Board, Llansamlet, UK

Marian Walker BSc MRPharmS
Joint Division Head, Substance Misuse, Berkshire Healthcare NHS Trust and Pharmacist, Clinical Team, National Treatment Agency for Substance Misuse, London, UK

Phil Wiffen MSc MRPharmS MFPHM(Hon)
Co-ordinating Editor, Cochrane Pain and Palliative Care Group,
Pain Research Unit, Churchill Hospital, Oxford, UK

Alan Willson BPharm MSc PhD MRPharmS
Director of Service Development, National Leadership and
Innovation Agency for Healthcare, Llanharan, UK

PREFACE

The aim of this book is to be a quick prompt for practising pharmacists, pre-registration trainees and students in the latter half of their course. It is designed as a book to help you in your everyday practice. It should support hospital and community pharmacists alike and will be of use when dealing with individual patients or when providing services such as advising doctors, be they GPs or consultants, on their prescribing.

We have revised the second edition in both content and scope, allowing us to bring in new areas for pharmacists, such as errors and prescribing. In the UK at present, suitably qualified pharmacists can prescribe with a doctor, and will soon be able to prescribe independently. In reality, as much of clinical pharmacy involves reproducing the prescriber's thinking, this has not required too much change to the book; however, we have revised issues such as relationship with the patient, and adherence support, with the prescribing role in mind. We have also developed the material on primary care prescribing, with two chapters setting out first strategy then practice. A new chapter on smoking cessation guides the pharmacist intending to provide this effective health promotion role. Taken together, the revisions reflect the significant developments to the pharmacist's role.

The book starts with a fundamental chapter on the nature of clinical pharmacy and is then split into four sections: Policy, Choice, Monitoring and management, and Reference.

POLICY

A large part of clinical pharmacists' influence has come from setting and influencing policy – deciding and getting agreement on what is the right thing to do. To do that effectively, you require an idea of what clinical pharmacy is, how to deliver advice to doctors, and a thorough knowledge of the evidence on which you are basing your recommendations.

CHOICE

Pharmacists influence the choice of drugs either by advising others on which drug or regime to use for a particular patient, or by choosing the appropriate drug themselves. These chapters deal with some common situations.

MONITORING AND MANAGEMENT

Once a drug has been prescribed it is only the beginning of what is often a long process of taking the drug. The patient's condition and what they want from drug treatment can vary over time and some form of monitoring and feedback is required. Some common situations and patient groups are included in this section.

REFERENCE

A repository of useful information that you may not be able to summon to the forefront of your mind just when you need it!

When preparing this book, we have kept in mind the excellence of the British National Formulary; we have tried not to duplicate any of its functions, so that the two books complement each other rather than compete.

The information in this book is as up to date and accurate as the authors can make it, but we hope you won't just look up a chapter for a quick fix – we want you to *evaluate* information and apply it dependent on the circumstances. If you have any doubts, check with other reference sources or another colleague.

ACKNOWLEDGEMENT

We would like to thank SafeScript Limited (Ch. 20) for permission to reproduce their copyright material.

2006

Nick Barber
Alan Willson

A philosophy of clinical pharmacy

N. Barber

What is clinical pharmacy trying to achieve? Unless we can answer this question we will have difficulty delivering and developing a service and convincing others of its value. In this chapter I will present you with a philosophy of clinical pharmacy; the rest of the book will help you deliver it.

The key point about clinical pharmacy is that it suggests what is *right* about therapy, so it involves *values* as well as *facts*. This is why clinical pharmacy has been so important in the development of pharmacy as a whole – it moves beyond our knowledge of facts about medicines and into the arena of how we should use that knowledge.

A BRIEF HISTORY LESSON

In tracing the development of clinical pharmacy in the UK, one sees parallels with the development of a religious sect as much as the development of a new way of practice. The early prophets developed clinical services in hospitals, educated prolifically to spread the gospel, and pushed back the boundaries of pharmacy. Most of us were fired by the belief that we could use our knowledge of drugs to help patients be better treated; what is more we used our skills to minimise the use of inappropriately expensive drugs. We were so successful that a whole series of clinical pharmacy services grew over a few years. But were they any good?

In the USA, clinical pharmacy had developed earlier than in the UK and researchers Hepler and Strand (1990) argued that clinical pharmacy was just a name for a series of services. There was no ideal against which we could measure it, so we could not really assess

2

A PHILOSOPHY OF CLINICAL PHARMACY
▶ WHAT ARE WE TRYING TO ACHIEVE?

clinical pharmacy. Unless we knew where we wanted to be, how could we know how close we were to our goal? And, if we didn't know how far we were from our goal, how could we assess clinical pharmacy services or, most importantly for our future, persuade others of their value? The solution Hepler and Strand suggested was pharmaceutical care – a *philosophy* on which, they argued, clinical pharmacy should be based. The essence of this philosophy (usually ignored in UK interpretations of it) was the morality (the definition of what is right) of the relationship between the pharmacist and the patient – it suggested that the pharmacist effectively contracted him/herself to the patient to serve the patient's needs.

While pharmaceutical care was a significant step in the development of clinical pharmacy, and is an attractive 'sound bite' to use when explaining a service to others, I tend not to use it. Its moral philosophy was, in my view, incomplete and, partly because of this, the term has been adapted to mean different things in different countries. Now it tends to be converging with the idea of medicines management (Barber 2001). In the rest of this chapter I'll explain what I think is the philosophy of clinical pharmacy and how its aims should be applied to your practice.

WHAT ARE WE TRYING TO ACHIEVE?

Clinical pharmacy services aim to improve prescribing, either through influencing what others do or by doing the prescribing ourselves. Our philosophy should therefore be rooted in a philosophy of good prescribing, a subject with a curiously sparse literature. I think our philosophy, the philosophy of clinical pharmacy, is to improve the quality of prescribing, and hence achieve the ends of good prescribing.

Good prescribing is a balance of three broad areas:

● *What the patient wants.* Health care starts with patients wanting something, and it is foolish to ignore or downgrade this. They may want treatment, or just reassurance. They may, or may not, articulate their wants. It is your job to take reasonable steps to establish what they are. Remember patients (i.e. all of us), have many wants, only some of which will be expressed and some of which may well be conflicting. We may not only express a want to get better but we will also want to keep other aspects of our life the same as well, for example to keep our job, play a sport or keep good relationships with our family.

● *Knowledge of the properties of the drugs.* These include their beneficial effects and side effects. It is important not just to know the effects on the population but also to be able to translate them to the likelihood of effects on an individual and to be able to predict the effects on those close to patients, such as their family. The properties of a drug include its physical properties. Is the 1 gram tablet too large for a frail old lady to swallow? Can a man with one arm nebulise his drugs? The cost of the drug should also be known, and some knowledge of the economics of its use.

● *The greater good.* This encompasses issues that are for the good of the population, or perhaps those people close to the patient. It encompasses a host of arguments and situations that may occur. The obvious one in any socialised health care system (such as the UK's National Health Service (NHS)) is that of containing the cost of treatment of an individual so that money may be saved to treat other individuals. However it may also include treating a patient who is a danger to those around, such as patients with certain infectious diseases, or one whose delusions make them dangerous. It may also encompass the greater good of the prescriber–patient relationship. Prescribers need to maintain a relationship with a patient in order to treat them, and will often make 'uncomfortable' prescribing decisions to maintain the relationship. They may, for example, maintain a subtherapeutic dose of a cheap drug because they know the patient strongly believes in its effects.

The situation is represented in Figure 1.1 (from Cribb and Barber 1997). In the centre, where all three areas overlap, prescribing is uncontroversially good. In the areas in which two aims are met, prescribing may be good but a rationale would have to be made for why one area is rejected. In the areas in which only one aim is met, it is very unlikely that prescribing would be thought of as good.

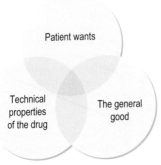

Fig. 1.1 Good prescribing is a balance of three broad areas.

This is all very well, but on which basis do we create our rationale, on which basis do we ignore or down-play one area? In these circumstances we fall back on the four principles of medical ethics, from which the above areas were partly drawn. The first is *beneficence* – doing good – and we aim to achieve this by making the drug have the clinical effect desired. The second is *non-maleficence* – not doing harm – in which we aim to reduce the chance and extent of harm by minimising errors and adverse events resulting from drug treatment. The third is *justice*, and in this case I'm taking the theory of distributive justice on which the NHS was founded – utilitarianism – which is often defined as providing the greatest good for the greatest number. Given that there is a fixed budget, we can treat more people if we keep costs down, and hence this is the moral authority behind cost reduction. The fourth principle respects *patient autonomy*, which means that patients can choose what their ends are and how those ends should be met. Patients always have a choice in what happens to them (even if that choice is to let the doctors do what they want) and we should recognise this and be responsive to it.

These are the four underlying principles on which clinical pharmacy should be founded. It will not be possible to achieve all the aims completely on all occasions, and debate is needed about situations in which conflicts occur; however they give a foundation to our practice and a way for us to discuss services between ourselves and explain them to others.

GETTING AIMS INTO PRACTICE

Aims are all very well but we need processes – pharmacy services – to make them happen. There are three points at which clinical pharmacy services are delivered to meet the aims of clinical pharmacy: before, during and after the prescribing decision.

- *Before*. This is achieved through the creation and influence of policy – deciding what is the right thing to be done by whom. This starts with licensing the drug and includes formularies, prescribing policies, guidelines, practices to reduce medication errors, and so on. It can also include educational methods such as feedback of prescribers' practice in comparison to others, for example through prescribing analysis and cost (PACT) data or by education, such as 'academic detailing'.
- *During*. Influencing the prescriber by affecting their knowledge, attitudes and priorities when prescribing. The pharmacist may be present at the time of prescribing and contribute to the decision-making process as part of a team. Alternatively, the pharmacist

may actually make the prescribing decision. At the time of writing, pharmacists in the UK are about to take on much wider prescribing roles.

- *After.* This involves monitoring, correcting error and improving the quality of prescribing. It can happen just after the prescription is written or as part of a regular medicines management process that goes on for years. Communication with patients is essential – checking how they are getting on with their drugs, what their needs are, offering help and advice to improve adherence where appropriate, and working towards accurate recording and transmission of information on their drug therapy (e.g. when transferring across the primary–secondary interface). Patients often get into non-adherent behaviour soon after starting a medication, so this is a good time to intervene.

BEING A GOOD CLINICAL PHARMACIST

What do you need to contribute to the above? First, you need to believe in a philosophy of clinical pharmacy and accept your professional and moral responsibility to deliver it and be accountable for your actions. This is easier said than done, and may make you unpopular at times – one needs to strike a balance between moral responsibility and professional suicide. Having said that, pharmacists have the power to influence drug therapy, and with that power comes responsibility; sometimes your responsibility is to argue against company or hospital policy, or a patient's wants. Second, you need the scientific knowledge to judge whether a prescribing decision is appropriate or not. This knowledge increasingly focuses on the relative weights of evidence, so you have to understand the strengths and weaknesses of the methods through which the evidence is obtained. These are, predominantly, clinical trials to assess effectiveness; pharmacoepidemiology to assess risk and pharmacoeconomics to understand costs and their relationships to outcomes. They must be accompanied by background knowledge of the ways by which we assess a disease and its progress, the characteristics of medicines, their mode of action, formulation, pharmacokinetics and method of delivery.

This leaves us one area to discuss, which is respecting the patient's choice. The key to this is establishing what patients want – the things they think important – and using your knowledge and communication skills to ensure, as much as possible within the principles outlined above, that they get them. One should also anticipate future choices patients may want to make – what if they feel worse on the medication? What if they can't fit the dosing interval into their lives? Information, guidance, making them aware of alternatives, and the encouragement to come back for further advice are the keys to this.

Finally, one needs to develop the skills necessary to deliver many of these services. Skills are learned through repetition and feedback; in developing the skill to ride a bicycle you wobble frequently and occasionally fall off before mastering it. Pharmacists need to have the space and support to do this and develop the skills through which they can deliver their service.

The contents of this book are there to provide some support for the philosophy of clinical pharmacy laid out in this chapter. We hope they help you become a better clinical pharmacist.

REFERENCES

Barber N 2001 Pharmaceutical care and medicines management – is there a difference? Pharmacy World and Science 23:210–211
Cribb A, Barber N 1997 Prescribers, patients and policy: the limits of technique. Health Care Analysis 5:292–298
Hepler CD, Strand LM 1990 Opportunities and responsibilities in pharmaceutical care. American Journal of Hospital Pharmacy 47:533–543

FURTHER READING

Beauchamp TL, Childress JF 2001 Principles of biomedical ethics. Oxford University Press, Oxford
Pendleton D, Schofield T, Tate P, Havelock P 2003 The new consultation. Oxford University Press, Oxford

POLICY

Prescribing in primary care

N. John, J. Hayes

Prescribing is a major clinical activity of the National Health Service (NHS). The cost of prescribing has grown to a total expenditure in excess of £7billion, with each member of the population now receiving an average of 12 prescription items per year (Maxwell and Walley 2003).

With legislative changes enabling other groups of professionals, including nurses and pharmacists, to prescribe, those attempting to manage primary care prescribing face a challenging future.

Receiving a prescription is the most common health intervention that patients encounter. Primary care organisations (PCOs) are concerned about:

- the financial risk of an increasing spend
- the clinical risks associated with poorly managed prescribing.

In the face of this, the prescribing adviser can feel like 'King Canute trying to stop the tide from coming in' (Audit Commission 2003); adopting a strategic approach helps you to show leadership by taking control and enabling the whole PCO to work together towards common goals.

- The process of developing the strategy will enable the organisation to understand and share the problems and agree the overall objectives at a corporate level.
- In PCOs, policies initiated by health care reformers have to compete with established ways of working and other initiatives. This may result in a gap between policy intent on the one hand and delivery on the other (Ham 2003).
- It is important when developing the strategy to consult widely and take on board comments, so that a sense of local ownership of the problems and possible solutions develops.

WHAT SHOULD THE STRATEGY CONTAIN?

ANALYSIS OF THE CURRENT POSITION

This should paint a picture of the pattern of prescribing in your PCO, and make comparisons with other areas, particularly those that are socioeconomically similar.

As well as basic information on overall costs and volume of prescribing, trends in the prescribing of high-growth areas should be mapped out. Include drug areas where National Service Frameworks and the National Institute for Clinical Excellence are encouraging growth, and also those drug areas where growth is discouraged, such as proton pump inhibitors.

The current set of prescribing indicators (PIs) should also be included, and comparisons made with other PCOs. The PIs should also be measured for each practice to highlight problem areas; these may be reported anonymously but will be helpful when targeting support.

Analysis of the current prescribing situation should also be accompanied by any relevant information regarding local baseline morbidity data.

STRATEGIC GOAL SETTING

Based on your analysis and taking into account national pressures and local patterns of prescribing, set out a vision for management of prescribing for the PCO as a whole, with strategic goals. As with all targets, these should be SMART (i.e. specific, measurable, achievable, realistic and timely).

HOW TO ACHIEVE THESE GOALS

The strategy should set out an implementation plan, with the aim of achieving a culture in your PCO of sustained sound management of prescribing. This can be achieved by recognising this as an ongoing change management process, with the prescribing advisers as 'agents of change'. Thus sustainable change only comes about when practices have appropriate systems in place, routinely used by clinical and support staff, and the advisers' role is to help practices achieve this themselves.

 Recognise that management of prescribing is really management of change.

BARRIERS TO CHANGE

Implementing any sort of change is not easy, and it helps to think about why this is. Common problems in every organisation include:

- Inertia
- Lack of time
- Fear of criticism
- Difficulty learning new skills
- Loss of job interest.

Knowing that influences on clinical practice are many and varied, a number of approaches are needed to improve performance. Evidence has shown that several interventions, using different components, are required, including educational initiatives, use of opinion leaders, peer review mechanisms, and financial and other incentives (Ham, 2003).

DISMANTLING THE BARRIERS TO CHANGE

No single act will transform prescribing. Instead a policy of adopting multifaceted interventions that contain individually effective components is more likely to be successful. Understanding what motivates professionals in their daily work is of particular importance, and remembering that the main motivation remains the desire to offer a high standard of service. Prescribing policies must be driven by quality, not cost-containment, if prescribers are truly to be influenced by PCOs.

The key to this is to get people engaged in the process and feeling that improvements are possible and achievable. Some of the mechanisms that are useful in the management of prescribing are as follows.

Supporting the development of effective teamworking in practices

Consideration should be given to how best to enable the whole practice to take on board this change management process, i.e. to create ownership of the change by the practitioners. It can be helpful to support the development of leadership in primary care by identifying key staff who can contribute, including:

- a GP lead for prescribing
- the practice manager.

These lead people should be instrumental in communicating prescribing issues and facilitating improvements within their practice. They should engage with the whole team, from GPs to reception staff, in the process of improvement. The role of the prescribing adviser is to support these key opinion-formers within practices. Working to support practices in this way enables clinicians to preserve professional autonomy in the achievement of high standards of care and to align management priorities with prescribers' own professional values. The offer of protected time or other resources to enable health professionals to work on prescribing issues can be the key to securing a high degree of cooperation. Links can also be developed with other practices in the PCO by, for example, putting on regular continuous professional development events or specific training. This facilitates communication of local good practice, sharing of data and sharing of problems, with possible solutions.

Budget setting

There is a clear intention to make the medicines they require available to patients at the least cost to the NHS. The need to get best value for money out of the drugs budget has been further emphasised by the amalgamation of the prescribing hospital community services and general medical services budgets. While there can be no legal limit on an individual GP's right to prescribe for a particular patient, any overspending on drugs budgets may have to be recovered from hospital and community services allocations.

It is fundamentally important that practices feel that the mechanism by which their indicative prescribing budget is set is fair, transparent, open and consistent. If there is a perception of a lack of any of these characteristics in their budget setting, practices may be very disinclined to work to stay within their allocation. There is no perfect way to set budgets that explains all the variation in prescribing costs. However, the factors that are important include demographic information on the number, age and sex of patients, and socioeconomic data on levels of deprivation, together with specific information such as the number of nursing-home patients, for whom prescribing costs are higher than average. Advice can be obtained from the Prescribing Support Unit in Leeds.

As well as gaining agreement from the PCO Board on budget setting, a communication exercise can help practices to understand their budgets and why they have received a particular level of uplift. To develop and maintain transparency and trust around budget setting, this exercise of speaking to each practice and dealing with their queries is best repeated annually during practice visits.

Incentive schemes

These can be helpful in motivating practices to improve prescribing, provided they are seen as achievable, given reasonable effort on their part, and reward a combination of efficient use of resources and good-quality prescribing. There is, however, some debate over the size and nature of the inducements needed to influence prescribing. Sullivan's (2002) view is that 'Firing silver bullets at prescribers may alter their behaviour, but a richer evidence base is needed to help primary care organisations aim more effectively'. Most incentive schemes now reflect the evidence that more than one technique is needed to change prescribing behaviour.

There should be wide local consultation before the introduction of any scheme, and ongoing communication with practices is again important, with in-year feedback provided on how they are doing.

Interface issues

Often consultants and trusts as a whole are unaware of the effect their prescribing decisions have on primary care prescribing patterns in their locality. It is important to build up good working relationships with local trusts to ensure that there is wide understanding of the implications of prescribing decisions and that processes are put in place to manage the local introduction of new drugs. This can be done via interface Prescribing Committees with joint representation from primary and secondary care, and also by links with other local professional committees.

It is helpful if such committees are supported by an interface pharmacist. They can critically appraise the evidence and provide reports on new drugs. Consultants making decisions may not have been trained in the skills of critical appraisal and be unfamiliar with the pitfalls. Collaboration with other prescribing committees can help to share the workload.

Such committees can also consider broader issues of medicines management, such as policies for prescribing at discharge and reuse of patients' own medicines.

Encouraging practice pharmacists and technicians to visit the local NHS trusts and spend time with clinical pharmacists/discharge pharmacists observing procedures can be beneficial and, similarly, hospital pharmacists will also benefit from spending time in general practice.

Collaboration with other primary care organisations

Partnership working between neighbouring PCOs can be an effective means of increasing influence. For example, a group of advisers can work together to agree a strategic approach to deal with particular issues, such as working with clinical networks that span many PCOs.

Relationship with the pharmaceutical industry

One choice that both primary and secondary care organisations will have is whether or not to work with the pharmaceutical industry. Tensions exist between the political desire to work with the industry in a partnership approach at a national level and the local picture of drug promotion, sponsorship of medical education and influence on prescribing patterns. It is important for health care organisations to have a formal policy that all staff, including non-medical and NHS managers, are aware of. For those organisations that choose to enter into partnership, a robust agreement is essential. The possible effect of such partnership approaches should not be underestimated – remember the 'halo' effect: being seen to work with you is often enough. Don't forget, medical education has been described as one of the most potent weapons in the marketing campaign (Cook 2001).

Issues for the strategy can include:

- Consideration of how medical education events can be financed without sponsorship
- If sponsorship is accepted, ensuring that more than one company is involved
- The prescribing advisor being the gatekeeper to the PCO, dealing with all industry enquiries
- Asking representatives to write in with issues that they would like to discuss
- Declaration of interests at Drugs and Therapeutics or other prescribing committee meetings
- Provision of incentives to practices with robust polices for working with industry
- Letting practices know how they should complain about inappropriate marketing.

The disadvantages of not engaging with industry are a lack of knowledge of what is going on and a lack of awareness of what is being said and promoted. Think of ways of overcoming this, such as e-mail discussion groups to enable rapid sharing of information, which can be sent to your GPs as 'holding information'.

RESOURCES NEEDED

Skill mix

The strategy should set out the staff needed to influence prescribing for each PCO. Consideration should be given to:

- developing the appropriate level of both strategic and operational support

- how both pharmacists and technicians can best be deployed
- the use of other advisers, such as doctors, nurses or dietitians
- the appropriate use of other expertise within the PCO, e.g. finance and planning departments
- adequate data analysis and administrative support for staff to enable them to concentrate on prescribing improvements.

Skills and knowledge required of staff

This chapter has focussed on the management of change as the means of achieving improvements in prescribing. All prescribing advisers' teams should therefore understand the human relations theory underpinning the management of change.

Similarly, they should have a sound understanding of the literature specifically related to achieving changes in prescribing, and the numerous factors that influence prescribers in their choice of drug.

A core competency for all prescribers and members of prescribing subgroups should be the ability to interpret drug advertisements and product promotional material critically.

Clinical knowledge is a clear advantage, but is not essential for all on the advisory team, as many changes in prescribing are concerned with improved systems rather than choice of drug.

In the context of providing prescribing advice, perhaps more important than clinical knowledge is the ability to understand study results, and to be comfortable describing or explaining absolute risks, absolute risk reductions, numbers needed to treat (NNTs), relative risk, relative risk reduction and odds ratios. An important point is that many health professionals, including local experts and opinion leaders, may not be up to date with some of these concepts. PCO prescribing advisers also need to think about how can they provide prescribers with timely, accessible, user-friendly product information.

'There should be shift of emphasis from the ability to cite acronyms and facile conclusions of the latest clinical trials, and instead reinforce the analytical skills necessary for critical assessment of an ever expanding stock of published work' – Bogarty and Brophy 2003

Prescribers should value the quality of the encounter they have with the PCO prescribing team and view the adviser as a credible opinion leader with whom they can build a long-term relationship, such that prescribing visits become established as traditional and accepted practice. This is supported by the research of Prosser and Walley (2003) looking at why GPs see pharmaceutical representatives. Meeting management and social skills are thus also important.

A further skill should be the ability to recognise the circumstances under which a business case is appropriate. 'In-year' and 'end-of-year' monies are almost inevitable and often initiate a bidding process. Prescribing initiatives will be competing with other priorities and so a business case that stands out is more likely to secure funding. A successful business case will be a result of a well-thought-out and structured idea coupled with timely, effective writing.

REPORTING MECHANISM

It is important to keep your board informed of progress with the strategy, as they will not like surprises – good or bad. So the strategy should set out how often reports on progress will be made to the board, and also what they will contain.

Aim to be realistic with these – a quarterly report may suffice, with key statistics presented and a progress report on target areas. The reports are really valued when produced by a team with, for example, input from the finance department and an information analyst, and produced with administrative support.

Presenting to the board is a two-way process, so treat any feedback given as valuable.

TO SUMMARISE

It is suggested that a strategic approach to managing prescribing in primary care is adopted, which enables clarification of:

- the current position
- the goals set
- barriers to achieving the changes needed to attain these goals, and how to overcome them
- the resources needed.

REFERENCES

Audit Commission 2003 Primary care prescribing. Audit Commission, London

Bogarty P, Brophy J 2003 Increasing burden of treatment in the acute coronary syndromes: is it justified? Lancet 361: 1813–1816

Cook J 2001 Effective medical education? Medical Education Practical Guide 6. Pharmaceutical Marketing 12: 14–22

Ham C 2003 Improving the performance of health services: the role of
   clinical leadership. Lancet 361: 1978–1980.

Maxwell S, Walley T 2003. Teaching safe and effective prescribing in UK
   medical schools: a core curriculum for tomorrow's doctors. British
   Journal of Clinical Pharmacology 55: 496–503

Prosser H, Walley T 2003 Understanding why GPs see pharmaceutical
   representatives: a qualitative review. British Journal of General Practice
   53: 305–311

Sullivan F 2002 Prescribing incentive schemes – more evidence is needed on
   how they work. British Medical Journal 324: 118

CHAPTER 3

Clinical directorates and the role of the pharmacist

A. Jacklin

Clinical directorates were widely introduced into the National Health Service during the mid to late 1980s in response to two major initiatives:

- *The resource management initiative.* This was a joint Department of Health and British Medical Association project to involve doctors in managing information and resources
- The White Paper *Working for Patients.* This introduced the purchaser–provider model of health care commissioning by which all hospital work would be paid for via contracts. Contracts were to be based on clinical activity.

Common to both of these changes was the need to involve doctors in management and to provide doctors with improved information and business support to enable them to manage their 'clinical business'.

Prior to the introduction of clinical directorates, doctors were already grouped together in clinical specialties but were not always integrated into other disciplines, particularly nursing and management. Directorates in many places were hence a strengthening of existing medical structures with the introduction of multidisciplinary working in directorate teams. A common initial structure for a clinical directorate (also known as care groups, clinical teams and various other names) is shown in Figure 3.1.

As directorates have developed, this structure has been further strengthened by the identification by directorate groupings of other

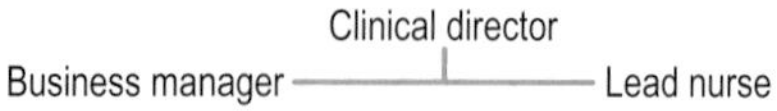

Clinical director

Business manager ——————|—————— Lead nurse

Fig. 3.1 The clinical directorate.

health care professionals, including pharmacists, so that commonly directorates will have a support team including:

- directorate pharmacist
- directorate finance officer
- directorate contracts/information manager.

The clinical director will be the budget holder for a number of budgets, which will include medical staff, nursing staff, drugs and equipment. S/he will be responsible for ensuring that expenditure within these budgets is managed and contained, and will need support and information in order to do this. Advising on drug budgets is hence an important role for directorate pharmacists but is not the only role clinical pharmacists have in supporting the directorate. The clinical director will be the lead clinician for clinical governance within the directorate.

HC(88)54, *The Way Forward*, in advocating clinical pharmacy, described the developing role of pharmacists in which skills are applied to medicine usage both at the 'policy-making level' and in the treatment of individual patients.

Prior to the introduction of clinical directorates, 'policy-making' contributions were often confined to only one or two senior pharmacists in each hospital. A hospital with multiple clinical directorates, each with an allocated directorate pharmacist, provides an increased number of opportunities for involvement in business decision-making.

WHAT IS A DIRECTORATE PHARMACIST?

The directorate pharmacist's role can be described as having four key elements:

- being a clinical specialist
  - know the literature relating to your directorate
  - have a working knowledge of current practice and protocols
- supporting clinical governance within the directorate
  - this will include clinical audit, protocol review and medication incident reporting
- monitoring drug expenditure
  - provide regular information and interpretation of drug expenditure, advise on how best to manage expenditure
  - predict and advise on changes

- supporting pharmacy
  - be a service ambassador for all pharmacy services
  - advise pharmacy of directorate service plans
  - train and educate other pharmacy staff in specialist area.

To perform well at a directorate level, pharmacists need to have knowledge and skills in a number of areas:

- clinical knowledge appropriate to directorate
- data handling/presentation/interpretation skills
- knowledge of local pharmacy systems, including computers
- knowledge of hospital organisation structure and management style
- knowledge of local commissioners and understanding of relevance of contracting round
- interpersonal skills appropriate for dealing with senior doctors, nurses and business managers
- knowledge of primary care organisation priorities locally
- knowledge of local procurement systems.

BUDGET MANAGEMENT

While a directorate pharmacist will be involved in many of the roles outlined above, most will be regularly involved in drugs budget support, which is described here in more detail. A budget-holder compares budget to expenditure and aims to spend less than the budgeted allowance. The basic questions to be answered when monitoring a budget are:

Q1 What is my budget position this month? Am I underspent, overspent or balanced?

Q2 By how much?

Q3 How does this affect my position year to date? Am I better off, worse off or the same?

Q4 By how much?

Q5 How different was this month from previous months this year/last year?

Q6 What is my predicted position at the end of the financial year?

Q7 How does this compare to last year?

The answers to these basic questions will establish whether a budget is a 'problem' or not and dictate the amount of further information and interpretation required.

Q8 What are the reasons for my under/overspend or balanced position?

Q9   Is this what we expected, or is it a surprise?

Q10   Which drugs, patients, doctors, therapeutic class (e.g. antibiotics), patient group, disease state are responsible for the over/underspend? (This is the biggest question to answer)

Q11   Do we think these were clinically appropriate?

Q12   What actions could or should we take? (e.g. restrict availability, define guidelines)

Q13   How many of the problems are recurring/non-recurring?

Q14   What does the year-end position look like after we take out the non-recurring elements?

Q15   What else are we aware of that will improve or worsen our position? (e.g. new drugs or change in use of existing drugs)

Q16   How can you/pharmacy help reduce/contain expenditure?

By asking these questions when preparing a report, which can be either verbal or written, for a clinical director, a directorate pharmacist will be able to target the requirements of the recipient.

The following section describes data that are likely to be available to a directorate pharmacist to help answer these questions. Before using any data it is imperative to have a full understanding of the systems (human, procedural and technological) used to capture data in order to be able to provide interpretation.

By understanding how the pharmacy computer system works and, more importantly, how your pharmacy uses the computer, you will know how best to make use of data available to you. You will also be able to interpret any apparent quirks by understanding the potential for errors or anomalies.

DATA AVAILABLE FOR EXPENDITURE INTERPRETATION

Pharmacy computer systems provide us with a large amount of data that need to be sorted and manipulated to suit the needs of a clinical director. Thought needs to be given to the relative advantages and disadvantages of presenting all of the data available.

In preparing reports a directorate pharmacist should consider the relevance and importance of showing:

- data to
  - consultant
  - specialty
  - directorate
- data by

  – inpatient
  – outpatient
  – day case.

Unless showing data by any of these groupings is relevant to the management of expenditure, then conciseness is lost and interpretation may be clouded – so don't subdivide into too many categories.

Merge pack size/formulations

Occasionally, different formulations/strengths will be used in different clinical indications and hence would be relevant to report separately; more often these data should be merged.

Top N

Showing doctors their 'top of the pops' is interesting but unless targeted to show relative change can be of limited repeated value. Often this is best saved for once- or twice-yearly snapshot reviews.

Level of detail

How many decimal points you report to will depend on the scale of expenditure; too much detail can be irrelevant and impair concise interpretation.

Similarly, grouping drugs by therapeutic class may be more meaningful than reporting individual drugs where there are no particularly high-cost drugs.

Other hospital data

The amount and quality of data available from the trust's patient information administration system (PAS) will depend very much on local circumstances.

Before beginning to use any PAS data it is always worth establishing how the directorate views the data. In many hospitals clinical directors have often expressed concerns about the:

● reliability
● accuracy
● interpretation
● timeliness
● usefulness

of data. If this is the case it may be best to avoid the use of such data.

If the data are well supported locally then activity and case-mix data may be useful to include in drug reports, for example to provide figures on average drug cost per outpatient attendance or average drug cost per patient spell.

CLINICAL GOVERNANCE

A directorate pharmacist will have an important role in supporting the medicines-related aspects of clinical governance. In many organisations clinical governance can be divided into three main groupings of work, all of which are relevant to medicines and hence to pharmacists:

- *Clinical audit.* The directorate pharmacist may provide guidance on areas suitable for audit to inform the audit programme as well as undertaking specific medicines-based audits
- *Clinical management guidelines and protocols.* The directorate pharmacist is ideally placed to provide drug expertise and play an editorial and publishing role for guidelines that include medicines
- *Clinical risk management.* Most trusts will have well-developed medication incidents reporting systems that record and report medication incidents at an organisational level. A directorate pharmacist can report on directorate-specific medication incidents at an appropriate directorate clinical governance committee. This ensures multidisciplinary review and ownership of incidents. Local action plans can then be developed to reduce the risk of future incidents.

INFORMATION TO SUPPORT A BROADER ROLE

Other information, both generated within pharmacy and available externally, can be used to facilitate activity in some of the broader roles described earlier.

Examples of such information are:

- *Clinical trials.* Depending on the number and size of trials, this may or may not be relevant or interesting
- *Drug information queries.* A review of these may form the basis of future clinical audit initiatives or individual patient reviews
- *Unlicensed drugs or indications.* Clinical directors may be interested in reviewing unlicensed use of medicines within the directorate
- *'Policy compliance' data*
  - for example, a review of outpatient 'scripts will reveal compliance (or not) with outpatient policies in addition to formulary compliance
  - a review of inpatient 'scripts will similarly review compliance with formulary and locally agreed protocols.

Information should be relevant, accurate, timely, concise, comparative, consistent, unbiased, unambiguous and, most important of all, practical/economic to produce and directed to action.

It is important, with such a mass of data that can be presented in many ways, that a focus is kept on the key issue: to sort, manage and present only data that are 'directed to action'.

It is always necessary to clarify the definitions of inpatient stays compared to day-case or regular day attenders to ensure interpretability of data. If in any doubt it is better not to use such data.

Drug licensing and safety

D. Erskine, S. Barnes

Pharmacists operate in an increasingly risk-sensitive environment and this is particularly relevant when we become involved with clinical trials, unlicensed drugs and providing advice on drug-induced adverse events. Recently, the Health and Safety Executive brought charges against two Metropolitan Police commissioners for failing to instruct their officers as to how to undertake a risk assessment before pursuing a suspect across a roof! The case was only dismissed after the jury was unable to decide whether or not the commissioners had failed to ensure their officers' health and safety by establishing the right working practices and proper training.

How long before a pharmacist is asked to produce evidence of the risk assessment s/he undertook before deciding not to advise a clinician that the drug s/he prescribed was being used outside the terms of the product licence, and the patient is now suing because of an adverse reaction?

It is probably true to say that our insurance premiums would fall considerably if we restricted ourselves to supplying medicines only to patients who met the exact criteria laid out in that product's summary of product characteristics (SmPC). However, given the current licensing processes, this is never likely to happen and as our fundamental role becomes ever more patient-focussed we will inevitably get involved in supplying medicines in situations where the implications of our actions are sometimes less than clear. Outlined below is a very basic overview of the issues a pharmacist should be aware of in dealing with these matters.

HOW A PRODUCT IS DEVELOPED

The process of drug development from molecule to product licence can take between 10 and 20 years and it has recently been estimated that this process costs in excess of £500 million to bring a product to market. This cost reflects the vast amount of data that is required by a licensing authority to demonstrate the safety and efficacy of that product in the intended population before a product licence is granted and also the fact that only one from every 5000–10000 molecules investigated actually makes it to market.

The stages of clinical trials are outlined below:

- *Preclinical testing.* The purpose of this phase is to evaluate pharmacodynamics, pharmacokinetics and toxicological properties of the product when administered to animals. The aims of toxicity studies are to establish a maximum tolerated dose prior to commencing phase 1 trials, and to identify target organ toxicity
- *Phase I studies.* These are the first trials of the treatment in humans and are usually concerned with determining pharmacokinetics and the acute side effect profile in a small number of healthy volunteers
- *Phase II studies.* These are small-scale studies, often involving 100–200 patients with the condition concerned. They are often used to estimate the best dose that should be investigated in larger trials
- *Phase III studies.* These trials are intended to provide the data necessary to determine the role of the drug in clinical practice. They usually involve many more patients, who are followed up for an appropriate length of time (often months or years) to determine long-term safety and efficacy. These trials usually involve the use of a double-blind design with either placebo or active comparators to minimise potential bias
- *Phase IV studies.* These are usually conducted after the drug has been marketed and are intended to provide data to clarify the adverse effect profile and clinical effectiveness when used 'in the real world'.

Some of the terminology used in clinical trial design is outlined in Table 4.1.

TYPES OF TRIAL DESIGN

Trial designs may be crossover or parallel group, placebo-controlled, active comparator or not controlled.

TABLE 4.1 Terminology used in clinical trials

Term	Meaning
Blinding/masking	A procedure in which one or more parties to the trial are kept unaware of the treatment assignment(s). Single-blinding usually refers to the subject(s) being unaware, and double-blinding usually refers to the subject(s), investigator(s), monitor and, in some cases, data analyst(s) being unaware of treatment assignments
Comparator	An investigational or marketed product (i.e. active control), or placebo, used as a reference in a clinical trial
Compliance	Adherence to all the trial-related requirements, good clinical practice requirements and the applicable regulatory requirements
Good clinical practice (GCP)	A standard for the design, conduct, performance, monitoring, auditing, recording, analysis and reporting of clinical trials, which provides assurance that the data and reported results are credible and accurate, and that the rights, integrity and confidentiality of trial subjects are protected
Independent data-monitoring committee	A committee that may be established by the sponsor to assess at intervals the progress of a clinical trial, the safety data and the critical efficacy endpoints, and to recommend to the sponsor whether to continue, modify or stop a trial
Independent ethics committee	An independent body, constituted of medical professionals and non-medical members, whose responsibility it is to ensure the protection of the rights, safety and wellbeing of human subjects involved in a trial and to provide public assurance of that protection by, among other things, reviewing and approving the trial protocol, the suitability of the investigators' facilities and the methods and material to be used in obtaining and documenting informed consent of the trial subjects
Informed consent	A process by which a subject voluntarily confirms his/her willingness to participate in a particular trial, after having been informed of all aspects of the trial that are relevant to the subject's decision to participate. Informed consent is

TABLE 4.1 Terminology used in clinical trials – cont'd	
Term	*Meaning*
	documented by means of a written, signed and dated informed consent form
Investigator's brochure	A compilation of the clinical and non-clinical data on the investigational product that is relevant to the study in human subjects
Multicentre trial	A clinical trial conducted to a single protocol but at more than one site and therefore carried out by more than one investigator
Protocol	A document that describes the objective, design, methodology, statistical considerations and organisation of a trial
Protocol amendment	A written description of a change(s) to or formal clarification of a protocol
Randomisation	The process of assigning trial subjects to treatment or control groups using an element of chance to determine the assignments in order to reduce bias

In crossover studies subjects act as their own control. Every subject takes each treatment in successive periods. For every treatment, baseline assessments must be made at the start of each treatment period and a washout phase must normally be allowed in between periods to avoid the effect of one treatment being carried over to the next period. The main advantage of crossover trials is that they require fewer patients than parallel studies. The main disadvantage is that there are very few diseases or interventions that lend themselves to this type of study – they are inappropriate for testing interventions that are:

● given as finite treatment courses
● given in conditions where the underlying disease is progressive
● given in conditions where the use of a washout period is not ethical.

In parallel studies, subjects are randomised to receive either the experimental treatment or the control treatment, which can be either an active drug or a placebo, depending on the trial design (Fig. 4.1). Use of a placebo group is intended to allow quantification of the effect of the active drug over and above any effect that might occur anyway (the placebo effect). An active drug is used as comparator either because

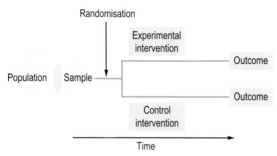

Fig. 4.1 Structure of a randomised controlled trial.

the researchers intend to demonstrate that the experimental drug is equivalent or superior to an existing 'gold standard' or because it is felt that the use of placebo would not be ethical. Randomisation should produce two populations, the experimental group and the control group, that are similar in every known and unknown respect. Any differences in outcome observed between the groups can then be attributed with confidence to the intervention.

In uncontrolled studies the medicine is given to all the participants and the results are described. The authors may try to set their findings in context by comparing their findings with other results reported in the literature. However, using these designs it is never possible to eliminate the impact of confounding variables. These studies tend to be restricted to phase II studies and to conditions where there is no other treatment available and it is considered unethical to compare the drug against placebo.

HOW THE PHARMACIST CAN CONTRIBUTE

In hospital the role of the pharmacist in clinical trials is well established. First, by using their knowledge of pharmacology and clinical pharmacy, they play a valuable role in helping ensure that ethics committees fulfil their required functions (described in Table 4.1). On a more operational level they provide vital support to clinical trial investigators in ensuring that drug-related trials meet good clinical practice (GCP) standards. Any pharmacist involved in any clinical trial should be aware of the standards required and these days this is usually ensured by having a pharmacy clinical trial standard operating procedure (SOP) for each trial being run at a particular centre. Pharmacists should never dispense a supply, destroy clinical trial supplies or implement a code break without first ensuring that their actions are completely in line with the procedures outlined in the SOP. In addition, they should make sure that all drugs started during the clinical trial are in line with the trial protocol and, if not, this should be brought to the attention of the study investigators.

A very useful resource in helping assess the perceived relevance of a clinical trial to practice is the European Medicines Evaluation Agency (EMEA) website (see Resources), which provides guidance on the types of study design and outcome monitoring required to support a licence application in particular therapeutic areas such as hypertension. This may be particularly relevant for pharmacists who are screening proposed clinical trial protocols on behalf of their ethics committee.

A good indication of how the data derived from the clinical trial programme influence discussions at the licensing authority can be obtained from the scientific discussion section for any product that has undergone approval via the EMEA (see Resources).

HOW MEDICINES ARE LICENSED

Medicines are licensed to ensure efficacy and safety and to allow scrutiny of the production facilities. In the UK, the Medicines and Healthcare Products Regulatory Agency (MHRA), formerly known as the Medicines Control Agency (MCA), is responsible for consideration of the data presented to them and the decision on whether to approve market authorisation (i.e. grant a product licence) and whether that authorisation should be restricted in any way.

Presently, the MHRA can act as a sole agency on behalf of the UK itself, as part of the European system known as the mutual recognition system, or as a rapporteur or co-rapporteur in the European Union (EU) centralised system. The national system is becoming less frequently used as more companies choose to get their products approved for use across Europe. In the mutual recognition system a drug company can choose which regulatory agency it would like to evaluate its product and the agency then evaluates that product on behalf of the other member states. Once the reference member state approves the product the other member states have 90 days to 'mutually recognise' it. If countries raise objections, the Committee for Proprietary Medicinal Products (CPMP – see below) acts as an arbitrator and each country can then issue its own marketing authorisation.

However the most commonly used route for marketing authorisation these days is the EU centralised system. This system is in fact already obligatory for all biotechnology products and it has been proposed, and agreed by the EU, that all new active substances should also be obliged to use this route. This would mean that, unless an agency was acting as part of the EU centralised system, only applications for generic products would be dealt with by individual regulatory agencies.

In the centralised system, the pharmaceutical company files an application with the European Medicines Evaluation Agency (EMEA), which passes it to the CPMP. Representatives from two member states are selected to consider the application on behalf of the CPMP – one of which can be selected by the pharmaceutical company (the rapporteur and co-rapporteur). The CPMP has up to 210 days to issue an opinion following receipt of the application. If a positive opinion is issued, the other member states have up to 28 days to respond. Any objections are considered by the CPMP and a recommendation is then made as to whether to permit an EU-wide licence. Once authorisation is approved, the EMEA publishes a European public assessment report (EPAR) on its website. After this has occurred the company is able to market the drug in any EU country, although it is not obliged to launch the drug in all EU countries.

It should be noted that, while drug companies are obliged to market products only within the terms of the product licence, clinicians are still able to prescribe them to any patient for whom they feel they are appropriate.

ORPHAN DRUGS

In order to encourage pharmaceutical companies to develop drugs to help diagnose, prevent or treat rare, life-threatening or very serious diseases, the EU has created the orphan medicinal product scheme. For a drug to be considered in this scheme the condition should have a prevalence of not more than 1 in 2000 of the general population. Companies developing such products may be helped by obtaining EU funds to help research the product, exemptions from the usual licensing fees and, probably most importantly from a company perspective, direct access to the EU centralised approval process and a guaranteed 10-year market exclusivity period, during which time directly competitive similar products cannot usually be placed on the market.

Applications for orphan products are dealt with by a subcommittee of the CPMP known as the Committee for Orphan Medicinal Products (COMP).

WHAT INFORMATION IS CONTAINED IN THE SUMMARY OF PRODUCT CHARACTERISTICS

The summary of product characteristics (SmPC) for over 3000 products that have marketing authorisation in the UK is freely accessible via the Electronic Medicines Compendium website. Similarly, the site allows you access to over 2000 patient information leaflets for these products. There are an estimated 12 000 changes a year to UK regulatory medicines information and, as this resource is updated daily, it should be regarded as the first-line resource when seeking information on any of the following:

- Approved indications
- Recommended doses and method of administration
- Contraindications
- Special warnings and special precautions for use
- Interactions with other medicines and other forms of interaction
- Use in pregnancy and lactation
- Effects on ability to drive and use machines
- Undesirable effects
- Overdose
- List of excipients
- Special precautions for storage.

Brief details of the trials used in the licensing application may also be presented within the SmPC. However, if the product has been approved via the EU centralised process, much more detail on the clinical data available is presented on the EMEA site as the European product assessment report (EPAR).

WITHDRAWAL OF A MEDICINE FROM THE MARKET

Once a company has launched a product it can choose to withdraw that product voluntarily from the market provided it has informed the licensing authority. Companies usually choose to do this for commercial reasons but may also do so for safety reasons to pre-empt adverse publicity arising from a product withdrawal instigated by a regulatory agency. As well as revoking marketing authorisation, the licensing authority also has the power to suspend or vary a product licence and in an emergency can suspend a licence with immediate effect for up to 3 months. Recently the MHRA, then the MCA, decided to revoke the licences for Epogam and Efamast. This was the first time that product licences had been revoked on the basis of lack of proven efficacy. All previous product withdrawals were the result of safety concerns.

WHAT ABOUT MEDICINES THAT ARE NOT LICENSED?

It is difficult to define simply 'what is an unlicensed medicine?' A medicine may be unlicensed for a variety of reasons, for example:

- 'off-label use' (anything not specified in the marketing authorisations, e.g. indications, doses, routes of administration, age groups, diluents)
- medicines imported from another country for a named patient (*Note*: these medicines may also not be licensed in that country or intended use may be outside of the terms of the marketing authorisation held in that country)
- extemporaneously prepared products for specific patients (e.g. total parenteral nutrition)
- products prepared under a 'specials' licence (e.g. liquid preparations for those with swallowing difficulties)
- cases where the marketing authorisation has been suspended, revoked or not renewed (the product may still be available either from the company or by importing, e.g. spectinomycin injection, tetracycline capsules)
- the product is not a medicine but is being used to treat a rare condition (e.g. for a metabolic disease)
- the product is being used in a clinical trial, unless trial use is in accordance with a UK marketing authorisation.

MHRA guidance states that the use of unlicensed/off-label medicines should be restricted to occasions where there are no suitable and equally effective licensed alternatives. Unsurprisingly, the reasons for such use, as with the forms of unlicensed medicines, are various, for example:

- licensed indications do not include well-proven uses (amitriptyline for neuropathic pain)
- variance in licence between brand and generic (e.g. omeprazole)
- use in individuals not covered by the marketing authorisation (e.g. children, pregnant or breast-feeding women)
- conditions in which there are no other treatments (sometimes in the absence of strong evidence).

UNLICENSED/OFF-LABEL DRUGS

Whether a medicine is licensed or unlicensed/off-label is significant. Whenever an unlicensed/off label medicine is prescribed, the prescriber is professionally accountable for any harm caused to the patient as a result of administration of medicines that is not caused by a defective product. The supplying pharmacist will also assume some liability, as part of their duty of care to the patient.

It is important that pharmacists are aware of their responsibility to patients, particularly in respect to unlicensed/off-label medicines where the quality, safety and efficacy of products may not be assured. The Royal Pharmaceutical Society of Great Britain Code of Ethics lays an obligation on pharmacists not to deviate from the prescriber's intention except when necessary to protect the patient. The quality of unlicensed and extemporaneous medicines is the responsibility of the pharmacist. Pharmacists therefore need to be able obtain sufficient information to make a value judgement on whether to supply to a patient or not. Obtaining sufficient information to be able to make this decision is not always easy; possible sources include:

- some information on off-label or unlicensed medicines considered standard therapy is contained within the *British National Formulary*
- the prescribing clinician should be able to support the use of the medicine
- although advertising the use of unlicensed/off-label medicines is prohibited by the MHRA, specific information relating to specific medicines can be made available by pharmaceutical companies or, for imported unlicensed medicines, by the import company. An import company may also be able to provide an English translation of the SmPC (or equivalent)
- use of unlicensed/off-label medicines is widespread in teaching hospitals and, following a specific request, any information they have on the intended use could be made available.

Pharmacists should ensure that:

- the prescriber is aware of the licensed status of the product and any possible consequences. How do you identify all off-label use? This can be difficult and is not always practicable but why/how medicines are being used is an essential aspect of the pharmacist's role, whether the medicine is licensed or not
- they keep adequate records when ordering and supplying unlicensed medicines
- they inform patients of unlicensed/off-label medicines. It can be confusing and worrying for patients to receive conflicting advice

from a product information leaflet and from a doctor/pharmacist when a medicine is being used off-label. In addition, for unlicensed medicines there may be very little written information available for the patient and so how sufficient information can be given to the patient for safe administration needs to be considered

- they are aware of the MHRA guidance on importation of unlicensed medicines into the UK. There can be delays in obtaining the medicine and the continuity of supply may not be assured – where this is the case this information should be communicated to both the prescriber and the patient.

PHARMACOVIGILANCE

Adverse drug reactions (ADRs) are common. It is estimated that they occur in between 10% and 20% of hospitalised patients and are responsible for about 5% of hospital admissions. The extent of ADRs in primary care is less well studied but there have been estimates that up to 2% of GP consultations may be due to suspected ADRs.

From the discussion above it can be seen that when a product reaches the market it will only have been tested in a limited number of highly selected patients. When it is used in patients with a range of other problems, taking a range of other drugs, a very different toxicity profile may become apparent.

The adverse event data that have been compiled during the clinical trial programme will be presented in the SmPC.

The need for formal procedures to detect the true adverse effect profile of a newly licensed medicine is obvious. It is a sobering fact that when a drug is licensed perhaps only 2000 people will have been exposed to it. Even assuming that the drug has not been implicated in any deaths during its development, we can only surmise that it shouldn't kill more than 15 people out of every 10000 that take it (i.e. death would be uncommon using the classification referred to in Chapter 15!). Recent examples of drugs that came to market only to be withdrawn after new adverse effects came to light include troglitazone, tolcapone, cerivastatin and, very recently, rofecoxib.

In the UK, probably the most widely recognised postmarketing surveillance scheme is the one coordinated by the Committee of Safety on Medicines (CSM), known as the 'yellow card' scheme. The yellow card scheme for spontaneous reporting of suspected ADRs was introduced in 1964 after the thalidomide tragedy highlighted the urgent need for routine postmarketing surveillance of medicines. Since then more than 500000 reports of suspected ADRs have been submitted on a voluntary basis by doctors, dentists, pharmacists, coroners, nurses and pharmaceutical companies under statutory obligations. A pilot scheme has also been created to encourage reports directly from patients using NHS Direct.

The CSM invites reports of all adverse reactions, that are thought to be related to administration of a 'black triangle' drug but only requires details of serious adverse reactions for established drugs. Serious reactions include those that are fatal, life-threatening, disabling, incapacitating or that result in or prolong hospitalisation and/or are medically significant or include congenital abnormalities. The CSM yellow card system should also be used for any unexpected or adverse reactions relating to unlicensed/off-label medicine use.

A black triangle is assigned to a newly launched product if that product:

- is a new active substance
- is a previously licensed substance that is contained in a new combination of active substances
- involves administration via a novel route or drug delivery system
- represents a significant new indication that may alter the established risk/benefit profile of that drug.

There is no standard time for a product to retain black triangle status. However, an assessment is usually made following two years of post-marketing experience and the black triangle symbol is not removed until the safety profile of the drug is well established.

The black triangle symbol should appear beside all relevant products listed in the British National Formulary, the Monthly Index of Medical Specialities, the Association of the British Pharmaceutical Industry *Compendium of Datasheets and Summaries of Product Characteristics* and in all relevant advertising material. The list is updated monthly and can be downloaded from the CSM website.

> ⚠ **The symbol beside a drug should be regarded as being analogous to your response to seeing 'L' plates on the car in front – some extra caution is required as you cannot quite predict what that driver might do.**

The CSM makes this data freely available on a website. This website allows you to access data on individual drugs which details:

- all the adverse reactions that have been reported to the CSM that have been associated with that drug (in disease-specific hierarchy)

- the total number of yellow cards that have been received for that drug
- the total number of fatalities that have occurred with each reaction.

Given the nature of the scheme it is always difficult to interpret these data. Firstly, the CSM asks for suspected ADRs so causality is not proven. Secondly, as the scheme is voluntary and the true exposure rate is not known, it is not valid to use the data to make estimates of incidence or make comparisons between drugs within a therapeutic class.

Using the data from the yellow card scheme and other reporting, the CSM obtains an ongoing picture of the safety profiles of therapeutic agents. They update prescribers to adverse effects and products that are causing concern through their regular newsletter *Current Problems in Pharmacovigilance*. Previous editions of this newsletter can be accessed via the CSM website.

Following product launch, other formal prescription event monitoring schemes may also be instigated to obtain a more accurate picture of the effectiveness and safety of a product in the wider population (typically over 10000 patients). The Drug Safety Research Unit runs a green card prescription monitoring system, whereby GPs who prescribe a targeted product are identified by prescription data and are sent a green reporting card.. They are encouraged to report any clinical events that have occurred while the patient has been taking the drug, or after they have stopped it. The studies are published in conventional medical journals. Recent examples include:

- Evaluation of the safety of bupropion (Zyban) for smoking cessation from experience gained in England in 2000 (European Journal of Clinical Pharmacology 2003; 59: 767–773)
- Evaluation of the safety of sildenafil for male erectile dysfunction: experience gained in general practice use in England in 1999 (British Journal of Urology International 2004; 93: 796–801)
- Safety profile of rofecoxib as used in general practice in England: results of a prescription-event monitoring study (British Journal of Clinical Pharmacology 2003;55: 166–174).

Pharmaceutical companies themselves often run similar schemes, but in that circumstance they should adhere to agreed guidelines that cover the safety assessment of marketed medicines (SAMM). These guidelines are basically in place to ensure that such trials have a legitimate clinical objective and are not merely a disguised form of promotion. The guidelines require that medicines in the study should only be prescribed when the doctor has already made a clear intent to treat.

Hopefully it should be clear that the only way the true adverse reaction profile of a drug can ever be established is to ensure that all relevant information is brought to the attention of the licensing authorities and the pharmaceutical company itself. As pharmacists we rely on these data to do our job properly and therefore it is incumbent on us to ensure that we contribute any relevant information we encounter in our practice.

 Pharmacists should ensure that they are familiar with the yellow card scheme, how to access the latest version of the black triangle list and what details are required in reporting a suspected ADR.

RESOURCES

Committee of Safety on Medicines website for details of CSM black triangle scheme and newsletters: http://medicines.mhra.gov.uk/aboutagency/regframework/csm/csmhome.htm

Committee of Safety on Medicines website to access reports of adverse events reported through the 'yellow card system': http://medicines.mhra.gov.uk/yellowcard_gov_uk/daps.html

Department of Health website for details of Research Governance Framework: http://www.dh.gov.uk/PolicyAndGuidance/ResearchAndDevelopment/fs/en

Drug Research Safety Unit: details of previous and ongoing post-marketing surveillance studies: http://www.dsru.org/main.html

Electronic Medicines Compendium for access to the most recent editions of SmPCs and PILs for a wide range of products with marketing authorisation in the UK: http://www.medicines.org.uk/

European Medicines Evaluation Agency website for EPARs, scientific discussions on approved products, guidance on the types of studies and outcomes considered appropriate for assessing medicines in a range of illnesses, product safety updates and details of the orphan product scheme: http://www.emea.eu.int/

Guild of Healthcare Pharmacists website: guidance on unlicensed medicines use in hospitals: www.ghp.org.uk

Medicines and Healthcare Products Regulatory Agency website for access to information about product withdrawals and guidance on supply of unlicensed medicines: http://www.mhra.gov.uk/index.htm

Royal Pharmaceutical Society of Great Britain (RPSGB) website: code of ethics and standards for pharmacists and professional standards factsheet: http://www.rpsgb.org.uk/

Evidence-based practice

N. J. Vetter

The phrases 'evidence-based medicine' (EBM) and 'evidence-based practice' (EBP) (not all health care is medicine) became popular in the 1990s following a movement to increase the scientific basis of health care. Those practising evidence-based health care aim to maximise the percentage of interventions used by them that have been shown, scientifically, to be effective.

EBP is defined as 'the conscientious, explicit and judicious use of current best evidence in making decisions about the care of individual patients'. The practice of EBP requires the integration of individual clinical expertise with the best available external clinical evidence from systematic research. Its philosophical base dates back to the sceptics of postrevolutionary Paris, the fathers of modern anatomy and physiology, Bichat, Louis and Magendie.

Evidence-based practice is not restricted to randomised controlled trials:

- **For diagnostic tests: a proper cross-sectional study of patients clinically suspected of harbouring the disorder is better**
- **For prognosis, a proper follow-up study of patients collected at an early point in the clinical course of their disease, a cohort study, is better**
- **Sometimes the evidence comes from the basic sciences, such as genetics or immunology.**

However, when asking questions about therapy we shun the non-experimental approaches, which often lead to false conclusions about efficacy. The randomised trial and systematic review of a number of those trials are the 'gold standard' for judging whether a treatment does more good than harm.

EVIDENCE OF EFFECTIVENESS

There is a hierarchy of evidence used to judge the strength of evidence on the effectiveness of health care interventions which is generally graded from top down as follows:

1. Systematic reviews
2. Randomised controlled trials
3. Non-randomised experimental studies
4. Observational studies
5. Expert opinion.

A *systematic review* is a summary of the literature (generally from a group of randomised controlled trials) in which evidence is systematically identified, appraised and summarised. The essential point is that a review should give enough information for others to be able replicate it.

A *randomised controlled trial* (RCT) is an experimental study whereby people with a certain condition are randomly allocated to one or more intervention or control groups. Properly performed it allows an unbiased estimate of an intervention's effectiveness.

Non-randomised experimental studies include those where people are allocated to treatment groups sequentially or by other methods known to the investigator. They may include *cohort studies*, where a group of people are tested for their characteristics then followed up over a period to see which of them become ill, and *case-control studies*, where people with a particular disease (the cases) are compared with another specially chosen group (the controls) and their past history is examined to test if the cases have some risk factor in common that is not found among the controls.

Observational studies are those where there is no control group, and may include before and after studies or direct comparison of a treated group with a non-treated group. *Expert opinion* relies on the teaching and experience of clinicians. This may be reliable or biased due to a clinician having experienced an atypical group of cases.

While it is generally accepted that systematic reviews of RCTs are more accurate than single RCTs, very large trials (megatrials) that give precise results are the best source of evidence, as meta-analyses of trials may be prone to publication bias if a number of negative-result trials have not been published, e.g. the use of magnesium after myocardial infarction was advocated in a meta analysis but found to be useless in the ISIS-4 mega trial and must be used with care (Egger et al 2001).

It must also be borne in mind that RCTs can ethically only be carried out if the investigators really believe both treatments to be equally effective, known as equipoise. As a result, many interventions with large, unequivocal effects, e.g. the introduction of penicillin, which massively reduced mortality, have never been formally scientifically tested in trials and are never likely to be. The same is likely to be true for comparing treatments for AIDS and other universally lethal diseases with a placebo (inactive substance, used to check if the patient will get better without intervention).

However, such major effects are rare and all new drugs are now tested for effectiveness using RCTs. Unfortunately, licensing requirements under the Medicines Act do not require that new preparations are tested against the best existing treatment and, because the main concern of the licensing authorities is about safety, not efficacy, the trials are often of short duration. Many drugs are only tested against placebos for short periods and so it is not clear whether the new treatment will be better than existing treatments, especially in chronic disease, where the long-term effects are important.

Medical procedures do not require licensing as such, but this may be changing as the National Institute for Health and Clinical Excellence (NICE), a government-sponsored body that checks on whether new treatments are sufficiently cost-effective to be allowed within the National Health Service (NHS), has set up a group to evaluate interventional procedures. These are procedures used for diagnosis or treatment that involve making a cut or hole in the body, entry into a body cavity or using electromagnetic energy (including X-rays or lasers) or ultrasound. NICE develops guidance on whether interventional procedures are safe enough and work well enough for use in the NHS. This guidance aims to protect the safety of patients and support clinicians, health care organisations and the NHS as a whole in the process of introducing new procedures. Many of the procedures that the programme investigates are new, but the programme also scrutinises more established procedures if there is uncertainty about safety or efficacy. This is not a mandatory licensing process at present but may become so in the future.

EQUIVALENCE, EFFICACY AND EFFECTIVENESS

Sometimes new drugs are tested against existing drugs not to demonstrate that one is better than another but to demonstrate that they are the same in order to gain a foothold in the market. Such trials are called equivalence trials and are open to many biases. A good critique of such trials is available (Jones et al 1996).

Most drug trials aim to test the efficacy or effectiveness of the therapeutic agent. Efficacy or explanatory trials test whether the agent works in the best possible circumstances; for instance, only males within a certain age range without any other major disease may be included in a study of hypotensive agents. Effectiveness or pragmatic trials test whether the agent works in ordinary practice so that all ages and sexes are involved and there are few, if any, restrictions to exclude those with other illnesses.

Both are analysed on an intention-to-treat basis; that is, all patients who are randomised are included in the final analysis, even if some receive a smaller dose or even if they had to stop taking the agent they were on because of side effects or simply because they were lost to follow-up. In the latter case as much information as possible is gathered, e.g. whether they are alive or dead.

DETECTING ADVERSE EFFECTS

 Very few drug trials are sufficiently large or are run for a sufficiently long time to detect all adverse drug events.

The detection of many adverse drug events depends on postmarketing surveillance and the reporting of adverse events thought to be linked to the drug once it has entered general use. However, when a drug has been used on limited numbers of people it is still possible to estimate the risk of a serious adverse event using a statistical formula derived from 95% confidence intervals. A 95% confidence interval is a range within which we are 95% certain the true population value lies, and is derived from a study of a sample of the population.

Suppose 100 people have tried a new drug (or had a new operation) and there have been no adverse events. What is the risk to a person taking the drug of having an adverse event? With our knowledge of confidence intervals we can say that we are 95% certain that the risk of an adverse event is no more than $3/n$ where n = number of people who have had the drug. Here $n = 100$ and $3/n = 3\%$. We are 95% sure that the risk of an adverse event after taking the drug is no more than 3%. The rule of $3/n$ is very useful when people ask about serious adverse events of new therapies.

MEASURES OF EFFECTIVENESS

How effective a treatment is can be expressed in many ways.

RELATIVE RISK AND ODDS RATIOS

These are measures of the risk of an event, either good or bad, occurring in a group that receives treatment A, versus the risk in a group receiving placebo treatment B. Suppose 80 of 100 people receiving A improve compared with 40 of 100 receiving B. The relative risk of improvement of A over B is $80/100 \div 40/100 = 2.0$, i.e. twice as many improve.

Sometimes a slightly different measure, the odds ratio, is used instead of the relative risk. Odds ratios are often used as they are easier to compute and, where there are reasonable numbers, approximate closely to the relative risk, but in theory the relative risk is the more accurate measure as it compares the rate of attack with the population at risk, not simply with another special group.

The following standard 2 by 2 table shows the difference in calculation between relative risk and odds ratio.

		Outcome		Total
		+	−	
Treated	+	A	B	A + B
	−	C	D	C + D
		A + C	B + D	A + B + C + D

A, B, C, D are numbers of people who are treated (+) or not (−) and have a dichotomous, good (+) or bad (−), outcome. The relative risk of a favourable outcome given treatment is $A/(A + B)$ divided by $C/(C + D)$. The odds ratio of a favourable outcome given treatment is A/B divided by C/D or $\dfrac{A \times D}{B \times C}$.

The 95% confidence interval for the above relative risk is 1.5–2.6, so that we can be 95% certain that the true effect of the drug is a 1.5 to 2.6 times improvement. 95% confidence intervals for relative risks and odds ratios that exclude 1.0 are statistically significant, i.e. $p < 0.05$.

IMPROVEMENT IN SURVIVAL OR REDUCTION IN SYMPTOMS

Suppose 100 people receiving drug A survive on average 80 months and 100 receiving drug B survive on average 40 months. The net average survival effect of drug A is 40 months and the 95% confidence interval from a 37.2-month survival advantage to a 42.8-month survival advantage. 95% confidence intervals for improvements in survival or symptom reduction that exclude 0.0 are statistically significant, i.e. $p < 0.05$.

NUMBER NEEDED TO TREAT (NNT)

In evidence-based practice the number of people that it is necessary to treat to produce (on average) one additional successful outcome is currently a useful measure of effectiveness. It is better to use it than relative risk because it gives more information by taking into account the baseline risk and is easier to explain to patients. In the above example, 80/100 people improved with drug A and 40/100 with drug B. The absolute risk reduction (ARR) with drug A is 80/100 − 40/100 = 40/100 or 0.4. The NNT with drug A to produce an additional successful outcome is the inverse of the absolute risk reduction (NNT = 1/ARR), here 1/0.4 = 2.5. This means that on average it is necessary to treat 2.5 people with drug A to make one of them better. By tradition, NNTs are usually rounded to the nearest whole number. Suppose a successful outcome occurred in 80/1000 with drug A and 40/1000 with drug B. The relative risk of improvement would still be 2.0 but the NNT would now be 25. Clearly NNTs give a better feel for how effective a drug is. It is also possible to calculate 95% confidence intervals for NNTs.

NUMBER NEEDED TO HARM (NNH)

This is analogous to the NNT but is a useful way of describing to patients problems related to side effects. It is computed as for NNTs but the outcomes are harmful events rather than successes.

GRAPHICAL REPRESENTATION

Meta analyses often demonstrate the effect size and confidence intervals of each of the individual studies and the pooled results in a graph are often referred to by those teaching critical appraisal skills as a blobbogram (Fig. 5.1).

The lines with dots in the centre represent four studies. The dots represent the odds ratios of the treatment relative to placebo in achieving a desired outcome. The length of the line represents the confidence interval around the odds ratio. The central vertical line represents an odds ratio of 1, i.e. no treatment effect. Two of the studies do not cross the line of no effect and demonstrate statistically significant improvement in outcome with treatment. In the other two studies the confidence intervals cross the line of no effect and while on average they are positive they are also consistent with the treatment having a negative effect. The diamond represents the odds ratio of the combined estimate of effectiveness in the meta-analysis.

EFFECTIVE INTERVENTIONS FOR INDIVIDUALS

So much for the principles of EBP. What happens when a clinician wishes to put EBP into practice with an individual patient? Trials tell us whether on average a group of people with a certain condition will

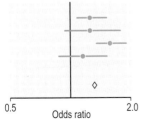

0.5   2.0
        Odds ratio

Fig. 5.1 A blobbogram.

be better or worse off with treatment, but not whether it is in the best interest of any one individual to accept treatment.

To make a decision for an individual further information is required. It is necessary to know: (a) how effective the treatment is (relative risks from meta-analyses or RCTs); (b) the risk to an individual patient of a particular age, sex, race, and with certain risk factors (should come from multivariate risk equations derived from cohort studies) of the event happening that it is hoped to prevent; and (c) the risk of harm from treatment (data on frequency of adverse events). Only if the reduction in absolute risk with treatment exceeds the risk of an adverse event is treatment worthwhile for the individual. It is often worthwhile treating individuals at high risk of illness but not often worth treating low-risk individuals. Some work has been done to explain an example of how to use these risks in practice (Glasziou and Irwig 1995).

SOURCES OF EVIDENCE

While there are an increasing number of systematic reviews available it will be a long time before reviews are ready for all but a sizeable minority of clinical problems. The following sources are particularly useful. Current internet addresses are provided on contact points (these may change).

National Institute for Health and Clinical Excellence

NICE was set up as a special health authority for England and Wales on 1 April 1999. Scotland has its own counterpart. It is part of the NHS and its role is to provide patients, health professionals and the public with authoritative, robust and reliable guidance on current best practice. The guidance covers individual health technologies (including medicines, medical devices, diagnostic techniques and procedures) and the clinical management of specific conditions.

The guidance for individual technologies comes in two phases. The first of these is an assessment of the technology arrived at by exploring the literature, including, where possible, unpublished literature, to examine the effectiveness of the technology. This will also include a cost-effectiveness evaluation in terms of the cost of the intervention to save one quality-adjusted life year or QALY. Thus, even if the technology is found to be effective, it may be rejected for use by the NHS if it is very costly for the good that it does. A general rule is that any treatment costing more than £20000–£30000 per QALY achieved is looked at very carefully before it is approved. NICE publishes all its findings as far as possible so that the deliberations it makes are all open to public scrutiny.

In addition, NICE produces guidelines on a wide range of subjects. These look at the treatment pathway overall, rather than just a component of it, as the appraisal committees do. NICE has also recently set up committees to look at public health interventions.

Internet address: http://www.nice.org.uk/

International Cochrane Collaboration

This group, set up in memory of Archie Cochrane, a great advocate of the use of RCTs, facilitates the creation, review and dissemination of reviews of the effectiveness of health care.

Internet address: http://www.cochrane.org/

NHS Centre for Reviews and Dissemination

The Centre for Reviews and Dissemination (CRD) produced two publicly available databases: (a) the Database of Abstract of Reviews of Effectiveness (DARE); and (b) the NHS Economic Evaluation Database (NEED). The NHS CRD also produces two printed bulletins: *Effective Healthcare* (along with Nuffield Institute) and *Effectiveness Matters*. Both papers contain copies of reviews.

Internet address: http://www.york.ac.uk/inst/crd/

Bandolier

These are paper copies of reviews and interpretations of statistical tests used in evidence-based health care. Bandolier is funded by the NHS Management Executive and Anglia and Oxford Regional Health Authority.

Internet address: http://www.jr2.ox.ac.uk/bandolier/

Evidence-Based Purchasing

This is produced by the research and development directorate of the NHS Executive.

Internet address: http://www.pasa.doh.gov.uk/evaluation

On-line databases

It is also possible to search databases (e.g. Medline, Embase) for RCTs where reviews have not been carried out. To ensure that your search strategy is comprehensive and scientific, consult a librarian for advice as amateur attempts generally only acquire 15–20% of the appropriate literature.

If you are asked to carry out a systematic review yourself, help is available in the form of a report (University of York and NHS Centre for Reviews and Dissemination 1996). Carrying out a systematic review is a daunting task not to be undertaken lightly or by the untrained. Librarians are often skilled in this work and can be of great assistance. However the general rule is: look for one off the shelf where possible, rather than starting your own from scratch.

Internet address for Medline: http://www.ncbi.nlm.nih.gov/entrez/query.fcgi

CRITICAL APPRAISAL

It is much more likely that you might be asked to carry out a critical appraisal of existing literature. Critical appraisal is a systematic method for assessing the scientific quality and relevance of the literature on a particular topic. Critical appraisal of a systematic review involves assessing whether the following steps listed have been carried out.

STEPS IN CRITICAL APPRAISAL OF SYSTEMATIC REVIEWS

- Is the review focused in terms of clearly describing
  - the population or types of patients studied
  - the intervention
  - the outcomes measured?

- Were the right types of study to answer the question included in the review?
  - RCTs to assess efficacy and effectiveness
  - controlled trials, postmarketing surveillance, adverse event reporting for side effects
- Were all the relevant studies included?
  - a comprehensive search strategy, i.e. include unpublished and foreign-language studies
- Were the decisions to include/exclude studies in/from the review reasonable?
  - specified inclusion/exclusion criteria described, preferably before results of study seen
  - do you agree with them?
- If the overall results have been summarised in a meta-analysis, was it reasonable to do so (i.e. combining the results of studies to form a group-averaged result)? Meta-analysis can be validly carried out when:
  - similar-type studies are compared (similar interventions, outcomes and populations)
  - the results of the different studies are clearly displayed
  - the reasons for differences in results are explicable
- Have the overall results been clearly displayed?
  - estimate of effect (odds ratio, mean, etc.)
  - confidence intervals for above
  - numbers needed to treat to produce one extra positive outcome
  - cost of producing one extra positive outcome.

> ⚠ **You need to form a clinical judgement about whether the benefits are worth the harm and the cost of the intervention.**
>
> **Remember other important outcomes will not have been measured. All interventions have multiple outcomes, which are time-dependent.**

GETTING RESEARCH INTO PRACTICE – IMPLEMENTING CLINICAL PRACTICE GUIDELINES

There is always a considerable delay in implementing the findings of research into routine clinical practice. The government has taken a lead in some specific areas by setting up National Service Frameworks (NSFs) for different groups of diseases or groups of people.

So far there are NSFs for cancer, coronary heart disease, mental health, paediatric intensive care, children, diabetes, renal, long-term conditions and older people. The NSFs suggest approaches to best practice for an effective service and the details and targets are based on the best available evidence.

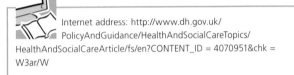

Internet address: http://www.dh.gov.uk/ PolicyAndGuidance/HealthAndSocialCareTopics/ HealthAndSocialCareArticle/fs/en?CONTENT_ID = 4070951&chk = W3ar/W

At the level of the individual clinician, however, there are still problems. There are many reasons for this, including clinicians' lack of awareness of research, which is hardly surprising given the volume of literature on any one topic. Textbooks may be written by individuals without recourse to systematic reviews and often contain outdated or erroneous material. For example, while definitive evidence of the effectiveness of thrombolytic agents in acute myocardial infarction was available in the early 1970s, most textbooks written in the 1980s omitted the topic and the therapy was not widely introduced until the 1990s. There is some evidence that training in EBP is problematic, even for pharmacists (Watson et al 2002).

One way to keep up with substantial changes in clinical practice is to subscribe to a journal that contains lists of reviews, such as *Evidence-based Medicine*, which is available on the internet.

Internet address: http://ebm.bmjjournals.com/

Clinical guidelines are increasingly used to implement EBP. It is important that the guidelines are themselves evidence-based. Some of the best evidence-based guidelines have been developed by the Agency for Health Care Policy and Research in the USA. The National Electronic Library for Health is a fount of much wisdom, including a useful section on medical news 'scare' stories and how much credence to give them.

Internet address: http://www.nelh.nhs.uk/

In order to reduce black spots where these criteria are not adhered to, the government has set up another umbrella organisation: the Healthcare Commission. It inspects the quality of health care across the public and private sectors. It inspects every NHS institution regularly on a rotation basis and can also be called in by the government if an NHS establishment has been shown to be not up to standard in its work. The process of ensuring good health care standards throughout a hospital or other health care facility is known as *clinical governance*.

The Healthcare Commission has the power to replace the management of an NHS unit and put in another team if things seem to be going badly; this includes adherence to NICE guidelines.

Internet address: http://www.healthcarecommission.org.uk/

An *Effective Health Care Bulletin* (**Nuffield Institute for Health 1996**) has produced a report on implementing clinical guidelines. The reviewers found that guidelines could change clinical practice and affect patient outcome but that the method of development and implementation affected the likelihood of successfully improving outcomes. Guidelines were more likely to be effective if they took into account local circumstances, were disseminated by an active educational intervention and were implemented by patient-specific reminders relating directly to clinical activity. Those intending to introduce clinical practice guidelines should read the reviews before starting.

Box 5.1 Pharmacy sources on the internet

This section on evidence-based practice has made much reference to what is available on the internet. *Since the internet is unregulated, addresses may change or new services may start up or existing ones stop.* At the time of going to press the following sources can provide valuable information to the clinical pharmacist (*Note:* searching via Google will usually find the source):

● Centre for Evidence-Based Pharmacy in Oxford: http://www.jr2. ox.ac.uk/pharmacy/
● Evidence-Based Pharmacy Regulation, part of the Cochrane Collaboration: http://www.jr2.ox.ac.uk/pharmacy/
● The Centre for Evidence-Based Pharmaco-Therapy at Aston University: http://www.aston.ac.uk/lhs/research/
● Pharmacy Update: evidence-based medicine questionnaire: http:// www.dotpharmacy.co.uk/groups/med/

REFERENCES

Egger M, Smith GD, Sterne JA 2001 Uses and abuses of meta-analysis. Clinical Medicine 1: 478–484

Glasziou PP, Irwig LM 1995 An evidence based approach to individualising treatment. British Medical Journal 311: 1356–1359.

Jones B, Jarvis P, Lewis JA, Ebbutt AF 1996 Trials to assess equivalence: the importance of rigorous methods. British Medical Journal 313: 36–39.

Nuffield Institute for Health 1996 Effective health care: implementing clinical practice guidelines. University of Leeds, Leeds

University of York and NHS Centre for Reviews and Dissemination 1996 Undertaking systematic reviews of research on effectiveness. CRD guidelines for those carrying out or commissioning reviews. University of York, York

Watson MC, Bond CM, Grimshaw JM 2002 Educational strategies to promote evidence-based community pharmacy practice: a cluster randomized controlled trial (RCT). Family Practice 19: 529–536.

CHAPTER 6

Pharmacoeconomics

R. Elliott

WHAT ARE HEALTH ECONOMICS AND PHARMACOECONOMICS?

Health economics applies economics to health and health care and considers the choices concerned with allocating scarce resources.

Pharmacoeconomics is the branch of health economics that is specifically concerned with pharmaceutical products and services.

THE ROLE OF HEALTH ECONOMICS AND PHARMACOECONOMICS

Containing the rate of increase in health care spending is a principal concern in health policy. 'Cost-effectiveness' is now an important criterion for selection of therapies by providers and purchasers of health care.

Health economics and pharmacoeconomics analyse the relationship between the costs and consequences of health care. This analysis of new and existing therapies is needed to inform decisions about allocating scarce resources. The method used to analyse this relationship is *economic evaluation*.

Pharmacists need to understand economic evaluations so that they can decide whether economic evidence can be included in the decision-making process by purchasers and formulary committees.

ECONOMIC EVALUATION

WHAT IS ECONOMIC EVALUATION?

> **Economic evaluation is the comparative analysis of the costs and consequences of two or more courses of action**

In Europe and the USA, economic evaluations of drugs are undertaken voluntarily by pharmaceutical companies to provide information for purchasers. In Australia and some provinces of Canada, companies have to include economic evaluation of their products in any application for reimbursement. In the UK, the National Institute for Clinical Excellence (NICE) uses economic evaluation to assist their decisions about the cost-effectiveness of alternative treatments.

COMPONENTS OF ECONOMIC EVALUATION

Principal components are costs and consequences (outcomes) (Fig. 6.1).

Costs

The inputs in an intervention are the resources used. The value attached to this resource use is the *cost*. Costs (Fig. 6.2) can be divided into:

- Direct costs: *Direct medical costs* occur within the health sector, e.g. drugs, laboratory tests and staff time. *Direct non-medical costs* are incurred by other parts of the public sector or by patients and families, e.g. travel costs.

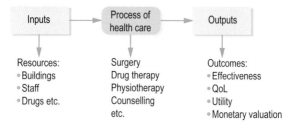

Fig. 6.1 Principal components are resources and outcomes

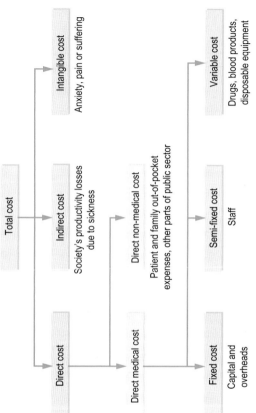

Fig. 6.2 Analysis of cost

- Indirect costs: relate to lost productivity of patients and families due to treatment, illness or death, e.g. time off work and premature mortality. Inclusion of indirect costs, e.g. cost of illness, in economic evaluation usually has a significant effect on conclusions.
- Intangible costs: cannot easily be measured, e.g. pain and suffering experienced by patients. Due to measurement problems they are often left out of an analysis.

Costs are also divided into:

- Fixed costs: incurred whether patients are treated or not. *Capital costs* occur when major capital assets are purchased, e.g. building a counselling room. *Overhead costs* include services such as lighting, heating and security.
- Semi-fixed costs: remain unchanged over a range of activity. Given sufficient changes in activity, they increase or decrease, e.g. staff costs.
- Variable costs: incurred from a patient's treatment, e.g. drugs, blood products and laboratory investigations.

Outcome measures

- *Effectiveness*: single measures of outcome, such as impact on survival (life years gained). Clinical indicators are also used (intermediate outcome measures), e.g. reduction in blood pressure
- *Health-related quality of life (QoL)*: a complex concept with many functional, social, psychological and cognitive and subjective components. QoL measures can be divided into:
  - *Disease-specific*: These measures have been developed for specific diseases, e.g. the Arthritis Impact Measurement Scale (AIMS) in rheumatoid arthritis
  - *Generic*: These measures are useful when looking at groups of patients who may have different illnesses, and can be used to compare health gains in different patient groups, e.g. the Nottingham Health Profile and the EuroQol
  - *Utility* is a measure of the relative preference for a specific level of health status. It can be directly measured or derived from generic QoL measures. It is expressed as quality-adjusted life-years (QALYs) or healthy year equivalents (HYEs). For example, 1 year in 'perfect health' = 1 QALY; 2 years in a health state valued as 50% 'perfect health' = 1 QALY
- *Expressing benefits as monetary values*: This is simple for some measures, such as loss of earnings, cost to the health service or social services for treatment and care. It is more difficult to attach

monetary values to disability, distress, uncertainty or threat to life. One method, 'willingness to pay', seeks to elicit how much an individual would be willing to pay to avoid an illness or obtain the benefits of a treatment.

TYPES OF ECONOMIC EVALUATION

Four types:

- Cost-effectiveness analysis (CEA)
- Cost-minimisation analysis (CMA)
- Cost–utility analysis (CUA)
- Cost–benefit analysis (CBA)

They measure inputs (costs) in the same way but differ in the type of outcome measure used (Table 6.1).

WHAT TO LOOK FOR IN AN ECONOMIC EVALUATION

Apply the following questions to identify strengths and weaknesses in published economic evaluations.

Was a well-defined question posed in answerable form?

The study should include justification of the economic analysis technique chosen. Assess whether the study compared both costs and consequences of alternatives. Make sure the viewpoint has been stated, e.g. 'From the viewpoint of this community trust, is it more cost-effective to initiate therapy of major depressive disorder in the community with an SSRI or a tricyclic antidepressant?', not 'Is treating depression worth it?'

The viewpoint, or *perspective*, of the study determines which costs need to be included, e.g. the cost to a hospital of initiating lipid-lowering treatment will be less than the cost to the whole NHS, which will also include primary care costs.

Ideally, the viewpoint should be societal. In practice, the viewpoint is usually that of the funder of the service, e.g. a trust, a community trust or the NHS.

Was a comprehensive description of the competing alternatives given?

Can you tell *who* did *what* to *whom*, *where* and *how often*? Assess whether any important alternatives have been left out (e.g. 'do

TABLE 6.1 Measurements of inputs and outcomes in different forms of economic evaluations

Form of analysis	Measurement of input	Measurement of outcome	Use of results
Cost–effectiveness analysis	Costs	Natural units (cases successfully treated, life-years gained, disease-free time)	Comparison of interventions with the same unit of benefit but a different magnitude: cost per unit of effect
Cost–minimisation analysis	Costs (often only direct)	No measurement within study	Cost comparison (lowest cost to achieve an identical result): cost per case
Cost–utility analysis	Costs	Quality-adjusted life years (QALYs), healthy year equivalents (HYEs)	Summary of multiple dimensions into one scale; comparison of treatments with initial different outcome measures: cost per QALY
Cost–benefit analysis	Costs	Monetary benefit	Cost minus benefit: cost–benefit ratio

Source: Kobelt 1996

nothing' or current practice); e.g. to assess the cost-effectiveness of a pharmacist-run anticoagulant clinic, comparison with an existing clinician-led clinic could be valid.

The treatment paths of the alternatives should be described. *Decision analytic* techniques are often used.

The principles of decision analysis are used to define the research question and express the intervention as a decision-analytic model, where we:

● characterise each uncertain event by a single number (probability)
● illustrate the decisions and uncertain events diagrammatically with a decision tree (decision-analytic model).

It will look something like the decision tree (also called a 'decision-analytic model') in Figure 6.3.

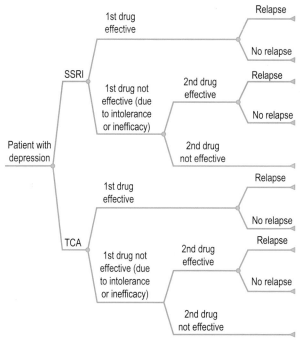

Fig. 6.3 Decision-analytic tool for antidepressant therapy

The second stage is to obtain economic and clinical evidence to apply to the decision-analytic model. In primary economic evaluation the data come from primary sources. This is either a prospective study attached to a randomised controlled trial or an observational study. In secondary economic evaluation, the sources of data are published evidence. Systematic review of economic and clinical data is used to find and assess information to combine with the decision-analytic model. The third stage involves the analysis of the incremental effect of an intervention on overall resource use and patient outcome, compared with alternatives.

Was there evidence that the programme's effectiveness had been established?

This is preferably done via randomised controlled trials. Sources of evidence need to be identified and justified.

> ⚠ **Is the evidence relevant to the economic evaluation (i.e. setting, patient group, treatment pathways, outcome measures used)?**
> **Are the trial treatment protocols relevant to everyday clinical practice?**

An economic evaluation of antibiotic treatment of community-acquired pneumonia (CAP) requires evidence of the efficacy of antibiotics used for CAP in patients likely to acquire CAP.

Assumptions of equal effectiveness of alternatives in cost-minimisation analyses should be stated.

Have all relevant costs been identified, measured and valued?

All resource use needs to be identified and measured, e.g. drugs, staff time. Methods used to measure resource use need to be described in detail, e.g. computerised dispensing records.

Costs should then be attached to resources used. The sources and methods of valuation of costs must be clearly stated. For example, market prices may be used for resource use such as drugs. Methods used to allocate resource use such as overheads must be reported. Make sure that costs have not been inadvertently counted twice, i.e. *double-counting*. This can happen when overheads are allocated.

'Top-down' costs, 'bottom-up' costs or charges?

Studies often use costs provided by accounting departments in the form of *average costs*, e.g. cost per day in hospital. These are *'top-down' costs*, which divide total running costs for a department by total number of patient-days. Average costs often over- or underestimate actual costs. Studies may use *charges* instead of costs. These are less accurate than costs because they usually include cross-subsidisation, which makes up for losses on one service by making a profit on another. *'Bottom-up' costs* represent the actual resource use associated with an individual patient's treatment. They are the most relevant in an economic evaluation because they are the most sensitive to treatment differences.

Some studies report only additional costs of the alternative under investigation. This is valid as long as all changes in resource use have been identified.

Have all relevant outcomes been identified, measured and valued?

Outcome measures should be identified and their selection justified. Those used are dictated by the study objective. For example, looking at the impact of lipid-lowering agents on survival means that long-term mortality is the outcome measure.

Intermediate outcome measures, such as infection rates, can be used as long as the study makes explicit the link to a final health outcome, e.g. survival or QoL.

Studies may report more than one outcome measure, e.g. reduction in blood pressure, myocardial infarction rates and QoL.

In cost–utility analysis, proven generic QoL measures should be used.

In cost–benefit analysis, accepted methods for attaching monetary values to benefits should be used, e.g. willingness to pay, contingent valuation.

Have costs and consequences been discounted?

Discounting is a technique that allows comparison between costs and consequences that occur at different times. In health care, costs often occur immediately, while benefits occur later. Discounting is not a correction for inflation. It reflects that we prefer to receive benefits now and postpone costs. It also reflects the returns that could have been gained if the resources were invested elsewhere, e.g. based on a discount rate of 5%, a cost of £1000 occurring in 1 year's time is considered to be worth only about 95% at present value, i.e. £950.

Discounting is done on an annual basis, so studies shorter than 1 year do not need to use it.

Office of Health Economics Recommendations for
Discounting (Kobelt 1996). Two methods should be used:

1. All costs and outcomes discounted at the prevailing rate
   recommended by the Treasury
2. All costs and monetary outcomes discounted at the Treasury rate
   (currently 3.5% per annum) but non-monetary outcomes not
   discounted.

Was an incremental analysis of costs and consequences of alternatives performed?

Incremental analysis is the preferred method of comparing the costs
and consequences of a health care intervention.

If one alternative is more effective and less costly, it is the *dominant* therapy. When one alternative is more effective, but requires
more resources, the cost required to achieve each extra unit of outcome
is calculated. This is the incremental cost-effectiveness ratio (ICER):

$$\text{ICER} = (\text{Cost}_{\text{Treatment 1}} - \text{Cost}_{\text{Treatment 2}})/(\text{Outcome}_{\text{Treatment 1}} - \text{Outcome}_{\text{Treatment 2}})$$

Should the ICER be big or small?

The larger the ICER is, the more money is required to buy each unit
of outcome. Therefore, as an ICER becomes bigger, the intervention
is said to be less cost-effective.

Cost-effectiveness planes

ICERs can be plotted on to a graph known as a cost-effectiveness plane
(Fig. 6.4). The difference in cost is plotted with the difference in effect.
Depending upon the results of the incremental economic analysis, the
ICERs can be placed in any one of the four quadrants:

- *north-east quadrant*: intervention is more effective and more
  costly
- *south-east quadrant*: intervention is more effective and less costly
- *south-west quadrant*: intervention is less effective and less costly
- *north-west quadrant*: intervention is less effective and more
  costly.

Was sensitivity analysis performed?

This examines the effect on the results of changes in key assumptions
or parameters. For example, what effect does it have if the effective-

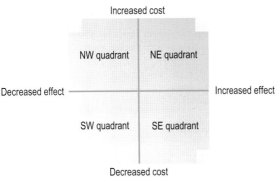

Fig. 6.4 The cost-effectiveness plane

ness of a treatment is doubled or halved, the incidence of side effects lowered or increased? It identifies which parameters or assumptions have the most significant effect on the outcome and stability of the results.

Make sure that the study has justified the choice and range of parameters to vary.

Did the discussion of the study results include all issues of concern to users?

Assess whether the study has dealt sufficiently with related issues such as ethical concerns and equity, generalisability and implementation.

Comparison with other studies should take into account differences in methods (e.g. which costs are included) and setting (e.g. patient groups). Published league tables of economic evaluations, such as cost per QALY league tables, should be interpreted and used with caution because of these differences.

A FINAL NOTE

The appraisal above assesses whether the results of an economic evaluation are valid. It is then necessary to ask:

 If the results are valid, would they apply to my setting?

GLOSSARY

Cost-effectiveness Efficient use of scarce resources

Decision analysis Explicit quantitative approach to decision-making under uncertainty

Direct medical costs Fixed and variable costs directly associated with a health care intervention

Effectiveness Therapeutic consequence of a treatment in real-world conditions

Efficacy Consequence of a treatment under controlled clinical conditions

Incremental cost-effectiveness ratio Additional cost of producing an extra unit of outcome by one therapy compared with another

Indirect costs Cost of reduced productivity resulting from illness or treatment

Intangible costs The cost of pain and suffering resulting from illness or treatment

Marginal costs The extra cost of one extra unit of product or service delivered

Sensitivity analysis Assessment of the robustness of study results through systematic variation of key variables

Utility A measure of the relative preference for, or desirability of, a specific level of health status or a specific health outcome

REFERENCE

Kobelt G. Health economics: an introduction to economic evaluation. Office of Health Economics, London, 1996

FURTHER READING

Byford S, Raftery J 1998 Economics notes: perspectives in economic evaluation. British Medical Journal 316: 1529–1530

Department of Health 1994 Guidance on good practice in the conduct of economic evaluations of medicines. National Health Service and Association of the British Pharmaceutical Industry, London

Drummond MF, Stoddart GL, Torrance GW 1997 Methods for the economic evaluation of health care programmes, 2nd edn. Oxford University Press, Oxford

Jefferson T, Demicheli V, Mugford M 1996 Elementary economic evaluation in health care. British Medical Journal Publishing Group, London

National Prescribing Centre 2000 An introduction to health economics. MeReC Briefing. Available online at:http://www.npc.co.uk/ MeReC_Briefings/2000/briefing_no_13.pdf

Palmer S, Raftery J 1999 Economics notes: opportunity cost. British Medical
  Journal 318: 1551–1552
Raftery J 2000 Economics notes: costing in economic evaluation. British
  Medical Journal 320:1597
Torgerson DJ, Raftery J 1999 Economics notes: discounting. British Medical
  Journal 319: 914–915

CHOICE

CHAPTER 7

The pharmacist as prescriber

J. Cantrill, I. Smith

In 1999 in the UK, a review of the prescribing, supply and administration of medicines became a catalyst to the introduction of pharmacist prescribing, in that it recommended that prescribing responsibilities should be extended to a wide range of health care professionals, including pharmacists. The Health and Social Care Act of 2001 provided the legal framework for the introduction of the extension of prescribing to include other groups of health care professionals.

Two categories of prescribers were defined:

- *independent prescribers* who would be responsible for the initial assessment of the patient and drawing up a treatment plan. The independent prescriber also has the authority to prescribe the medicines required as part of the plan
- *supplementary prescribers* (then referred to as 'dependent' prescribers) who would be authorised to prescribe for patients whose condition had been diagnosed or assessed by an independent prescriber, within the parameters of an agreed clinical management plan (see Box 7.1).

For many years pharmacists have been trained in skills such as communication and professional decision-making. Indeed, these skills are used daily when counter prescribing or providing prescribing advice to doctors and nurses. The requirements for both supplementary and independent prescribers include formal training, assessment and supervised practice. Robust continuing professional development is also

Box 7.1 Components of a clinical management plan

- Diagnoses
- Aims of treatment (or therapeutic objectives)
- Medical history
- Medication allergies and intolerances
- Indications for drug therapy
- Plans for review and monitoring
- Process for reporting adverse drug reactions
- Guidelines to support clinical management plan
- Criteria and process for referral

essential to ensure that pharmacists continue to develop the skills and competencies that are required to deliver this increased responsibility. The competencies for pharmacist supplementary prescribers have been identified by the National Prescribing Centre (2003).

At the time of writing the new prescribing roles have yet to develop, so we have based this chapter on counter prescribing in community pharmacy, although the principles are general and will be applicable to other prescribing roles.

INFORMATION GATHERING

Information gathering is a key skill in any aspect of a pharmacist's role and is an essential component of prescribing. Pharmacists as prescribers have to make or review the diagnosis of the patient. In addition to effective questioning, physical examination and diagnostic tests may be required for some patients. The pharmacist will also need to take a comprehensive medical and medication history and document their findings.

COMMUNICATION SKILLS

QUESTIONING STYLE

When gathering information from any patient, a pharmacist needs to consider the structure and the types of question that they ask. There are two types of question, open and closed; both have advantages and disadvantages.

- *Open questions* (which often begin with how, when, where, why, what and who or even 'tell me about . . .') give the patient an opportunity to speak freely and may provide more in-depth information and even elicit information the interviewer did not expect. However, this may be time-consuming and may not allow the interviewer to explore specific areas. If the interviewer asks too many open questions the information may lack clarity and the interviewer may also lose control of the interview. Open questions may also produce information that is difficult to analyse and record.

- *Closed questions*, which require a yes/no or limited answer, take less time and less thought in answering and are useful in identifying specific, predetermined information. However, this style may be frustrating for the patient who has information they want to divulge, and can shut down the flow of information, resulting in misleading answers or conclusions. If too many closed questions are used the interview may feel more like an interrogation.

In good professional–patient dialogue, the questioning strategy should be a balance of question types. One strategy is to funnel the conversation. This means starting with open questions such as 'Tell me about your indigestion?' and then using closed questions to probe for more specific information or to test understanding of the subjective words a patient might use, such as 'sometimes', 'often', 'bad', etc.

The skilled interviewer should also be aware of the problems involved in the use of leading or multiple questions. Leading questions do as they say and lead the patient to the answer and this can produce misleading or even false information; 'The pain isn't too bad today, is it?' Multiple questions are one or more questions joined together: 'When did you last have indigestion and how long did it last?' They can cause the interviewee confusion, not knowing which question to answer. As well as adopting an appropriate questioning style, the pharmacist should give patients time to formulate their answer, particularly when a difficult question is being asked.

LISTENING AND OBSERVATION SKILLS

The pharmacist should assimilate both the verbal and non-verbal messages being transmitted. That way the pharmacist will not only get information about the patient's condition but may gain insight into the patient's anxieties, beliefs and expectations.

Listening skills are important in ensuring understanding of the verbal message. Active listening requires concentration and the removal of distractions and barriers. It is essential that communication takes place in a professional environment that encourages the patient to participate in an honest and open exchange of information. The location, layout and general appearance of the room or area used for the consultation will affect the communication process. It will need to offer an appropriate level of privacy and freedom from interruptions. Remember that by using the principles of communication the pharmacist can help to make the environment less threatening, in particular, by paying attention to their proximity and orientation to the patient.

The patient should have the pharmacist's full attention. Summarising what you understood the patient to have said back to the patient is a useful technique when the patient has given a lot of information. It also aids concentration and listening, as well as recall of information, and the patient may use the summary to clarify, correct or even offer more information: 'So, I would just like to summarise what you have said to me so far. The first time you had indigestion was . . , etc. . . . Have I understood what you said correctly?'

Taking notes can be helpful in documenting and focusing on information received but can also hinder the flow of information. However, notes will require to be made during the interview, particularly when receiving large amounts of information. The pharmacist can be summarising verbally at the same time as writing. The notes can also be used as signposts to indicate that one section of the interview is complete and the pharmacist is moving on to explore another area, particularly when taking a complete medical and medication history. Time should be planned at the end of the consultation for the review and completion of any documentation to avoid losing important information.

MEDICAL HISTORY TAKING

Obtaining a comprehensive medical and medication history is a key component of safe and effective prescribing. Independent prescribing and counter prescribing may require a complete history. For supplementary prescribing, a history may already have been produced when the diagnosis was made by another prescriber. A complete medical history contains the following elements, as outlined in the *Oxford Handbook of Clinical Medicine* (Longmore et al 2004):

- *Presenting complaint (PC)*: What is the nature of the problem for which the patient is seeking advice/help? One way to focus the patient and to start the interview is to ask an open question: 'Tell me about your indigestion?' or 'What made you come for advice about your indigestion today?'
- *History of presenting complaint (HPC)*: These are a series of questions to find out more about the nature of the condition: 'How long have you been suffering from indigestion?' 'How often does it occur?' 'Are you aware of anything that causes it?'

- *Past medical history (PMH)*: This is a series of questions to find out about any relevant medical history that may impact on the diagnosis or prescribing decision: 'Have you ever had a stomach ulcer in the past?' 'Have you any heart problems?' (angina may form part of the differential diagnosis), 'Do you have high blood pressure?' (a contraindication/caution for some antacids)

- *Medication*: To ensure that a complete medication history is taken it is important to identify not only the patient's past and present prescription medication but also their non-prescription treatments (including complementary and herbal treatments) and their use of alcohol, recreational drugs and tobacco. The nature of any allergies or drug intolerances should also be documented in this section.

- *Social and family history (SH/FH)*: Questions about the patient's family's health can be used to assess their risk of disease (e.g. of heart disease) or as part of a diagnosis. Taking the time to understand something of the patient's life and social context helps to develop the pharmacist–patient relationship. It may also elicit factors that influence the choice of medicine for them. For example, questions about the level of support at home can aid when making a treatment or prescribing decision, in that some elderly people may have difficulty administering liquid medicines themselves.

DIAGNOSIS/DIFFERENTIAL DIAGNOSIS

Having completed the history, the pharmacist will need to make or confirm the diagnosis. Information gathering is only one part of the clinical reasoning process and the skilled prescribing pharmacist will have to consider the differential diagnosis.

Hypothetico-deductive reasoning is one of a number of methods of reaching a differential diagnosis. The practitioner produces a list of possible causes (hypotheses) for the symptoms presented by a patient, e.g. a patient complaining of 'indigestion' might have angina, peptic ulcer, hiatus hernia, etc. Once the practitioner has produced this list, more information is usually gathered either to support or reject each hypothesis. When the list of hypotheses cannot be shortened further this becomes the working or differential diagnosis. All the time that information is being gathered through questioning, examination or tests, it is checked against the list of hypotheses and if the data are not supportive of the hypothesis then that hypothesis is rejected. If the data support the hypothesis then it remains on the list. The pitfall for beginners is in not generating enough hypotheses and narrowing the list too quickly, i.e. jumping to conclusions from incomplete data. For example, just because a patient has a past history of peptic ulcer, 'indigestion' should not automatically be assumed to be gastric in origin.

DANGER SYMPTOMS (WARNING FLAGS) AND HIGH-RISK GROUPS

When gathering information to review the diagnosis it is also important to consider any 'warning flags'. These are pieces of information that may be indicative of a more sinister condition or a change in the disease. Examples of such 'warning flags' are weight loss without a reason or the appearance of blood in stools, which may signify a gastric carcinoma.

There are a number of patient groups that may be considered at higher risk, in particular, the elderly and the very young. Therefore, when producing a list of hypotheses one important factor must be the patient's age. For example, there may be more concern if a 75-year-old patient presents with indigestion for the first time than if the patient is 30 years old. It will change the probabilities of the likely hypotheses and may require more robust investigation or rapid referral. Other groups for whom decision-making is a more complex process are those with multiple pathologies and medication, those with renal or hepatic impairment and pregnant or breast-feeding women.

MANAGEMENT OPTIONS

Having arrived at a working diagnosis, the next step is to discuss management options with the patient. The discussion should focus on establishing shared aims (therapeutic objectives). For example, a patient presenting with indigestion may want relief of their symptoms as quickly as possible, and prevention of a recurrence. The therapeutic objectives can be achieved through prescribing (POM, P or GSL), advising (lifestyle changes) and/or referring the patient. When deciding on an appropriate management plan for a condition this should be done in a structured and rational way. The World Health Organization document *A Guide to Good Prescribing* (World Health Organization 1994) outlines the principles for ensuring effective management of a condition.

RATIONAL PRODUCT SELECTION

The drug treatment should be based on the balance of benefits and risks (using best available *population* evidence) and the information

---

Box 7.2 Assessing the risks and benefits of treatment

Benefit assessment for a drug or medicine should include:

- Efficacy
- Dosage form
- Treatment schedule
- Treatment duration

Risk assessment for a drug or medicine should include:

- Cautions and contraindications
- Side effects
- Pharmacokinetic and pharmacodynamic profile
- Interactions
- Abuse potential

---

you have gathered during the medical history taking (the *individual patient*) (Box 7.2).

When prescribing, some of these decisions may already have been made, especially if formularies or guidelines have been adopted or when working within an individual clinical management plan. If not, then prescribers should develop a personal formulary of first-line treatments for the conditions for which they frequently prescribe. In considering these issues it should be remembered that guidelines are not rules and that sometimes a patient's circumstances may mean that it is appropriate to prescribe outside the guidelines. It is also important to remember that effective disease management does not always require medication and that drugs may be only one component of the management plan.

The regime of the treatment selected will then be tailored to meet the needs of the individual patient and the therapeutic objectives. This will also include decisions about the formulation, route of administration, dose frequency and schedule, duration of treatment and the quantity to be prescribed or sold. This will obviously depend on current treatment recommendations but may also be driven by any requirement to monitor and follow up the treatment.

PRODUCT-SPECIFIC ADVICE

Particularly with the first supply of any medication, it is essential to tell the patient about their medication. Key information is:

What does the drug do?

- What is this treatment expected to do (in line with the therapeutic objective) and how long will that take?
- What problems and side effects might be encountered? (the patient will also need to understand any monitoring requirements)
- How can side effects be recognised and what action should then be taken? Will they be short- or long-term?

How do I use this medicine?

- How should the medicine be taken or used?
- What supporting information is available? (product information leaflets, advice sheets, compliance aids, etc.)
- When should I take it and what should I do if a dose is missed?
- Special storage requirements
- What should I do with any unused medicine?

The requirement for giving the patient enough information about their treatment is paramount in maximising the benefits of treatment. The amount of information may be considerable and the prescriber will be required to make a judgement about how much information the patient can assimilate.

The information should be divided by the prescriber into:

- must knows
- should knows
- could knows.

As a minimum, the 'must knows' should be achieved. Finding out how much the patient already knows and building on this will help in getting the information across. Breaking the information into logical chunks and summarising and testing the understanding of the patient, as much as possible, will also help. Using patient information leaflets supports but does not replace the need for effective counselling. Effective counselling is a time-consuming and potentially lengthy process. Consideration should be given as to when is the best time for this to take place.

MONITORING AND PATIENT FOLLOW-UP

Making a diagnosis and selecting a suitable treatment option is not the end of the prescribing process. It is essential that the patient is monitored to ensure that the therapeutic objective is met and undesired effects are minimised.

Monitoring can be a prescriber- or patient-led action plan. *Prescriber-led* would be the prescriber requiring the patient to revisit after a certain time or having monitoring tests conducted at specified time intervals. *Patient-led* monitoring would be by informing patients how they should monitor their condition and what action they should take if the condition does not improve or if side effects occur. If the treatment is expected to cure the presenting problem, e.g. *Helicobacter pylori* eradication, patient-led monitoring would be appropriate, requiring the patient to return only if the symptoms are not resolved after treatment or there is a later recurrence. Chronic conditions, e.g. gastro-oesophageal reflux disease, will tend to require prescriber-led review, specifying clearly when the patient should return for follow-up.

There are a number of possibilities when considering the outcome of the monitoring process. One outcome could be that the treatment was effective and achieved the therapeutic objective. In this case, the medication might be stopped or it might be continued (for a chronic condition) with further monitoring. Although the objective may have been achieved, another essential component of review is to ensure that other problems, e.g. side effects, have not arisen. Alternatively, it might not have achieved the therapeutic objective and this will prompt further action, including:

● reviewing the diagnosis
● reviewing the therapeutic objective
● re-assessing whether the medication was appropriate
● identifying any reasons why the patient may not have complied with the medication.

REFERRAL

Referral to another practitioner can be necessary for a number of reasons, such as further investigation or specialist advice. If a patient is being treated as part of a clinical management plan then the referral criteria will be explicitly stated. If the pharmacist decides to refer the patient at any stage in the prescribing process it needs to be done effectively. Urgent referral may require direct contact with another practitioner. Less urgent referrals may be facilitated by sending written information either with the patient or directly to the practitioner or, ideally, through the use of shared patient records.

REFERENCES

Longmore M, Wilkinson IB, Rajagopalan S 2004 Oxford handbook of
   clinical medicine. Oxford University Press, Oxford
National Prescribing Centre 2003 Maintaining competency in prescribing: an
   outline framework to help pharmacist supplementary prescribers.
   Available online at: http://www.npc.co.uk/publications_a_h.htm
World Health Organization 1994 A guide to good prescribing. WHO, Geneva.
   Available online at: http://whqlibdoc.who.int/hq/1994/WHO_DAP_94.11.
   pdf

Pain

P. Wiffen

The International Association for the Study of Pain defines pain as: 'An unpleasant sensory and emotional experience associated with actual or potential tissue damage, or described in terms of such damage'.

Pain is always subjective. Each individual learns the application of the word through experiences related to injury in early life. Accordingly, pain is that experience we associate with actual or potential tissue damage. It is unquestionably a sensation in a part or parts of the body but it is also always unpleasant and therefore also an emotional experience.

Many people report pain in the absence of tissue damage or any likely pathophysiological cause; usually this happens for psychological reasons. There is usually no way to distinguish their experience from that due to tissue damage, if we take the subjective report. If they regard their experience as pain and if they report it in the same ways as pain caused by tissue damage, it should be accepted as pain. This definition avoids tying pain to the stimulus (www.iasp-pain.org).

NOCICEPTIVE PAIN

Nociceptive pain is pain that occurs when nociceptors are stimulated. This is normal pain in response to injury of the body. It discourages the use of injured body parts and thereby extending the injury further. This pain normally responds to conventional analgesics such as paracetamol, non-steroidal anti-inflammatory drugs (NSAIDs) and opioids.

NEUROPATHIC PAIN

Neuropathic pain is that pain initiated or caused by a primary lesion or dysfunction in the nervous system. The pain is often triggered by an injury, but this injury may or may not involve actual damage to the nervous system. The pain frequently has burning, lancinating or electric shock qualities. Persistent allodynia, pain resulting from a nonpainful stimulus such as a light touch, is also a common characteristic of neuropathic pain. The pain may persist for months or years beyond the apparent healing of any damaged tissues. This type of pain often does not respond to standard analgesics and may respond to unconventional analgesic treatments such as antidepressants and anticonvulsants.

MEASURING PAIN

There are good, validated scales for assessing pain. These are usually based on assessment of both pain intensity and pain relief when analgesics are used. Both visual analogue scales – a line moving from 'no pain' to 'worse possible pain' or categorical scales using words such as 'none', 'slight', 'moderate' or 'severe' are employed, often together. They can be useful to monitor progress in patients who are suffering from pain.

GENERAL PRINCIPLE

Once an analgesic has been chosen, it is good practice to increase the dose steadily until either pain relief is achieved or side effects are experienced. This should be undertaken within the licence for that particular agent. Some of the recommendations made in this section – particularly those for neuropathic pain – are outside the licensed indications for those medicines. You should therefore apply due care when recommending such treatments in the course of your clinical pharmacy duties.

Numbers needed to treat (NNT), usually with 95% confidence intervals (95%CI), are provided where available. For a definition of NNT, see Chapter 5. The NNTs presented here have been derived from systematic review or large randomised controlled trial evidence.

ACUTE PAIN

In surveys, as many as 87% of hospitalised patients (both medical and surgical) reported pain of moderate or severe intensity at some time during their admission. Unfortunately, many such patients have to wait for pain relief even if they have asked for it.

DENTAL PAIN

Dental pain, especially extraction of molars, can be intensely painful. Ibuprofen 400 mg is the most commonly prescribed analgesic and is effective, NNT 2.2 (2.1–2.4). Dihydrocodeine remains popular with dental prescribers but is much less effective.

PERIOD PAIN

Period pain (primary dysmenorrhoea) responds to NSAIDs and paracetamol, although quality evidence is limited. Oral contraceptives are also used, although again evidence is sparse.

POSTOPERATIVE PAIN

The requirement for postoperative analgesia varies widely due to the operation performed and patient perception of pain. Regimes should therefore be tailored to the patient.

PARENTERAL ANALGESIA

Patient-controlled analgesia has become common practice. It is usually based on morphine. There is no real advantage in terms of achieving pain relief over intermittent administration by the clock except that busy ward staff don't have to worry about the next dose. Pharmacists should be familiar with the pumps used on their own wards and ensure that safeguards are in place to prevent inadvertent overdosing. A continuous background infusion of opioid should not be provided, as it can lead to overdose.

ORAL ANALGESIA

Oral medication may be sufficient for minor operations and can be useful once patients are mobilised. NSAIDs and/or paracetamol are usually the medicines of choice.

LEAGUE TABLE

One of the advantages of NNTs is their ability to support league tables comparing analgesics. Table 8.1 has been developed by the team at the Oxford University Pain Research Unit and is based on single-dose acute pain studies. All these studies are placebo-controlled and the NNTs are for greater than 50% pain relief. It should be remembered that effectiveness is not the only parameter for choosing an analgesic and co-morbid conditions need to be carefully considered.

MUSCULOSKELETAL PAIN

ORAL NSAIDs

These have a role to play and can effectively control musculoskeletal pain. NNTs from single-dose studies can be used to give an indication of effectiveness in a regular dosing scenario. The cautionary note below about the adverse effects should be carefully considered. Not all NSAIDs have the same adverse effect profile.

TOPICAL NSAIDs

Topical NSAIDs are effective at treating both strains and sprains and musculoskeletal pain. They have the advantage of a better side effect profile than oral NSAIDs. In acute pain, the NNT for greater than 50% reduction in pain is 3.8 (95% CI 3.4–4.4). Ketorolac performed better but most topical NSAIDs perform well.

COX-2 NSAIDs

While these are probably as effective as older NSAIDs, they do have a cleaner side effect profile in terms of gastric irritation. Caution is needed in patients with a history of cardiac disease.

CHRONIC PAIN

OPIOIDS IN CHRONIC NON-MALIGNANT PAIN

There is a place for strong opioids in chronic non-malignant pain. However it is important that patients are adequately assessed in terms of their pain and also suitability for opioid treatment. This assessment usually requires the services of experienced pain clinicians.

TABLE 8.1 The Oxford league table of analgesic efficacy (commonly used analgesic doses)

Analgesic	Number of patients in comparison	At least 50% pain relief (%)	NNT	Lower CI	Higher CI
Valdecoxib 40mg	473	73	1.6	1.4	1.8
Valdecoxib 20mg	204	68	1.7	1.4	2.0
Diclofenac 100	411	67	1.9	1.6	2.2
Rofecoxib 50	1900	63	1.9	1.8	2.1
Paracetamol 1000 + codeine 60	197	57	2.2	1.7	2.9
Parecoxib 40mg (intravenous)	349	63	2.2	1.8	2.7
Diclofenac 50	738	63	2.3	2.0	2.7
Naproxen 440	257	50	2.3	2.0	2.9
Ibuprofen 600	203	79	2.4	2.0	4.2
Ibuprofen 400	4703	56	2.4	2.3	2.6
Naproxen 550	500	50	2.6	2.2	3.2
Ketorolac 10	790	50	2.6	2.3	3.1
Ibuprofen 200	1414	45	2.7	2.5	3.1
Piroxicam 20	280	63	2.7	2.1	3.8
Diclofenac 25	204	54	2.8	2.1	4.3
Pethidine 100 (intramuscular)	364	54	2.9	2.3	3.9
Morphine 10 (intramuscular)	946	50	2.9	2.6	3.6

TABLE 8.1 The Oxford league table of analgesic efficacy (commonly used analgesic doses) – cont'd

Parecoxib 20 (intravenous)	346	50	3.0	2.3	4.1
Naproxen 220/250	183	58	3.1	2.2	5.2
Ketorolac 30 (intramuscular)	359	53	3.4	2.5	4.9
Paracetamol 500	561	61	3.5	2.2	13.3
Paracetamol 1000	2759	46	3.8	3.4	4.4
Paracetamol 600/650 + codeine 60	1123	42	4.2	3.4	5.3
Paracetamol 650 + dextropropoxyphene	963	38	4.4	3.5	5.6
(65 mg hydrochloride or 100 mg napsylate)					
Aspirin 600/650	5061	38	4.4	4.0	4.9
Paracetamol 600/650	1886	38	4.6	3.9	5.5
Tramadol 100	882	30	4.8	3.8	6.1
Tramadol 75	563	32	5.3	3.9	8.2
Aspirin 650 + codeine 60	598	25	5.3	4.1	7.4
Paracetamol 300 + codeine 30	379	26	5.7	4.0	9.8
Tramadol 50	770	19	8.3	6.0	13.0
Codeine 60	1305	15	16.7	11.0	48.0

Source: reproduced with permission from Oxford University Pain Research Unit.

TREATMENTS FOR NEUROPATHIC PAIN

There are many unconventional analgesics that are used for neuropathic pain. Generally these pains do not respond to conventional analgesics but it is sensible to try them first.

The most common neuropathies seen in clinical practice are postherpetic neuralgia, trigeminal neuralgia and diabetic neuropathies.

Antidepressants

There is good systematic review evidence for the effectiveness of tricyclic antidepressants. The best evidence is for amitriptyline, with an NNT of 2 (95%CI 1.7–2.5) to achieve at least moderate pain relief compared to placebo. Limited evidence exists for other tricyclics. If a patient gains some benefit from these medicines but finds the adverse effects problematic, it is worth switching to another drug in the class. In clinical trials, approximately 20% of participants dropped out because of unacceptable adverse effects.

Selective serotonin reuptake inhibitors (SSRIs) are gaining ground in the treatment of neuropathic pain. The evidence for effect is still poor because of a lack of quality studies. However, in patients who cannot tolerate tricyclics they are worth a trial of treatment.

Anticonvulsants

Carbamazepine and gabapentin are common choices for treatment. Carbamazepine is the cheapest, although gabapentin has been actively promoted and has a wider licence for pain. Carbamazepine has an NNT of 2.5 (95%CI 1.8–3.8) and gabapentin an NNT of 2.9 (95%CI 2.2–4.3). Both can produce drowsiness as a significant adverse effect. Generally, doses should be started low and steadily increased until either pain relief or adverse effects are experienced. It should be noted that doses used in some of the clinical trials of gabapentin were above the licensed dose.

Capsaicin

Topical capsaicin can be effective in patients with a range of neuropathies who can tolerate its application. The NNT is 4 (95%CI 3–7.5).

Other medication

Clonidine, baclofen, dextromethorphan and ketamine are among a long list of other medicines that are tried in the treatment of neuropathic pain. These require specialist knowledge before use.

CANCER PAIN

OPIOIDS

The key elements are:

- by the mouth
- by the clock
- by the ladder
- for the individual
- with attention to detail.

The analgesic ladder

It should not be assumed that all cancer pain requires treatment with opioids. The World Health Organization analgesic ladder consists of three levels starting with paracetamol or other non-opioids such as NSAIDs, then moving to the addition of an opioid such as codeine together with paracetamol, finally moving to a strong opioid if pain persists or increases (Fig. 8.1). A proportion of patients with cancer-related pain can be successfully treated with levels 1 or 2.

Morphine by mouth remains the mainstay of treatment for cancer pain. Patients can be started on sustained-release formulations and the dose generally increased by 30–50% until relief is achieved (or there are intolerable side effects). Some 60% of patients will not require more than 200 mg per day. Upper doses in trials have been over 2 g and a proportion of patients do require high doses. Constipation and nausea are common adverse effects and suitable treatment to deal with these should be supplied when morphine is initiated.

Diamorphine is useful parenterally because of its high solubility. It is unavailable in many countries.

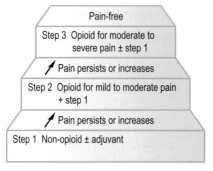

Fig. 8.1 The analgesic ladder.

Other strong opioids such as hydromorphone and oxycodone are also used but have little advantage over morphine. Pethidine has no role to play in modern pain relief. It has a short duration of action and one of the metabolites can induce fitting.

Fentanyl patches are increasingly used. Steady-state levels are achieved after 36–48 hours so rescue medication will need to be supplied for at least the first day or so. The plasma half-life after removal of the patch is almost 24 hours. Patches should be replaced every 72 hours. Replacement patches should be placed at a different location on the body from the original with a time gap of about 7 days before the original space is used again. Discarded patches still contain fentanyl, so care is needed in disposal. Fentanyl is generally less constipating than morphine.

Opioid rotation, whereby opioids are switched to enhance analgesia and reduce adverse effects, is currently in vogue. There is, at present, little quality evidence to support this approach.

NON-STEROIDAL ANTI-INFLAMMATORY DRUGS

This class of medicines has an important role to play in cancer pain, either as single agents or alongside opioids. There is little evidence to inform choice so preference and adverse effect profiles should be considered. Ibuprofen is a good choice.

Bone metastases

NSAIDs often provide good analgesia, although morphine may be needed alongside. Bisphosphonates have some effect on the pain of bony metastases but are not first-line therapy. There is good evidence for the benefit of radiotherapy in reducing the pain associated with bone metastases.

Adverse effects of NSAIDs

A US study has shown that the death rate related to NSAID use is higher than that from cervical cancer, asthma or malignant melanoma. Regular oral use of NSAIDs should be accompanied with some form of gastric protection. Studies have shown that, of patients who take NSAIDs for more than 2 months without gastric protection, around 1 in 150 will suffer a bleeding ulcer and around 1 in 1200 are at risk of dying from a bleeding ulcer.

MIGRAINE

Surveys suggest that approximately 5% of men and 16% of women are migraine sufferers. The triptans have greatly improved the treatment of migraine, with sumatriptan 6 mg injection providing the best NNT, at approximately 2. Oral triptans do reasonably well, with rizatriptan 10 mg having an NNT of 3 and zolmitriptan 5 mg an NNT of 3–4. All NNTs are for headache response at 2 hours. Aspirin 900 mg with metoclopramide 10 mg has a similar NNT to zolmitriptan 5 mg. Sumatriptan 100 mg has an NNT of approximately 4. Lower doses of the triptans do not do so well and are probably a false economy.

PAIN IN CHILDREN

Postoperative surveys in children have shown that 75% usually suffer at least some pain and 25% have moderate to severe pain. Generally, pain is poorly managed, especially in accident and emergency departments. Pain in neonates is another poorly studied area. Recommendations and doses are beyond the scope of this chapter and readers are referred to specialist formularies such as those produced by Guy's Hospital and Alder Hey Hospital.

USEFUL RESOURCES

There are some excellent resources available on the web; some key ones are listed here:

Bandolier (www.ebandolier.com) has a great deal of good material on pain

The International Association for the Study of Pain (www.isap-pain.org) has useful glossaries for pain terms

The Cochrane Library is available in many countries as a national provision. Within the UK it is available in most medical libraries and also via the National Electronic Library for Health (www.nelh.nhs.org)

Anti-infectives

W. Lawson, M. Gilchrist

Anti-infectives, as with all medications, need to be used carefully to optimise their efficacy, avoid toxicity and minimise costs. Of increasing concern is the morbidity and mortality attributed to the development of antimicrobial resistance. Approximately 80% of anti-infective use is in primary care, with the remaining 20% in secondary care, although use is more highly concentrated in a confined environment (Standing Medical Advisory Committee Sub-Group on Antimicrobial Resistance 1998). Approximately a third of hospital patients are receiving anti-infectives at any time. Expenditure on anti-infectives in the hospital setting accounts for between 10% and 30% of the total drug budget (Standing Medical Advisory Committee Sub-Group on Antimicrobial Resistance 1998).

The importance of the prudent use of antimicrobials has been highlighted by a number of key documents published by the Department of Health, most recently a document entitled *Winning Ways – Working Together to Reduce Healthcare Associated Infection in England* (Department of Health, Chief Medical Officer 2003). The document recommends that antibiotic prescribing is supported by clinical pharmacists. Action points on how to tackle the problem of increasing resistance include the use of antibiotics only where existence of infection is highly apparent, prophylaxis only where benefits have been shown, and use of narrow-spectrum agents wherever possible. The role of the clinical pharmacist in promoting rational prescribing of antimicrobial agents includes the development of evidence-based guidelines. These require regular updating, auditing and adaptation based on local sensitivities. Further roles include switching intravenous (IV) agents to the oral route as soon as practical, together with education of prescribers (Cooke 2003). Working in a multidisciplinary team with microbiologists, infectious diseases specialists, infection control teams, pharmacists and prescribers is essential to optimise anti-infective use.

SELECTION AND USE

In individual patient care, the selection and use of anti-infective agents depend upon the following factors:

- Clinical assessment
  - Diagnosis and determination of likely source of infection
  - Localisation/dissemination of the infection
  - Potential severity of the infection
  - Patient's underlying condition and vulnerability
- Bacteriological assessment
  - Presumed pathogen(s), initially by inference, subject to laboratory confirmation (Fig. 9.1)
  - Sensitivity of the organism to different anti-infective agents, including local variations
- Pharmaceutical assessment
  - Choice of agent and dose regimen
  - Suitability of route of administration
  - Potential toxicity and drug interactions associated with anti-infective agents
- Pharmacokinetic assessment
  - Penetration of antibiotic to site of infection
- Prescribing policies
  - Evidence-based policies
  - Local restricted antibiotic policies
  - Cost of treatment.

Each of these criteria will now be addressed in more detail.

CLINICAL ASSESSMENT

Sources of infection may be exogenous (organism acquired from an outside source) or endogenous (migration of flora from normal body site of residence). Portal of entry or primary locus of infection (skin and soft tissues, lungs, gastrointestinal and urinary tracts) is sought from history and examination (Boxes 9.1 and 9.2).

Confounding factors: **Corticosteroid use may mask signs of infection. Drugs, including some anti-infectives (e.g. rifampicin), may cause febrile reactions.**

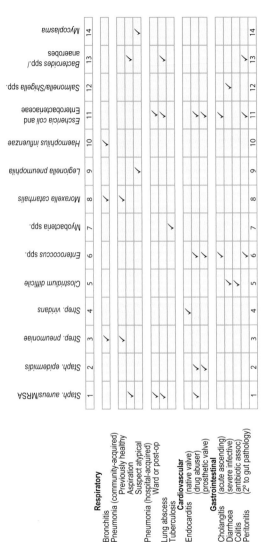

Fig. 9.1 Some common infections and likely pathogens.

	Anaerobic cocci	Staph. aureus	Staph. epidermidis	Strep. pyogenes and Group B Strep.	Strep. pneumoniae	Enterococcus faecalis	Clostridium spp.	Neisseria meningitidis	Neisseria gonorrhoeae	Haemophilus influenzae	Escherichia coli and Enterobacteriaceae	Bacteroides spp./ anaerobes	Spirochaetes	Chlamydia spp.	Pasterella spp.
	1	2	3	4	5	6	7	8	9	10	11	12	13	14	15
Skin/ soft tissue/ bone															
Cellulitis/ erysipelas		✓		✓											
Lyme disease													✓		
Toxic shock syndrome		✓													
Bite (animal)	✓	✓													✓
Bite (human)	✓	✓		✓											✓
Acute osteomyelitis/ septic arthritis		✓		✓											
Central nervous system															
Bacterial meningitis: elderly					✓						✓				
Infant <2 months				✓				(✓) rare			✓				
Child 2 months–12 years					✓			✓		✓					
Young adult					✓			✓	In young adults ✓						
Brain abscess					✓							✓			
Ear, nose and throat															
Otitis media, acute			✓		✓					✓					
Sinusitis			✓		✓					✓					
Tonsillitis			✓	✓											
Quinsy			✓	✓											
Genitourinary															
UTI (lower) / cystitis		✓	✓								✓				
Pyelonephritis (acute)			✓								✓				
Prostatitis (acute)			✓								✓				
Epididymo-orchitis									✓						
Gonorrhoea									✓						
Non-specific urethritis														✓	
Pelvic inflammatory (acute)									✓			✓			
Device related															
Long lines (Hickman)		✓	✓			✓					✓	✓			

Fig. 9.1, cont'd

Box 9.1 Signs and symptoms of infection

Patient

- Temperature higher than 37.5°C (perhaps afebrile in uncomplicated/localised infections)
- Tachycardia: heart rate more than 90 beats per minute
- Tachypnoea: respiratory rate more than 20 per minute.
- Hypotension
- Hyperglycaemia (especially if diabetic)
- Local signs of inflammation/purulence

Laboratory

- Increased C-reactive protein
- White blood cells greater than 12.0 (or less than 4.0) × 10^{-9}/l
  Polymorphocytosis in bacterial infection/ lymphocytosis in viral infection

---

Box 9.2 Signs and symptoms of infection in patients with central nervous system infections (lumbar puncture)

- Decreased cerebrospinal fluid (CSF) glucose
- Increased CSF white blood cells
- Increased CSF protein

Patients at risk

The number of patients who acquire infections during the course of a hospital stay is increasing. These are known as hospital-acquired infections (HAIs) or nosocomial infections. Health care-associated infection affects an estimated one in 10 NHS hospital patients. The cost of hospital-acquired infection in England was stated in 2000 to be as much as £1 billion per year (National Audit Office 2000).

The development of HAIs can be due to a number of factors, including:

- *Patient-associated*: Those at higher risk include immunocompromised patients, transplant recipients, patients receiving chemotherapy or high-dose steroids, patients on artificial ventilation, diabetics and those undergoing complex surgery procedures. Additional risk includes change of patient's flora on admission to hospital
- *Therapeutic interventions*: Presence of medical devices, e.g. indwelling catheters, prostheses, intravenous feeding lines

- *Organisational*:
  - Low nurse-to-patient ratios
  - Lack of isolation facilities
  - High bed occupancy and movement of patients within the health care setting
- *Environmental*:
  - 'Dirty' hospitals
  - Reuse of instruments
- *Behavioural*:
  - Substandard hand-washing, cleaning and hygiene standards.

HAIs characteristically involve a greater diversity of microorganisms, including Gram-negative organisms, which are becoming inherently more resistant to antibacterials when compared to community-acquired infections. The commonest sites of HAI are urinary (23%), lung (22%), wound (9%) and blood (6%) (Emmerson et al 1996). In debilitated patients HAI can lead to:

- Disseminated intravascular coagulation
- Acute respiratory distress syndrome
- Septicaemic (endotoxic) shock.

Methods for combating HAIs target their source, reservoir or mode of transmission include:

- Optimal infection control and hygiene standards
- Control of antibiotic policies
- Surveillance systems and feedback
- Organisational support, including effective information technology support
- Continuing education and updates.

BACTERIOLOGICAL ASSESSMENT

The appropriate sample should be requested by the patient's team and sent to the microbiology laboratory for processing.

Endogenous infection involves the contamination of normally sterile tissues by organisms known to colonise body spaces above the diaphragm (typically Gram-positive bacteria) or below the diaphragm (typically Gram-negative bacteria). Anaerobes are often present in the gut.

- Clinical diagnosis leads to best guess of source of infection and likely pathogen(s) (Fig. 9.1)
- Before treatment, samples should be taken depending on site of infection (blood, sputum, midstream urine (MSU) or catheter stream urine (CSU))

- After sampling, empirical treatment should be started on basis of best-guess pathogen(s), taking into account local sensitivities (Fig. 9.2)
- Culture and in vitro sensitivity results guide continuation or modification of regimen.

Culture and sensitivities of organisms usually take 24–48 hours. Sensitivities for tuberculosis require up to 6 weeks because of their slow growth.

A positive culture may not always signify infection but may represent colonisation by the organism or contamination of the sample. Comparative spectra of some anti-infective agents are shown in Figure 9.2.

PHARMACEUTICAL ASSESSMENT

Choice of agent

Initial recommendations should be based on 'best guess' (Fig. 9.3). Choice should then subsequently be reviewed as soon as these results are available. Rational use of anti-infective agents should be evidence-based and adapted to local sensitivity patterns. Ideally, specimens should be taken prior to commencement of anti-infectives.

Although effective dosing with a single agent is the preferred strategy, a combination of agents may potentially be used:

- Bactericidal (kill the organism) + another bactericidal agent may be synergistic
- Bacteriostatic (prevent replication of organism) + bacteriostatic agent may be additive
- Bactericidal + bacteriostatic agent may be antagonistic, therefore should be avoided.

Examples of combinations that are used in clinical practice include:

- Treatment of endocarditis, where a lower dosage of gentamicin can be used with benzylpenicillin because of their additive activity.
- Prevention of resistance emerging during treatment, e.g. antitubercular chemotherapy or oral treatment of methicillin-resistant *Staphylococcus aureus* (MRSA) with rifampicin and trimethoprim
- Avoidance of high doses to reduce risk of toxicity, e.g. systemic antifungal therapy with flucytosine and amphotericin.

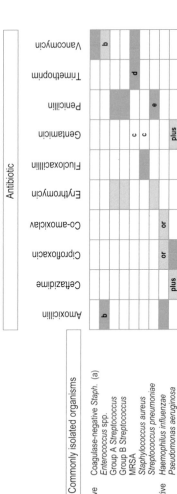

Fig. 9.2 Suggested empirical antibiotic choices based on the organism isolated or suspected.

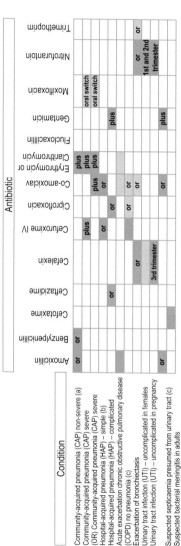

Condition	Amoxicillin	Benzylpenicillin	Cefotaxime	Ceftazidime	Cefalexin	Cefuroxime IV	Ciprofloxacin	Co-amoxiclav	Erythromycin or Clarithromycin	Flucloxacillin	Gentamicin	Moxifloxacin	Nitrofurantoin	Trimethoprim
Community-acquired pneumonia (CAP) non-severe (a)	or	or							plus					
Community-acquired pneumonia (CAP) severe						plus			plus			oral switch		
(OR) Community-acquired pneumonia (CAP) severe								plus	plus			oral switch		
Hospital-acquired pneumonia (HAP) – simple (b)						or								
Hospital-acquired pneumonia (HAP) – complicated				or				or			plus			
Acute exacerbation chronic obstructive pulmonary disease (COPD) no pneumonia (c)	or						or	or						
Exacerbation of bronchiectasis							or	or						
Urinary tract infection (UTI) – uncomplicated in females					or		or						or	or
Urinary tract infection (UTI) – uncomplicated in pregnancy					3rd trimester								1st and 2nd trimester	or
Suspected septicaemia presumed from urinary tract (c)								or			plus			
Suspected bacterial meningitis in adults	or													

NB Treatment depends on site and severity

Choice for empiric therapy:

- ▇ First choice
- ▒ Second choice

a. If penicillin or macrolide allergic use moxifloxacin
b. If penicillin allergic use erythromycin OR ciprofloxacin (beware of ciprofloxacin's poor cover versus *Strep. pneumoniae*)
c. Nitrofurantoin useful if infection confined to urine and if CrCl > 60ml/min. If penicillin allergic, discuss with microbiology

Fig. 9.3 Empirical antibiotic choices based on condition recommended.

- Check medical and drug history for possible contraindications/interactions.
- Check for previous allergic reactions and look for current signs. Allergies to anti-infectives are common.
- Confirm true allergies, where possible, as opposed to side effects and ensure they are clearly documented or reported.
- Drug interactions are common and preventable. Check the patient's current medication, including any over-the-counter medication
- Check present renal and hepatic status for contraindications, monitoring or dosage adjustment.

Suitability of route (Box 9.3)

Oral administration with suitable dosage is the preferred route where possible.

Where the IV route is necessary, the duration should be kept to a minimum, switching to the oral route as soon as possible. This should minimise the risk of IV line-associated infection and potential prolonged hospital stay. If the drug is to be administered via a feeding tube, ascertain the site of absorption of the drug relative to location of the tube to avoid potential drug degradation.

Choice of dose regimen (Fig. 9.3, Box 9.4)

Use of inadequate doses of anti-infectives: subtherapeutic dosing is a common cause of treatment failure.

Box 9.3 Intravenous to oral switch of anti-infectives, also referred to as step-down or sequential therapy

Suggested criteria for intravenous to oral switch include:

- Patient able to tolerate oral fluids and swallow
- Heart rate less than 100 beats per minute over preceding 12 hours
- Temperature 36–38°C for at least 24 hours
- White blood cell count between 4 and 12 × 10^{-9}/l
- Suitable agent available orally.

Box 9.4 Doses of anti-infectives

- Ensure adequately high doses
- Check doses are being given at the correct dose interval (an anti-infective prescribed to be given at the 8 am, 12 noon and 6 pm drug rounds is unlikely to be as effective as when it is given 8-hourly)
- Consider any dose-related toxicity (such as renal, hepatic, haematological or central nervous system effects)
- Assess renal and hepatic function and where necessary adjust doses accordingly
- Duration of parenteral therapy can affect outcome and cost of treatment.

The concentration of anti-infective at the infection site needs to be higher than the concentration required to kill the infecting organism (bactericidal) or to prevent the infecting organism replicating (bacteriostatic).

The optimal use of an appropriately chosen anti-infective agent depends on adjustments to the dose, the route and the duration of administration to suit the individual patient and condition. These additional decisions contribute to the overall effectiveness and cost of a treatment episode.

PHARMACOKINETIC ASSESSMENT

Confidence in the efficacy of an anti-infective agent requires achievement of effective concentrations at the site of infection. The selected agent must be able to penetrate the site of infection. For example, to treat an infection that is located in the central nervous system, e.g.

meningitis, the drug must penetrate the blood–brain barrier. In order to do this the drug must be lipid-soluble. Other drugs may require high concentrations at their site of action, e.g. in the treatment of osteomyelitis. Antibiotics do not readily penetrate into some abscesses, pus or collections because of their location; such cases may require surgical intervention.

PRESCRIBING POLICIES (Box 9.5)

There is a large armoury of anti-infective agents available, many with similar spectra of activity. Specific antibiotic policies should be adapted locally to assist with the appropriate selection and ensure that treatment is not prolonged unnecessarily. Local policies can be adapted from national guidelines where available and a multidisciplinary group, including microbiology, infectious diseases, pharmacy and the parent speciality, must review policies at regular intervals. The parent speciality is particularly important, as this ensures that the speciality

---

Box 9.5 Antibiotic prescribing policies

- Policies are usually general statements of hospital strategy
- Guidelines refer to specific conditions
- Formularies are lists of available agents

Antibiotic guidelines can include:

- First-choice agents available for any prescriber
- Restricted choices, e.g. for multiple-resistant organisms
- Reserved antibiotics for life-threatening conditions or where first-choice agent has failed

The last two options may require approval from microbiology or infectious diseases.
   Various methods can be used to implement restricted/reserved policies, including:

- Therapeutic substitution
- Requirement for prescription to be rewritten after specific number of days
- Applying sticker over administration boxes requesting microbiology approval
- Automatic stop orders
- Discussion with microbiology or infectious diseases

adopts and takes ownership of the policy. Such antibiotic policies prevent inappropriate and indiscriminate use of agents, in a cost-effective manner, and may bring about a reduction in the emergence of resistant organisms.

EVALUATION AND MONITORING

After initiating therapy with the chosen antibiotic(s), clinical signs should be monitored to determine if the infection is resolving (Box 9.6). Signs of improvement include changes in laboratory parameters such as a decrease in C-reactive protein (CRP), white blood cells, temperature and a normalisation of blood pressure and heart rate (Box 9.7). Drug levels and renal monitoring should be carried out where appropriate (Box 9.8).

Where combinations of antibiotics are used, ensuring that appropriate agents are prescribed avoids duplication of antimicrobial cover. Where IV agents are available orally, suggesting a switch is recommended. This is not only more acceptable for the patient and makes better use of nursing time, but also reduces the risk of developing a line-related infection.

Box 9.6 Clinical monitoring

Laboratory
- White blood cell count – ensure decreasing and within reference range
- C-reactive protein – ensure decreasing and within reference range

Observations
- Pulse (less than 90–100 beats per minute)
- Temperature – ensure temperature is normalising and patient remains afebrile
- Blood pressure (ensure blood pressure is returning to baseline)
- Respiratory rate and oxygen saturations
- Glucose control
- Symptomatic improvement (e.g. improvement in weakness, dyspnoea, anorexia, malaise, headache, delirium, pain, fever and chills)
- Physical examination signs (e.g. chest sounds, local redness, swelling, induration, suppuration, peripheral stigmata such as skin rashes)

Box 9.7 Laboratory monitoring

- Inflammatory markers: C-reactive protein and white cell count
- Biochemical markers, including sodium, potassium and magnesium, for signs of depletion/excess, and increasing creatinine and urea for drug toxicity relating to declining renal function
- Raised erythrocyte sedimentation rate and shift in the blood film
- Cultures and sensitivities (cultures take 24–48 hours on average – or, in the case of tuberculosis, weeks – for results)

Box 9.8 Therapeutic drug monitoring

- Therapeutic drug monitoring optimises efficacy and minimises toxicity of aminoglycosides, parenteral vancomycin and flucytosine
- Vancomycin: pre-dose (trough) levels, (5–10 mg/l) should be taken prior to the third or fourth dose, then twice weekly provided renal function remains stable (peak levels are also monitored in addition for endocarditis)
- Gentamicin: using divided daily dosing regimes, monitor 1 hour post-infusion 5–10 mg/l (3–5 mg/l for endocarditis) and pre-dose (trough) levels less than 2 mg/l (less than 1 mg/l for endocarditis). Some hospitals use extended daily regimens, e.g. 5–7 mg/kg 'daily', if sepsis. Local guidance should be used for levels and subsequent dose calculations
- Tobramycin: using divided daily dosage regimes, monitor 1 hour post-infusion less than 10 mg/l and pre-dose (trough) less than 2 mg/l. Some hospitals use extended daily regimens, e.g. 7 mg/kg daily. Local guidance should be used for levels and subsequent dose calculations
- Amikacin: 1 hour post (peak) infusion less than 30 mg/l and pre-dose (trough) less than 10 mg/l. Some hospitals use once-daily regimens (15 mg/kg). Local guidance should be used for levels and subsequent dose calculations

In taking all aminoglycoside or vancomycin blood levels, recording the time when the sample is taken in relation to the time of the last dose is imperative for interpretation of the results.

SPECIAL CONSIDERATIONS

MICROBIAL RESISTANCE

The increasing availability and use of anti-infective agents have been accompanied by rising levels of antimicrobial resistance. However, local patterns of resistance vary widely. Emergence of resistance has affected a range of different organisms, with the following presenting particular clinical problems:

- *Staphylococcus aureus* – commonly beta-lactamase producers and methicillin-sensitive (MSSA) and methicillin-resistant (MRSA). A large proportion of bacteraemias in hospitals are now MRSA and it is also becoming a problem in the community
- Enterobacteria, e.g. Acinetobacter, Klebsiella, Escherichia, Proteus. In hospitals the emergence of these potentially highly resistant Gram-negative organisms is becoming a problem as there are few agents available to treat them if pathogenic
- *Streptococcus pneumoniae* where there is increasing resistance to penicillin
- *Enterococcus faecalis* and *E. faecium*, the former often sensitive to amoxicillin, the latter often resistant to vancomycin, i.e. vancomycin-resistant enterococci (VRE), for which there are only a small number of agents available for treatment.

ANTIMICROBIAL PROPHYLAXIS (Box 9.9)

Examples of medical prophylaxis:

- Splenectomy
- Tuberculosis
- Dental prophylaxis for a damaged heart valve.

Examples of surgical prophylaxis:

- Appendectomy
- Tonsillectomy
- Laparotomy.

Prophylaxis is usually only required during the perioperative period (immediately before and during the procedure if prolonged) to ensure adequate concentration.

Antibacterial use beyond 24 hours constitutes treatment and should be discouraged in the absence of signs of infection.

TREATMENT OF ACUTE SEPSIS

Fever occurs as a result of release of endogenous pyrogens due to infection. Bacteriologically undiagnosed episodes of acute sepsis require the use of a single agent or a combination of agents to provide broad-spectrum cover against Gram-positive and Gram-negative aerobes

---

Box 9.9 Antimicrobial prophylaxis: important considerations

Timing

To maximise efficacy and minimise the development of surgical site infection, it is essential that the dose is administered up to half an hour prior to induction of anaesthesia.

Additional doses may be given for prolonged operations or where major blood loss occurs, although evidence is insufficient to make a general recommendation.

Dosage

Depends on:

● Potential pathogen and its sensitivity
● Required serum and tissue concentration
● Serum half-life of antimicrobial.

Route

The intravenous route is the most reliable for providing effective serum concentration of an antimicrobial.

If, however, high tissue concentrations are achieved orally, the antibiotic has good penetration to the desired site of action and the patient has no impaired absorption, this route could be used.

(beta-lactam + aminoglycoside) with additional metronidazole (for anaerobic cover). There are other non-antimicrobial agents that may also be considered (e.g. activated protein C).

IMMUNOCOMPROMISED PATIENTS

As new therapies and drugs have been developed over the past few decades, there are an increasing number of patients who may be classified as immunocompromised. This may be due to underlying disease, e.g. malignancy, immunosuppressant treatment regimes, and/or setting (such as in intensive care/high-dependency units). Patients with human immunodeficiency virus (HIV) infection are at particular risk of bacterial, fungal and protozoal infections. Profound immune suppression resulting in 'opportunistic' infections can severely affect the patient's capacity to eradicate an infection and often necessitates vigorous prolonged therapy with multiple anti-infective agents. Certain patient groups, e.g. bone marrow transplantation and HIV-positive, require suitable prophylaxis for infections such as *Pneumocystis jiravicii* (formerly *carinii*) pneumonia (PCP) and herpes simplex virus.

ANTIFUNGALS

FUNGAL INFECTIONS

Fungi can cause three types of disease:

- infections (mycosis)
- mycotoxicoses
- allergic reactions.

Type of infection

The main fungal infections of clinical importance are mycoses. These can be subclassified into three types:

- superficial infections of the skin with yeasts and infection of keratin of the skin, hair and nails with filamentous fungi (known as dermatophytes), causing ringworm
- subcutaneous infections
- systemic infections, which can spread throughout the body and are often serious; these occur most frequently in immunocompromised patients whose host defence system is impaired.

Type of antifungal agents for systemic infections

The three main groups of antifungals have different modes of action.

- *Polyenes*, e.g. amphotericin, including lipid formulations, interact with ergosterol in the fungal cell membrane, puncturing the cell wall and resulting in lysis. They are fungicidal
- *Azoles*, e.g. triazoles (itraconazole fluconazole) and second-generation azoles (voriconazole). They inhibit CYP-dependent enzymes, which are important for the synthesis of the ergosterol, the major steroid component in the fungal plasma membrane. They are fungicidal/fungistatic.
  Voriconazole indications:
  – Invasive aspergillosis
  – Serious infections caused by *Scedosporin* spp., *Fusarium* spp.
  – Invasive fluconazole-resistant *Candida* spp. (including *Candida krusei*)
  Voriconazole formulations: It is available intravenously and orally
- *Echinocandins*, e.g. caspofungin inhibit beta (1,3) glucan synthetase, which is required for cell wall synthesis in fungi but not in mammalian tissue. This results in the inhibition of growth of branching hyphae. They are fungistatic

Caspofungin indications:
– Invasive aspergillosis either unresponsive to amphotericin or itraconazole or in patients intolerant of amphotericin or itraconazole
– Invasive candidiasis
– Empirical treatment of systemic fungal infections in patients with neutropenia

Casofungin formulations: It is available intravenously.

REFERENCES

Cooke J 2003 Antimicrobial management: the role of clinical pharmacist. Hospital Pharmacy 10: 392–400

Department of Health, Chief Medical Officer 2003 Winning ways: working together to reduce healthcare associated infection in England. Department of Health, London. Available online at: http://www.dh.gov.uk/ PublicationsAndStatistics/Publications/PublicationsPolicy AndGuidance/PublicationsPolicyAndGuidanceArticle/fs/en?CONTENT_ ID = 4064682&chk = Vqjhyn (accessed 26 April 2006)

Emmerson AM, Enstone JE, Griffin M et al 1996 The second national prevalence survey of infections in hospitals – overview of results. Journal of Hospital Infection 32: 175–190.

National Audit Office 2000 The management and control of hospital acquired infection in acute NHS trusts in England. National Audit Office, London. Available online at: http://www.nao.org.uk/publications/nao_reports/ 9900230.pdf (accessed 26 April 2006)

Standing Medical Advisory Committee Sub-Group on Antimicrobial Resistance 1998 The path of least resistance. Department of Health, London. Available online at: http://www.dh.gov.uk/PublicationsAnd Statistics/Publications/PublicationsPolicyAndGuidance/ PublicationsPolicyAndGuidanceArticle/fs/en?CONTENT_ ID=4009357&chk=87ei43 (accessed 28 April 2006)

FURTHER READING

Elliott TSJ, Foweraker J, Gould FK et al 2004 Working Party of the British Society of Antimicrobial Chemotherapy. Guidelines for the antibiotic treatment of endocarditis in adults: report of the Working Party of the British Society of Antimicrobial Chemotherapy. Journal of Antimicrobial Chemotherapy 54(6): 971–81

British Medical Association and Royal Pharmaceutical Society of Great Britain 2006 British National Formulary, 51st edn. BMA and RPSGB, London

Smoking cessation

A. McCoig

INTRODUCTION

We are all facing a unique and historical opportunity. Let us live up to the greatness of this moment and over the coming days find the solutions we need to save our peoples from the death and suffering brought on by tobacco.
Dr Gro Harlem Bruntland, Director General of the World Health Organization, Intergovernmental Negotiating Body on the WHO framework convention on tobacco control at its sixth session – Geneva, Switzerland 17 February 2003.

The Department of Health, in common with all health care organisations, has long recognised the fact that smoking is the single most preventable form of illness and premature death. At the end of 1998, the Labour government published a White Paper entitled *Smoking Kills*. The document is 100 pages long and represents the first major comprehensive government initiative to tackle the issue of smoking amongst the population of the UK.

The document is an all-encompassing strategy that not only sets out the framework principles to provide smokers with an NHS-based smoking cessation service but also lays out intentions to de-normalise smoking in society. In the foreword, there is a promise to set in motion a publicity campaign that will 'shift attitudes and change behaviour'. The promise of an advertising ban made in 1998 only became a reality in 2003 following a European directive. In 2005, for the first time, the

Belgian Grand Prix Formula 1 racing event was cancelled, as the Belgian government will not allow the overt tobacco companies' promotional material to be screened on television or printed in media coverage. This bold governmental step bodes well for future official attitudes, at least in Europe.

The White Paper recognised the huge cost that smoking imposes on the country both financially and to society at large. Treating the effects of smoking comes at a huge price. The White Paper put the cost to the NHS at £1.7 billion annually. The risks to health are well documented, but resulting deaths can be due to many reasons apart from the obvious cause of cancer. Unambiguous and identifiable cancers caused by tobacco smoking are (Simpson 2000):

● lung cancer
● oral cavity cancers and cancer of the larynx
● cancers of the gastrointestinal tract (oesophagus, stomach, pancreas)
● cancers of the bladder and kidney
● leukaemia.

Excessive death rates have also been recorded among smokers with certain cardiovascular diseases such as:

● ischaemic heart disease
● myocardial degeneration
● aortic aneurysm
● arteriosclerosis
● cerebral thrombosis.

In addition to these disease categories, other important lung diseases other than cancer have been found to be caused or exacerbated by tobacco smoke. Chronic obstructive pulmonary disease (COPD) is affected directly by smoking and passive smoking. Smoking accelerates the progression of the disease as measurable by lung output (forced expiratory volume in one second, FEV_1) and capacity. As with other degenerative diseases, there is no recovery of affected tissue.

The government's attention was also targeted at passive smoking and the clear risks to people who either lived or worked with smokers, in particular children. The highlighted quote from the White Paper is: '17 000 hospital admissions in a single year of children under 5 are due to their parents smoking' (Royal College of Physicians of London 1992). In addition to this, there was also a recognition that many smokers were from poorer backgrounds and demonstrated health inequalities. The connection was made between low educational achievement, poverty and smoking prevalence. The government formally recognised what community pharmacists had experienced over a long period of time since the launch of nicotine replacement therapy (NRT); many poorer smokers were reluctant to part with their cash for a product with a higher price tag than cigarettes, or indeed any form of smoking cessation service. Although logic should determine otherwise, the sound financial argument for purchasing an NRT product in order to save money in the medium and long term does not impress many smokers addicted to a 'cheaper' product. At the time of the publication of the White Paper, the cost of 20 cigarettes was about £2.50. This has nearly doubled in the last 5 years, whereas NRT has remained at around £16–18 for a week's supply. In 1998, a week's supply of NRT was roughly equivalent to seven packets of 20 cigarettes. The price of NRT has now halved compared to the cost of 140 cigarettes.

The White Paper was therefore important for community pharmacists. This was the moment that the government formally recognised the importance of NRT for people wishing to quit. There was a clear commitment made to make NRT available on the NHS, providing that support for the quitter would also be on hand in the form of a health service-based professional counsellor. The slight sting in the tail in this section for community pharmacy was that there was also a pledge made to examine the possible relaxation of licensing requirements for the retail sale of NRT. The arguments in favour of this relaxation were put forward to mirror and counterbalance the ease in which cigarettes could be purchased at almost any retail outlet. This deregulation subsequently followed in 2001, when most forms of NRT were recategorised from pharmacy-only (P) status to general sales list (GSL). However, the case for appropriate use of NRT with counselling support had been made previously (Raw et al 1999) and was finally accepted as one of the main strategies of grappling with the quitters' desire for an NHS-based service. The World Health Organization stated in May 1999 that 'NRT should be part of the core treatment package offered to all smokers'.

Pharmacists have always been widely recognised as easily accessed health care professionals operating in a neutral environment with a high degree of public confidence. Perversely, although general practitioners also enjoy a similar degree of respect, they have not displayed a widespread enthusiasm for allocating time to counselling smoking patients. A qualitative study (Butler et al 1998) of patients' perceptions of the role of doctors' advice in quitting smoking found that doctor–patient relationships could be damaged if doctors routinely advised all smokers to quit. Recent other reports (Anon 2003a) indicate that GPs are 'too busy' to find the time necessary to advise and counsel would-be quitters to stop and that some consider this activity unrewarding, annoying and ineffective.

Pharmacists, on the other hand, play a critical role in smoking cessation, according to the Health Development Agency (Anon 2003b) and evidence of their contribution to public health in this field has been recently documented by two published reports (Anderson et al 2003a, b). Community pharmacists with the appropriate specialist training, therefore, have a unique role in smoking cessation in that they can avoid some of the difficulties experienced by the patient–doctor relationship and can offer NRT at the same time as the counselling episode.

COUNSELLING THE 'QUITTER' – PHASE 1

The use of the noun 'patient' could be inappropriate, as many smokers are often without any underlying medical condition and present with no pathology or symptoms of ill-health. Some professional quit counsellors prefer to use the term 'client', which they feel is more appropriate to the situation. Either way, a pharmacist can choose the language to suit any particular situation and some prefer simply to say 'customer'. For the purposes of this exercise, I will choose to use the word 'client' as this is the terminology used by my local primary care trust.

The first step with all clients is to establish where they are in terms of intention. There are several psychological areas that can be occupied by a smoker in relation to their addiction. As with all drug addictions (and nicotine is no different), there can be considerable denial employed by the client as to the hold that their habit has over their perceptions of behaviour and quality of life expectations. A simple everyday example of behaviour to illustrate risk assessment is to ask whether or not the client wears a seat belt when travelling in a car. If the answer is 'no' – then how are the risks to health from smoking perceived in relation to the risk of major injury in a vehicle road accident? If the answer is 'yes' – why is there a desire to end one life-threatening situation and not another? These questions will reveal a considerable amount of information about the client's attitudes to health behaviour and whether or not the client is ready for a change in lifestyle.

Above all, it is important to be relaxed, welcoming and give the appearance of being non-judgemental. Early impressions, as with any human contact, are lasting ones, particularly as the client may feel intimidated or be experiencing nervous anticipation coupled with guilt or shame. Almost everyone who puts themselves forward for counselling is sufficiently motivated at least to take the first tentative steps. In this initial phase, there are a number of key questions that should be raised:

- If you want to stop smoking, why?
- What are your concerns about quitting?
- Is this desire to quit a personal decision or have you been pressurised or persuaded by someone else?
- Have you tried to stop before and, if so, how many times and for how long were you successful on each occasion?
- How much does your smoking habit cost in daily, weekly or yearly terms?
- How did you feel about yourself when you were a non-smoker and what were the benefits to you and your immediate family, colleagues and friends?
- Why did you start again?

The other more challenging question to put to the client is to ask them to summarise what they enjoy about smoking. The answers to these questions should enable you to determine the level of honesty, commitment and motivation that is being presented.

Other models of the quitting process are essentially the same as the diagram in Figure 10.1. One manufacturer's website (www.nicotinell.com) suggests a comparison with building blocks for the smoker, starting with a bottom-up approach to the process of preparing to quit. The client is given a series of exercises to complete at each stage of the process. In preparing to quit, the steps are given as:

- Understanding commitment
- Choosing how to quit
- Setting a quit date
- Making a public commitment
- Contracting with others.

Once a determination is made by the client, setting a quit date is a vital part of the programme. Hesitation on this commitment is a sure indication of lack of self-confidence in tackling the underlying addiction and the client should be advised to return when s/he is more certain of the ultimate objective. Going public with this commitment is another step in ensuring that close family members, friends and colleagues are aware of the client's determination. Surprising amounts of support are usually forthcoming from these associates, and this is often a key ongoing motivational factor; it also drives up the desire to stay stopped and avoid embarrassment through relapse.

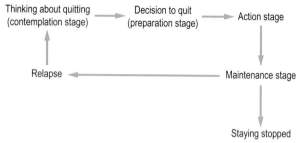

Fig. 10.1 Model of behaviour change (Prochaska & DiClemente 1984).

COUNSELLING THE QUITTER – PHASE 2

Once a decision has been made and the quit date agreed on, the client should be made aware of the preparations necessary to become a non-smoker. A comparison should be made with sterility, in that there are no degrees of 'sterile'. One is either a smoker or a non-smoker – there is no in-between position. The occasional cigarette or 'puff' must be classified as relapse and it should be stressed that cessation means the end of all forms of tobacco from the quit date onwards. Helpful tips about changing routine behaviour and managing coping skills are:

- Removing and destroying all material supporting the habit, e.g. cigarette lighters, ashtrays, matches
- Replacing previous smoking episodes with fruit, raw vegetables such as carrots and celery, or chewing gum
- Keeping fruit juice or cold water in the refrigerator to keep the palate 'fresh'
- Making all living and working areas 'smoke-free' and dissuading other smokers from smoking in your immediate area
- Going 'public' with friends, family and colleagues
- Avoiding visiting places associated with the previous smoking habit, e.g. pubs
- Asking for 'no smoking' areas in restaurants and hotels *or* being prepared to leave the situation
- Keeping a diary of success and money saved
- Establishing a financial reward or personal goal such as a holiday
- Timing the craving period – this will usually last only 60 seconds
- Actively considering relaxing techniques or herbal remedies for stress and irritability

- Encouraging contact between counselling sessions in times of crisis or stress.

At the start of the quit programme, the immediate short- and medium-term benefits of cessation should be explained in full. This can be initiated by performing a carbon monoxide test in the pharmacy (a CO monitor is an essential tool for all smoking cessation counsellors). Invariably, the client will have been smoking within the previous few hours and the monitor will give a reading in excess of 10 ppm of carbon monoxide in the exhaled breath. An association with car exhaust gases is an appropriate health hazard comparison.

Short- to medium-term benefits include:

- Within 20 minutes, blood pressure and pulse rate will return to normal
- Within 8 hours, oxygen levels return to normal and carbon monoxide levels in the blood reduce by half, resulting in improved energy levels
- Within 24 hours, the mucus in the lungs will start to clear
- In 2 days, there will be enhanced smell and taste
- In 3 days, respiration becomes easier as the bronchial tubes relax
- After 2 weeks, the cardiovascular system starts to improve
- Within 3–9 months, lung function increases by up to 10% (depending on age and general underlying health).

Long-term benefits are:

- At 1 year, the excess risk of death due to coronary heart disease is reduced by 50%
- At 2–3 years, female smokers have reduced their risk of a heart attack to the same level as non-smokers
- By 10 years, the risk of death from all smoking-related causes returns to almost the same as non-smokers
- At 2006 pricing levels, a 20-cigarette per day habit is converted into an annual saving of about £1800.

With younger quitters, the health reasons for stopping smoking appear to be, in spite of proven logic, a secondary consideration to personal appearance, emotional relationships and the amount of money spent on tobacco. A shorter summary would be simply to focus on 'love and money', as many young people can be better motivated by highlighting the damage that smoking may inflict on their image. Sporting personalities can be useful peer models when drawing comparisons.

Completing forms is part of everyday NHS record-keeping. Although record-keeping has not been a significant part of any pharmacy contract work to date, keeping accurate records of quit-smoking clients is essential for two important reasons. The first is to ensure that payments and fees are reimbursed by the local PCT – a rather obvious necessity. The second is to provide evidence of activity and results to both the PCT and the Department of Health. Figure 10.2 shows the various quit rates among male and female smoking cessation clients in one quarter of 2003.

COUNSELLING THE QUITTER – PHASE 3

Assuming that there is a committed and motivated individual willing to embark on becoming a non-smoker, the forms have to be completed (Fig. 10.3). Record-keeping is an essential part of the service, as has already been stated. Pharmacists should ensure that these records are kept confidential and that, in the absence of the main pharmacist, the locum should be briefed on what to expect when clients appear for subsequent sessions and further supplies of NRT.

The current service model in my area allows for 4 weeks of NRT to be supplied against the vouchers illustrated in Figure 10.3. Currently, Croydon is piloting an 8-week scheme in one of the deprived areas of the borough where adult smoking rates are well above the national average (43% as opposed to 28%). There is sufficient anecdotal evidence to suggest that a longer course of NRT in line with manufacturers' recommendations would increase the quit rates after 2 months.

After the first session with the client, which should last approximately 30 minutes, there will be an explanation about subsequent visits and follow-up. The client should be made aware of the need to 'touch base' within 3 days of the first appointment to ensure that the chosen

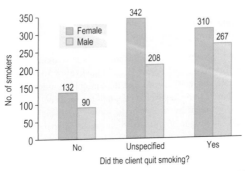

Fig. 10.2 Data on 4-week quitters by gender, for the year 2002/03.

Stop Smoking Service
Client Record Form

Croydon **NHS**
Primary Care Trust

Adviser Name: _____   Case No: [ ][ ][ ][ ][ ][ ]

Client Details

Last Name: _____   [ ][ ][ ][ ][ ][ ]

Title: _____   Mr/Mrs/Miss/Ms/Other _____

First Names: _____

Date of Birth: [d][d] [m][m] [y][y]

Address: _____

Sex: [M] [F]

_____

Home Tel: _____

Mobile: _____

Post Code: [ ][ ][ ][ ][ ][ ][ ]

Best Time to Contact: [AM] [PM] [EVE]

Ethnic Group: [ ][ ] (use code list in Handbook)

Pregnant? [Y] [N]   EDD: _____

GP: _____

GP Postcode: [ ][ ][ ][ ][ ][ ]

Address: _____

Fig. 10.3 Croydon Primary Care Trust Stop Smoking Service Client Record Form (reproduced with permission of Croydon Primary Care Trust).

Initial Consultation

No of cigarettes/grams tobacco per day:

How long has the client smoked? [ ] yrs

Previous Quit Attempts? [Y] [N]

How many? [ ] [Y] [N]

Most recent attempt:

When? [m] [m] [y] [y]

Has the client used the Croydon Service before? [Y] [N]

Medical History:

Current Medication:

QUIT DATE AGREED: [ ][ ][ ][ ][ ][ ] [m] [m] [y] [y]

Exempt from Charges? [Y] [N]

CO Reading: [ ] %/ppm

NRT: [ ] Voucher issued? [Y] [N]

Buproprion [ ] Willpower [ ]

Adviser Signature: _____

Client Signature: _____

Date: _____

Fig. 10.3, cont'd

Follow-Up

Clients taking NRT should be reviewed on Day 3 of the quit attempt. Clients prescribed Bupropion should be reviewed on Day 11. It is recommended that follow-up dates are planned at the initial meeting, and documented in your client file.

Four Week Follow-Up: This must take place no earlier than **28** days and not later than **42** days after the quit date.

Date of Review

Was the quit date changed?   Y   N   New Quit Date:

Date of Last Cigarette

CO

_____ %/ppm   Client Signature: _____

as reported by client

If client lost to follow-up, please state what attempts you have made to establish contact:

Phonecalls   Dates: _____

_____   Letter: Date

Adviser Signature: _____   Date:

Distribution: white copy to PCT within 3 weeks of setting quit date; yellow to PCT within 3 weeks after follow-up; blue to be retained by Adviser

Fig. 10.3, cont'd

form of NRT has proved satisfactory in use and that the quit date was adhered to as agreed. Following on from this brief encounter, the client should be given three firm dates and times for the next three appointments, at which times a further week's supply of NRT will be given. At the end of the 4-week period, the client is asked to sign off the client form and a CO monitor reading is taken to ensure that the lungs are smoke-free. You can offer to take a CO reading at each appointment and this should be considered for most clients, as it is a proven method of demonstrating the measure of short-term health gain.

CHOICE OF NICOTINE REPLACEMENT THERAPY

The choices available for smoking cessation are well-documented:

- Transdermal patches
- Gum
- Lozenges
- Micro-tabs
- Inhalator
- Nasal spray.

Transdermal patches are available in two types and three strengths. The first type is the 24-hour patch (21 mg, 14 mg and 7 mg available over a 24-hour period), which should be recommended initially for all smokers who crave their first cigarette immediately upon waking in the morning. This type of patch is also indicated for those who wake during the night occasionally and smoke in order to relax for further sleep periods. For those smokers who can normally go without their first tobacco contact until at least 1 hour after waking, the 16-hour patch (15 mg, 10 mg and 5 mg) should be recommended. In most cases, the highest strength should be given to quitters in the first week, as the amount of available nicotine from the transdermal patch will be below any levels achieved by smoking. It should be borne in mind that smokers almost always underestimate their rate of smoking and even those who claim to smoke only five or six cigarettes a day inevitably increase this rate on social occasions or at the weekend.

My own experience is that the patch transdermal delivery system is the most convenient and effective way of ensuring high compliance with NRT. Once the patch is applied, smoking must not take place and removal does not immediately facilitate a sudden decrease the nicotine blood level. Counselling the client will ensure that they have a clear understanding of this mode of action and basic pharmacology. Other forms of NRT, although mimicking the actual smoking nicotine 'highs', do not either ensure similar nicotine blood levels to smoking or encourage natural compliance. However, lozenges, gum and micro-tabs can be very useful for maintenance and supplementing the patches at times of withdrawal difficulty and craving. They can also be useful 'step-down' tools after the initial treatment period with patches. Micro-tabs can also be considered for pregnant women if the product license and dosing are interpreted correctly.

Some clients relate to the inhalator, which can be a useful tool for occupying the hands and address some of the behavioural habits associated with cigarette-holding. However, the inhalator is not my first choice of NRT as drawing sufficient amounts of nicotine into the buccal cavity can be difficult and the association with hand occupancy is one of the habit aspects that needs to be broken.

Gum and lozenges can give rise to gastric disturbance and a burning mouth when used in sufficient quantities to achieve the necessary blood levels of nicotine to suppress withdrawal symptoms. My own experience is that women tend not to comply particularly well with oral forms of NRT, although they can be useful for some male clients.

The most effective form of achieving higher nicotine blood levels is with the nasal spray but the unpleasant stinging sensation that most users experience will prevent proper compliance.

All manufacturers provide a wealth of useful support materials, including leaflets, personal progress charts, free telephone help lines, squeezy stress 'toys' and websites for quitters. All of these should be provided at the first appointment and supplemented with official public health materials that explain the reasons for quitting and why the NHS is investing in the service.

FOLLOWING-UP THE CLIENT

It must be realised that, although success rates have dramatically improved since the introduction of pharmacy-based smoking cessation services, the long-term quit rate is still fewer than 30% of all clients passing through the service. A well-used expression taught in many training sessions for pharmacists is that one should always tell the clients to 'Never give up giving up'. Some clients will achieve success at their first attempt but the majority need two or more efforts to meet the personal challenge of tackling their nicotine addiction. They should be encouraged to return whether or not they are successful and to maintain contact with the pharmacy. Some pharmacists fear that they may lose these clients as customers if they fail under their guidance but, in reality, most clients strike up a lasting relationship with their tutors despite their apparent failure. If they are encouraged correctly and the environment is kept friendly and informal, they will return when they are ready for another attempt at quitting. One thing is certain – the first attempt at quitting will remove the capacity for the smoker to recover the same level of denial about their addiction and associated habits if smoking is taken up again.

Those that are successful at the 4-week appointment should be encouraged to keep in touch and visit the pharmacy on a need-to basis. I have many clients who come through the door simply to boast that they are still non-smokers months and even years later. The rather embarrassing question they occasionally ask is 'How long has it been now?' and I am often at a loss to remember the original quit date. However, almost all quitters are able to quote the hour, day and date of their last cigarette. That memory indicator is a sign of how important quitting has been in their personal life and outlook. It is also a powerful motivator for encouraging more smokers to use the service and for pharmacists to become involved in bringing about the most important decision in some people's lives.

REFERENCES

Anderson C, Blenkinsopp A., Armstrong M 2003a The contribution of community pharmacy to improving the public's health. Report 1: Evidence from the peer-reviewed literature 1990–2001, 2nd edn. PharmacyHealthLink and the Royal Pharmaceutical Society of Great Britain, London. Available online at http://www.pharmacyhealthlink. org.uk/

Anderson C, Blenkinsopp A., Armstrong M 2003b The contribution of community pharmacy to improving the public's health. Report 2. Evidence from the UK non peer-reviewed literature 1990–2002. PharmacyHealthLink and the Royal Pharmaceutical Society of Great Britain, London. Available online at http://www.pharmacyhealthlink. org.uk/

Anon 2003a GPs too busy to advise on smoking. Pharmaceutical Journal 270: 355.

Anon 2003b Pharmacists play 'critical' role in smoking cessation. Pharmaceutical Journal 270: 260

Butler CC, Pill R, Stott NC 1998 Qualitative study of patients' perceptions of doctors' advice to quit smoking: implications for opportunistic health promotion. British Medical Journal 316: 1878–1881

Prochaska JO, DiClemente CC 1984 The transtheoretical approach: crossing traditional boundaries of therapy. Dow Jones-Irwin, Homewood, IL

Raw M, McNeill A, West R 1999 Smoking cessation: evidence based
   recommendations for the healthcare system. British Medical Journal 318:
   182–185
Royal College of Physicians of London 1992 Smoking and the young: a report
   of the working party of the Royal College of Physicians. RCP, London
Simpson D 2000 Doctors and tobacco: medicine's big challenge. Tobacco
   Control Resource Centre at the British Medical Association, London

MONITORING AND MANAGEMENT

CHAPTER 11

Medication error

N. Barber, A. Willson

BEING FREE FROM ERROR

The most successful strategy for ensuring that any system is free from error is to make it your policy that errors do not occur. That way, no one will be on the lookout for errors and, should any feeble individual stray from your policy, they can be dealt with through the disciplinary route. A more sophisticated version of this strategy is to acknowledge that mistakes happen outside your sphere and to establish your role as righting these wrongs. In the case of pharmacy, it helps to label the errors as prescribing, administration or compliance errors so that there can be no doubt that they are not happening in the pharmacy.

If you find that strategy attractive, you need read no further. If you prefer to measure your success in other ways, read on. In this chapter, we will suggest some ways of thinking about error, what are the known causes of medication error and what strategies can be useful to mitigate or avoid error.

RELIABILITY

Tom Nolan and Don Berwick of the Institute of Healthcare Improvement in the USA have developed the idea of reliability. How many defects are there when a task is repeated several times? They have developed a way of expressing the order of magnitude of reliability:

- Level 1: 10^{-1} – 1 defect in 10 tries
- Level 2: 10^{-2} – 1 defect in 100 tries
- Level 3: 10^{-3} – 1 defect in 1000 tries.

The categorisation is helpful because it avoids differentiating between small differences. A 6% or 26% error rate is still broadly Level 1. Processes that rely on humans performing single steps commonly exhibit Level 1 error rates. Our usual strategies for countering human error (writing protocols and checklists, enhanced training or exhortation) may improve the rate to Level 2.

Multiple-step processes are still less reliable, particularly if the steps are carried out in isolation from one another and there is no reconciliation or feedback route.

In the case of medication, most processes must be thought of as multiple-step. For a patient to receive the right dose of the right prophylactic antibiotic at the right time before a surgical procedure, there are at least six steps (Fig. 11.1).

It is even possible to break down individual steps: having the right drug available involves at least six further steps. The point is that, if the reliability of medication is judged by outcome of the whole process, it is prone to a compound error rate well within Level 1. From the patient's point of view, it is not reassuring to know that we cannot guarantee that we can get something as important as this right even close to most of the time.

This way of thinking about reliability and error is less comfortable than the denial method. It means that defects are happening in all hospitals, community pharmacies and homes on a regular basis – several times every day.

There are other ways of looking at systems and error. Your organisation may have bought in to a particular approach. The common tools include Six Sigma, Lean, Kaizen and Juran. It would be foolish (and probably prone to litigation) to choose here between these methods. They all have a useful role but they all share a quality-driven approach that assumes that things can and do go wrong. Success depends upon being clear on the desired outcome, being rigorous in checking what is achieved and seeking change through small-scale improvement. The Nolan approach described here has been developed for health care. It is very pragmatic and readily available, but any of these approaches will do!

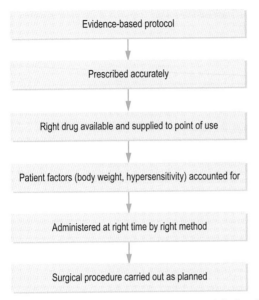

Fig. 11.1 Steps in prescribing and administering a prophylactic actibiotic before a surgical procedure.

SYSTEMS AND HUMANS

The world of health service improvement is full of quotations and one-liners. Perhaps the most famous is 'Every system is perfectly designed to achieve the results it achieves'. This means that error should be seen as a system problem. If a human has made an error, that should be considered as a result of the system. The reaction must be 'How do we learn?' and not 'Who is to blame?'

The strategy for avoiding or reducing error is:

- Be clear on what you are trying to do
- Agree how you measure quality and reliability
- Assume that there are errors and look for them – do not rely just on passive reporting
- Actively measure the errors through audit, inspection and by asking everyone involved (especially the patient) – think whole process, not just your part of the process
- Try out methods for reducing error and measure their effect – learn and change

- Reliability is improved by taking steps out of the process, not by adding them
- Reliability is improved by taking people out of the process, not by adding them.

FREQUENCY OF MEDICATION ERROR AND HARM

In order to know the frequency of errors you first need to know what a medication error is: a surprisingly contentious issue. We also need to separate an error from the issue of harm to the patient. Most medication errors do not result in harm; much of the harm caused by drugs is not the result of error. Many people confuse these issues. For example, if a drug is prescribed correctly and the patient is harmed by a known side effect, this can be called an adverse drug reaction or an adverse drug event but is not an error. Table 11.1 separates out these terms.

It is easy to get hysterical about errors by defining an ideal standard of practice and then showing that most people do not reach it. This helps no one. The word 'error' is more helpful if kept for deviations from normal practice and policy (unless normal practice/policy is bad).

The common sorts of error are prescribing errors, dispensing errors, errors in drug administration (hospitals, care homes), errors in medicine-taking (non-compliance or non-adherence – dealt with in Ch. 14), and errors at the interface between types of care, usually errors in transmission of information about medicines between primary and secondary care.

Drug administration errors are actions that deviate from the prescription or local policy. Prescribing error can be defined as a failure to decide on a suitable medicine (dose, formulation, etc.), or failure to produce this as a correct prescription (unclear writing, selection error

TABLE 11.1 Medication errors and harm to the patient

Term	An error	Causes harm
Medication error	Yes	Perhaps
Iatrogenic harm	May be	Yes
Adverse drug reaction	No	Yes
Adverse drug event	May be	Yes
Avoidable adverse drug event	Yes	Yes

on the computer, etc.), when compared to normal practice. Prescribing error can be a tricky area, as doctors, particularly GPs, may choose to write a prescription that is not pharmacologically correct, having balanced this with other decisions about the patient (e.g. the need to preserve a relationship with them).

HOW OFTEN DO MEDICATION ERRORS OCCUR?

It is hard to tell exactly: the frequency of errors depends strongly on the definitions used and the method of error detection. For example, spontaneous reporting may only detect 1 in 100 or 1 in 1000 of the errors detected by an expert observer. Prescribing and administration errors probably occur in around 5–10% of acts. We have little information on rates of error in administering drugs in care homes (although it is seen as an area of concern) or in transmitting information between primary and secondary care (but the frequency is probably, like non-adherence, between 10% and 50%). Dispensing error rates are largely unknown, as there are few studies, but the rate that reaches the public is probably between 1% and 0.1%.

HOW OFTEN DOES HARM OCCUR?

Surprisingly rarely. Perhaps 1 in 100 to 1 in 1000 errors lead to patient harm; however this depends on several factors, including what is considered to constitute 'harm'. There are certain factors that increase the likelihood that a patient is harmed, for example:

- Toxic medicines with a narrow therapeutic index, e.g. warfarin, methotrexate, strong opiates, strong potassium chloride injection
- Route of drug administration
- Extent of exposure to the error (repeated errors worse)
- Resilience of the patient – frail patients are more likely to be harmed
- Necessity of the medicine to health, e.g. it may be keeping the patient alive
- Poor safety culture – hence errors are more likely to be made and less likely to be detected.

WHY DO ERRORS OCCUR?

Studies of errors in organisations have discovered similar issues, and these have been organised into theories by psychologists. Their approach can be summarised as follows:

People make errors, either intentionally or unintentionally. The reasons why they make an error may be related to what is happening to them at the time, and to the organisation around them.

To understand why errors occur we need to understand all these factors. Once the cause is understood, solutions can be identified. Each of these factors is described in more detail below.

Intentional errors

These are also called *violations*. The person making them knows the right thing to do; however, they decide to 'cut corners', usually because this will save time and they think it is a safe thing to do. When we knowingly break the speed limit we are making an intentional error.

Unintentional errors

These are of two types:

- We know the right thing to do, we intend to do it correctly, but our brain 'hiccups' and we do the wrong thing. These are also called *slips* and *lapses*. We may simply do the wrong thing, thinking it is right (*slip*), such as trying to open the door to our house with our work key. Alternatively we may intend to do the right thing but get distracted and forget to do it (*lapse*)
- We think we know the right thing to do, but we are wrong; hence we make a bad plan, then carry it out, e.g. not knowing that a drug should have the dose adjusted in renal failure and hence prescribing the normal dose for a patient who has renal failure.

Error-producing conditions

At the time when an error happens there are usually factors that are more likely to make errors happen:

- Individual staff factors (tiredness, etc.)
- The team
- Working conditions
- Technology
- Systems of work.

Organisation

The culture of the organisation is also an important factor. Does it take errors seriously? Is it encouraging their reporting, linked to a process of learning and change, or is the organisation ignoring errors, sometimes driving people to achieve goals in spite of safety warnings?

DEFENCES

There are 'defences' that are there to stop errors causing harm, ideally by stopping them reaching the patient. Pharmacy is one such mechanism; others are the internal feeling that something is wrong, or the design of systems of work so effective checks are built in, or removing dangerous things, or using technology designed to stop errors happening. No defences are perfect – they are like a safety net with holes in: they work most of the time but will fail sometimes. Most serious harm that resulted from errors has been in cases in which there were minimal defences or in which, unusually, several defences all failed.

This framework is very powerful. It provides a guide for the investigation of error. Why did the person act in that way: a 'brain hiccup', a lack of knowledge? What were the contributing factors – the systems of work, the work group, poorly designed technology? And were they doing what the organisation had driven them towards, such as sacrificing safety for productivity? All these issues require different actions to stop them happening again.

STRATEGIES FOR STOPPING ERRORS

The first element to this is identifying where systems could be made better; the second element is working with people to create effective change. There are two approaches to identifying how systems could be made safer, prospective and retrospective; both of them should be followed. Prospective hazard analysis studies the system, identifies areas of risk and allows you to plan how to make the system safer. At the time of writing, research is being conducted to identify the best technique(s) for health care. However, as some of the more hazardous elements relating to medicines are listed above in the section on harm, it is clear that these should already be a focus for designing safer systems and methods of practice.

Retrospective analysis involves studying errors that have happened, so that the system can be made safer. It can involve just listing errors and near-misses (errors that were detected and stopped) looking for trends (e.g. dispensing errors coming from 'look-alike' drugs), or it can involve detailed investigation of errors – usually those that have caused serious harm. The detailed investigation is usually called 'root cause analysis'. There are several ways of doing it, and using the above understanding of the causes of errors is one way. The problems with root cause analysis are that it is very time-consuming, that it requires trained staff, that there is no single 'root', and that, if harm resulted from a 1 in 1 000 000 chance, much resource may be put into reducing the chance of a very rare event happening again.

PEOPLE AND CHANGE

We have acknowledged that error is usually about systems and talked about how errors happen and what they are. But when we need to rectify error, there is usually a need to do that through changing the actions of someone else. In other words, we try to blame the process not the person, but then we come up against the fact that the process consists of people. Fortunately, there are strategies for improving the chances of success with these interactions.

ONE-OFF INTERVENTIONS

The simplest interventions are when you need to correct an error or provide advice at some point in a process. Perhaps there has been a wrong dose prescribed or a patient factor has not been taken into account. A useful acronym is S-BAR:

Situation – What has happened and why are you making the intervention?
Background – What are the relevant surrounding facts?
Assessment – What are the options and the factors to be considered?
Recommendation – Be clear about whether and what you are proposing as action.

Like most acronyms, it is an aide mémoire rather than a rigid procedure. It may be more than is required in some situations. On the other hand, it safeguards against an intervention being rejected because it was poorly structured.

This style of intervention relies on people behaving in a logical way. The structure minimises the chance for failed communication. However, this is a less than ideal way to transact business. As Davis Balestracci says: 'Logic + Humans = Change? Think again! Change would be so easy if it weren't for all the people.'

A general strategy should be to reduce the need for one-off interventions. That can be approached through strategies for stopping errors, as described above, or by developing effective links with those who are involved in the same processes as you are.

DEVELOPING EFFECTIVE LINKS

There are several reasons why it is difficult to set up effective links. It is worth understanding them in order to minimise their effect.

Work is carried out in departments or silos. When there are problems, we blame the person up the line or down the line and even develop myths about why they are acting as they are. But most people (by far the majority of people) think they are doing their best. So there is great scope for misunderstanding and even conflict. This is hardly fertile ground for trying to sort out errors or preventing them from happening.

Because people are not machines, our actions are heavily influenced by our beliefs. And our beliefs are based on our experiences. If our experience of a person is that they are always giving us problems, we are less likely to trust their advice than someone we work alongside and who shares our values. Prescribers who have had good experience of working with pharmacists in the past are more likely to respond well to a new link with a pharmacist.

Finally, everyone has needs. We need to live, to have good relationships, to feel important and to have variety. When we seek to influence someone else, we may threaten their needs. The introduction of a prescribing protocol is a case in point. It may be driven by very laudable motives of cost-saving, improved efficacy or simplification of process. But it may be resisted if it reduces a prescriber's ability to try out new medicines, threatens their perceptions of status or conflicts with an undertaking they have given to a third party.

What are the strategies to overcome these difficulties?

- Decide who is in your production line. You need to give priority to those people who are regularly up or down the line from you
- Find out what they are trying to do and what they hold dear. Spend some time in their department, at audit meetings, seeing them conduct the other parts of their process
- Encourage members of staff to gain practical experience in one another's departments
- Find out what their problems are. You will have far greater success in achieving your needs if you help them achieve theirs
- Work out the best time, place and person to target your attention
- Think through your rationale and express it in shareable terms. Is it to reduce harm, increase efficacy, reduce delays, reduce waste or improve equity? If it cannot be justified in terms of these dimensions, why would anyone share your concern?
- Start by sharing an analysis of the problem. Starting with the solution can be irritating and is risky if you do not know all the salient facts

- Avoid unnecessary conflict. Get sanction to overwrite common and minor prescribing aberrations without the need for bothering busy people. This avoids squandering goodwill
- Agree methods for follow-up. How will actions be monitored and further decisions made?

CHAPTER 12

Prescription monitoring

R. Batty, K. Brackley, revised by B. D. Franklin

MONITORING PRESCRIPTIONS

Ideally, pharmacists would be able to review all of the information available for every patient, including their current condition and previous medical history, and play a major role in tailoring their drug therapy. Unfortunately, there is rarely enough time to do this. It is therefore important that pharmacists develop skills of problem detection and prioritisation using readily available information such as the prescription, talking to the patient, their appearance and other circumstantial evidence of drug-related problems.

Most prescriptions are seen on the hospital ward or in the community pharmacy. This chapter summarises structured approaches for prescription monitoring for each of these locations. These are intended to form the basis for discussion rather than authoritative documents.

PRESCRIPTION MONITORING ON THE HOSPITAL WARD

During their regular visits to the wards, pharmacists need to provide an efficient service that is of benefit to patients. Observing the patient, reviewing the prescription chart and talking to him/her allows the pharmacist to identify drug-related problems. This may lead the pharmacist to check specific information in the patient's notes or elsewhere. The following describes this approach to prescription review.

INFORMATION SOURCES

It is assumed that the prescription sheets and observations such as temperature and blood pressure are kept at the end of the patient's bed. The pharmacist visits each bed in turn, either on their own or as part of a multidisciplinary team, observing the patient, talking to him/her and reviewing the charts at the end of the bed. The pharmacist would not scrutinise the case notes or the nursing notes routinely; this is done only if the initial screen indicates a need to do so. It is assumed that the pharmacist understands local prescribing procedures.

> **You will not have time to look in every patient's notes, so look for pointers to certain diseases and refer to case notes to confirm your suspicions as to the diagnosis. Pointers may include: (1) appearance of patient; (2) diet; (3) other drugs (such as calcium carbonate or erythropoietin in renal patients; vitamins B and C strong intravenous (IV) injection in liver patients; furosemide in congestive cardiac failure).**

THE SCREEN

The approach can be summarised using the LANOT (Look Around, New drugs, Old drugs, TTAs) checklist (Batty & Barber 1991), which is summarised in Box 12.1. Each stage will now be discussed in more detail. This explanation is not exhaustive and there will be many other examples of questions that could be asked at each stage.

Box 12.1 LANOT prescription monitoring checklist for ward pharmacists

Look around

Before you look at the prescribed drugs, ask yourself the following questions.

1. Has the patient more than one prescription sheet? (e.g. separate IV, cytotoxic, total parenteral nutrition (TPN), variable dose).
2. Ward name/consultant/junior doctor – do they give clues as to the disease the patient may be suffering from?
3. Age and weight of patient – have they any implications for dose?
4. Diet – does it indicate renal failure, obesity, liver failure, patient unable to swallow solids?
5. What is the patient's appearance (jaundiced, oedematous, cyanosed, breathless or unconscious)? What is their race?

Box 12.1 LANOT prescription monitoring checklist for ward pharmacists – cont'd

New drugs
For each drug prescribed, ask yourself the following questions.

1. Is this the most effective drug for the disease? Is there a less expensive but equally effective drug available?
2. Is the dose and/or frequency appropriate, particularly with regard to renal and hepatic function, age and weight of the patient?
3. Is the form or route the most appropriate (e.g. consider sustained-release tablets with nasogastric tube, oral/IV/rectal bioavailability, etc.)?
4. Does the patient have a documented allergy to the drug or to a drug with a similar structure?
5. Will the drug interact with other drugs the patient is receiving, either to antagonise or duplicate a pharmacological action?
6. Does the patient have another disease that would contraindicate or caution the use of the drug?
7. For a drug to be given by the IV route – is it compatible with the infusion fluid? Is the duration of infusion appropriate? Is it compatible with other drugs it might mix with in the drug tubing or cannula?
8. Has the drug been added to treat a symptom caused by another drug (e.g. the addition of an anti-emetic may be because the patient is nauseated by theophylline, potassium chloride or digoxin toxicity)?
9. Is there anything in the diet that will affect drug therapy, or vice versa?
10. Do we stock it? Is it in the formulary?

Old drugs
For drugs already in the patient's regimen, the following questions should be asked.

1. Does the patient have a sufficient supply?
2. Is the drug still needed (especially anti-infectives)?
3. Is the drug working?
4. Does the dose need modifying?
5. Is the patient receiving the drug (check administration record)?
6. Is there a relationship between the drugs the patient is taking and information noted at the end of the bed?

TTAs
For discharge prescription (TTA) drugs, the following questions should be asked.

1. Are inpatient details the same as TTAs? If no, are the differences reasonable?
2. Does the patient still need the items?
3. Has steady state been achieved?
4. Are items from all prescription sheets included?

Source: Batty R, Barber N 1991 Prescription monitoring for ward pharmacists. Pharmaceutical Journal 247: 242–244

1. Look around

The patient's environment should be considered. This can give important clues about the patient, the types of disease(s) they may be suffering from, drug handling and/or administration problems.

Has the patient just been admitted?

Drug histories and patients' own drugs may need to be checked for newly admitted patients, according to local policies.

Has the patient more than one prescription sheet?

A drug on one prescription sheet may interact with a drug on another sheet. Sometimes duplication of therapy can occur, such as an antibiotic prescribed intravenously on one sheet and orally on another. If the prescription sheet has been rewritten, it may need to be checked against the old one to ensure that no transcription errors have occurred.

Ward name/consultant

A patient on a liver ward may have abnormal handling of drug eliminated by hepatic metabolism. It may also be advisable to avoid hepatotoxic drugs. Similarly, a patient under the care of a renal specialist may have impaired renal function, necessitating dosage adjustment of some drugs.

Age and weight of the patient

Neonates often have poor hepatic and renal clearance and absorption via the gastrointestinal tract may be variable. The elderly may have declining organ function and altered organ sensitivity.

Diet – does it indicate a patient problem?

Special dietary requirements are sometimes listed among the end-of-bed information and altered fluid, protein, sodium and/or potassium requirements may indicate liver or renal disease. Restrictions in fluid or electrolytes may necessitate the review of drugs that affect these.

What is the patient's appearance?

A patient who has 'nil by mouth' signs or is vomiting may need drugs to be administered by a non-oral route, while a patient with a nasogastric tube may need oral drugs administered as liquids. Certain races may have altered drug handling, e.g. some black people with hypertension do not respond well to angiotensin-converting enzyme (ACE) inhibitors.

2. New drugs

Is this the most effective drug for the disease?
The drug should be the most effective for the disease, considering other concurrent disease, other prescribed drugs, age, known drug allergies, hepatic and renal function, convenience and cost.

Is the dose and/or frequency appropriate?
The dosage regimen should be appropriate for the patient's age, weight, hepatic and renal function. Concomitant drugs may affect dose.

Is the form and/or route the most appropriate?
The form and route should be appropriate for the patient. A patient with a nasogastric tube will require liquid forms of oral medicines. Sustained-release formulations may need to be changed to immediate-release preparations given more frequently in patients who are unable to swallow the sustained-release preparation whole.

Does the patient have a documented allergy to the drug?
The choice of drug may be influenced by an allergy to the drug or one of a similar structure.

Will the drug interact with other drugs?
Some drugs antagonise the effects of others while some duplicate and enhance the effects of other drugs. Any such drug interactions should be managed so that the dose of each drug is appropriate. Alternatively, the pharmacist can recommend changing one of the drugs to an alternative from a different drug class, or changing the time of administration where the interaction is related to chelation (such as for oral ciprofloxacin and iron salts).

Has a drug been added to treat a symptom caused by another drug?
The adverse drug effect should be assessed and a decision taken as to whether it is better to change to another therapy rather than introduce a drug to treat the adverse effect.

Is there anything in the diet which will affect drug therapy or vice versa?
Where food can affect the absorption of a drug, the drug should be given at an appropriate time in relation to meals. Where the diet restricts the intake of a particular nutrient, e.g. sodium, a drug formulated to have none or low levels of that nutrient may need to be chosen. Many soluble tablet formulations contain high levels of sodium.

Is it prescribed clearly and unambiguously?

If there is any possibility for confusion over the drug, dose, route or formulation intended, this should be clarified with the prescriber and the prescription amended accordingly. For example, prescribing 'one tablet', 'III tablets', or using abbreviations is ambiguous and can lead to errors.

Are any other drugs needed?

For example, heparin or low-molecular-weight heparin may be needed for the prophylaxis of thromboembolism in surgical or immobile medical patients. Gastroprophylaxis may be needed in at-risk patients prescribed non-steroidal anti-inflammatory drugs (NSAIDs).

Is a supply needed?

Once the above questions have been answered, a supply of the drug should be initiated if required, according to local policies.

3. Old drugs

Is the drug still needed?

Some drug therapies should be continued for life, while others need be given for a short period, often as a course. Sometimes a patient is continued on therapy long after the 'course' has finished.

Is the drug working?

The response to the drug should be assessed to ensure that it is adequate and appropriate. If it is inadequate or causing unacceptable side effects, the dose and/or the drug should be changed.

Does the dose need modifying?

Sometimes the dose of a drug needs adjusting as therapy continues. This may be a dose increase because the drug induces its own metabolism (e.g. carbamazepine) or a decrease following a loading dose (e.g. oral amiodarone).

Is the patient receiving the drug?

The administration record section of the prescription sheet may indicate that the patient is not receiving the drug. Failure to follow the prescribed regimen may be a reason for an inadequate response. The reasons for non-administration should be followed up. If appropriate, alternative ways of ensuring the drug is given should be offered.

Is there a relationship between the drugs the patient is taking and the information at the end of the bed?

The end-of-bed information can give indication of some common side effects of drugs such as altered bowel habits, nausea and vomiting. Such effects should be assessed and managed appropriately.

Does the patient have a sufficient supply?

For medication that is not administered from ward stock, ensure that there is a sufficient supply on the ward.

4. TTAs

For discharge prescriptions (TTAs), check that no transcribing errors have occurred between the inpatient and TTA prescription charts.

Are any compliance aids needed?

Patients may require reminder cards to help them remember which doses to take at which time. Others use multicompartment compliance aids to help them take their medication. For patients prescribed the latter, check that the patient can open the box and that mechanisms are in place to fill them following discharge.

PRESCRIPTION MONITORING IN THE COMMUNITY

Like prescription monitoring in hospital, monitoring in the community should be patient-focused. The patient's condition and therapy should be considered as a whole. Items presented singly for dispensing should not be viewed out of context of the patient's entire regimen, including over-the-counter (OTC) medicines and complementary therapies.

This presents several challenges in the community as, unlike colleagues in hospital, community pharmacists do not have ready access to patients' medical records and the pharmacist may only see the patient's representative.

INFORMATION SOURCES

Although access to GP-held records may be limited, the community pharmacist has three valuable information sources available.

Patient medication record (PMR)

In addition to the record of dispensed medicines, information about the indication for each medicine should be elicited from the patient or prescriber. This, and additional information, can be built on during successive encounters if necessary.

OTC medicines purchased for the patient should be recorded wherever possible, as these can provide valuable information about the effectiveness or side effects of prescribed therapy. For example, a patient buying regular laxatives who is taking co-dydramol may require a review of their analgesic therapy. In order to maximise the PMR, information should be recorded in an easily used format. It should include a profile of:

- patient's current therapy
- indications for the use of each medicine
- past medication history
- allergies
- any personal information such as age and weight, special diets
- any other relevant medical information such as hepatic and renal function
- pharmaceutical care issues such as preferences for plain lids, use of compliance aids.

The patient

Talking to the patient is an essential step in determining what medicines they are currently taking. This may vary from the regimen recorded on both GP and pharmacy records.

Talking to the patient and *probing* can determine:

- *what* medicines (prescribed and purchased) they are taking
- *how* they are taking them
- *why* there are variations from the expected regimen
- *what* medicine-related problems they are experiencing (including any side effects)
- *what* measures they have taken themselves (if any) to overcome any medicine-related problems.

Personal knowledge

A community pharmacist will build up considerable knowledge of the patient and local prescribing preferences, which will assist in the review process.

When access to GP-held records is possible, these may supplement pharmacists' knowledge of the patient. Discussion with the GP may yield the same information. If the prescriber is not willing to release this information, a signed consent from the patient may be necessary. Ideally, the GP and pharmacist can work together as part of the health care team to optimise therapy. To achieve this, face-to-face meetings on a regular basis may be beneficial.

PRIORITISING

Ideally, a community pharmacist would review the therapy of each patient. However, time constraints make this difficult, so prioritising of patients is important. Patient groups such as the elderly, the housebound and those on multiple medication should be targeted.

Once the available patient information is collected, therapy should be reviewed. The following adaptation of LANOT (Batty & Barber 1991) could be used as a guide for both new and existing drugs.

- *Is the patient still taking the drug?* The regular prescribing and dispensing of a drug does not ensure that it is being taken or taken as intended. Likely adherence can be determined by talking to the patient.

- *Is therapy still required for an indication?* Some drug therapies should be continued for life, while others need to be given for a short period, often as a course. Sometimes a patient is continued on therapy long after the course has finished, e.g. a patient still taking an NSAID intended for short-term use after a back injury 6 months ago.

- *Is the drug still working?* The response to the drug should be assessed to ensure that it is adequate and appropriate. If inadequate or causing side effects, the dose and/or drug should be changed.

- *Is this the most effective drug for this indication?* The drug should be the most effective for the disease, considering other concurrent disease, other prescribed drugs, age, known drug allergies, hepatic and renal function, convenience, patient preference and cost. Does current evidence show that there is a less expensive but equally effective alternative available? Does current evidence show that medication should be added to the regimen? For example, a steroid inhaler needs to be added to bronchodilator-inhaler-only therapy when the patient requires the bronchodilator more than once a day.

- *Are the dose and frequency appropriate?* The dosage regimen should be appropriate, particularly with regard to renal and hepatic function, and age and weight of the patient. Concomitant drugs may affect dose.

- *Is the timing of doses appropriate?* The timing of some drugs is critical for maximum effectiveness, e.g. the timing of long-acting nitrates to allow for nitrate-free periods.

- *Is the dosage form the most appropriate?* The dosage form should be appropriate for the patient, drug and condition treated, e.g. modified-release calcium channel blockers – is the frequency correct for specific preparation? Has a modified-release analgesic formulation been prescribed for occasional use?

- *Does the patient have a documented allergy?* Does the patient have a documented allergy to the drug or to a drug with a similar structure?
- *Will the drug interact with other drugs?* Will the drug interact with other drugs the patient is receiving (prescribed and purchased), either to antagonise or duplicate a pharmacological action? If your computer highlights an interaction, how significant is it for *this* patient? For example, in a patient prescribed warfarin and aspirin – is the patient taking regular low-dose aspirin or using larger doses intermittently for analgesia?
- *Any contraindications?* Does the patient have another disease that would contraindicate or caution the use of the drug, e.g. use of a beta-blocker in an asthmatic patient?
- *Has the drug been added to treat a symptom caused by another drug?* The adverse drug effect should be assessed and a decision taken as to whether it is better to change to another therapy rather than introduce a drug to treat the adverse effect, e.g. omeprazole prescribed to treat NSAID-induced dyspepsia.

REFERENCE

Batty R, Barber N 1991 Prescription monitoring for ward pharmacists. Pharmaceutical Journal 247: 242–244

CHAPTER 13

Primary care prescribing: practical approaches

J. Vincent

With the government's goal to modernise the National Health Service (NHS) to meet the needs of patients, primary care organisations have been placed at the centre of delivering health care services. They have assumed the lead role for assessing and commissioning appropriate services to meet the health needs of their patients.

It is now well recognised that medicines form the most common medical intervention in the UK. As a consequence, medicines management and medication reviews have become a significant area of work for primary care organisations.

The modernisation agenda and the increasing focus on medicines management have resulted in the emergence of primary care pharmacists. These individuals are becoming key members of primary care organisations, with roles contributing to the development of local health service delivery in addition to leading the effective management of medicines within the health community. Several key publications have been developed by the National Prescribing Centre, which will support pharmacists in these roles.

The first, *Competencies for Pharmacists Working in Primary Care* (NHS Executive and National Prescribing Centre 2000), provides detail on a core competency framework that can be used by individuals and organisations to help identify development and training requirement for those pharmacists undertaking the broad range of primary care pharmacists' roles, i.e. practice-based, local co-ordinator and strategic lead. The document also provides details of those postgraduate courses that may be relevant to primary care pharmacists.

The second document, *GP Prescribing Support: a resource document and guide for the new NHS* (National Prescribing Centre 1998), defines the phrase 'prescribing support' and gives a detailed breakdown of the potential roles for primary care pharmacists. The document provides a 'comprehensive' resource aimed at those individuals concerned with delivering effective medicines management and, although published in 1998, contains relevant background and supporting information for those already involved in or about to embark on a prescribing support role.

The National Prescribing Centre is an NHS organisation formed in 1996 by the Department of Health following a review of centrally funded support for prescribing and medicine use. Its aim is to: 'facilitate the promotion of high quality, cost effective prescribing and medicines management through a co-ordinated and prioritised programme of activities aimed at supporting relevant professionals and senior managers working in the modern NHS'. The National Prescribing Centre website (www.npc.co.uk) is a rich resource for all involved in delivering effective medicines management. Of particular use is the electronic current awareness bulletin; this provides links to published evidence, policies, guidelines drug evaluations and other documents relevant to prescribing and medicines management. The statement of scope and sources provides links to other websites of interest.

It is acknowledged that medicines management is a major part of the clinical governance agenda; however, effective management of medicines will also contribute to the financial position of the primary care organisation. While the primary care drugs budget is in essence managed by the primary care organisation, it is in reality a health community agenda. In developing a medicines management strategy, it is critical that consideration is given to a secondary care element. How might this be achieved? And why indeed should it be even considered at all?

The Audit Commission Report *A Spoonful of Sugar* (Audit Commission 2001) cites the fact that up to 18% of primary care prescribing is initiated in secondary care, with a further 40% indirectly influenced by consultant choices. It is therefore apparent that working in isolation could have significant implications for the primary care organisation, and thus the health community. To support an integrated primary and secondary care approach to prescribing, consideration should be given to:

- developing an effective joint primary and secondary care prescribing advisory group or area prescribing committee; the role of this committee would be to provide strategic direction for prescribing locally

- appointment of an interface pharmacist, this individual should ideally work for both the primary care organisation and adjacent secondary care organisation. Their role is key to managing prescribing effectively and it is crucial that they are well known to the primary care organisation GPs and the secondary care consultants
- involving the interface pharmacist in the work of the primary care organisation, i.e. develop their competencies as a practice-based pharmacist. This will enable them to gain clearer understanding of the issues which underpin the local medicines management strategy
- involving GPs in the secondary care groups, whether at the strategic or the more practical specific grass-roots level. This encourages greater understanding of the pressures in each sector
- developing effective mechanisms for managing the introduction of new drugs into secondary care. When evaluating the impact of a new drug, the implications for primary care must be considered
- developing a joint approach to working with the pharmaceutical industry
- avoiding where possible the use of 'loss leaders', the implications of secondary care initiating therapy are significant. Patients often feel that, because the consultant has commenced therapy, then they must continue to receive it. Joint policies on selected areas of prescribing should be considered
- consideration of develoment of rotational training posts between primary and secondary care. As a minimum, encourage directorate pharmacists to spend time working in practice with the prescribing support team
- raising awareness and developing a joint action plan for managing key areas, e.g. statins and anti-platelet therapies.

PRIMARY CARE PRESCRIBING STRATEGY

The development of a primary care prescribing strategy is described in detail in *Primary Care Prescribing: A bulletin for primary care trusts* (Audit Commission 2003). Core to the delivery of the elements of the strategy will be the prescribing support team. These individuals will need to develop strong working relationships with the GP practices, and this must include the primary care organisation's strategic lead, not just the prescribing support pharmacists. These relationships need to include all GPs within the practice, the practice nurses and the practice staff.

Changing prescribing behaviour is not just about using or recommending the use of alternative products. It will involve the development of a culture that will require changing individuals attitudes to prescribing, their ingrained belief and certain behaviours. How can this be achieved effectively?

Evidence suggests that a combination of approaches is most effective and include:

- practice visits and use of printed material
- interactive face-to-face educational meetings
- educational outreach
- audit and feedback with discussions with peer group.

It has been shown a combination of three or four of these approaches has been most successful. Several papers have been published that look at implementing guidance and influencing prescribing behaviour. It is clear from these that there is ongoing belief that one of the significant influences on prescribing behaviour is the pharmaceutical industry and it has been suggested that primary care organisations should therefore look at the methods they use and consider developing these skills within the advisory team. Thus, when visiting practices to discuss a specific change, the prescribing team should provide the practice with background information linked to the most recent evidence and include a range of tools to support the practice in achieving the change. These could include:

- practice letters
- patient information
- search strategy to identify practice population
- read codes
- computer prompts
- training sessions with practice staff.

Face-to-face contact with GPs through a variety of scenarios has been shown to be the most effective way of delivering changes to the management of prescribing, to support this:

- The prescribing strategy should detail the level of practice support available and required by the primary care organisation
- The strategic lead pharmacists must target the support appropriately using pharmacist and technicians to maximum benefit and aimed at delivering effective change in prescribing behaviour
- Avoid using pharmacists in tasks that can be delegated by ensuring there is an appropriate skill mix within the team, i.e. to ensure access if possible to administrative support and data analyst
- The team must integrate with, and should be viewed as a key member of, the GP practice team. Working in isolation in an office will not affect positive influences on prescribing behaviour.

Often something as simple as sitting with the receptionists will identify other areas for potential improvement, e.g. repeat prescribing

- Use alternative professionals where possible, to target areas outside pharmacists' specialist areas, e.g. dietitians, stoma care/incontinence nurses
- Monitor the interventions made; record any significant interventions, ensuring regular feedback to aid practice and primary care organisation learning.

At practice level, regular meetings with the advisory team will facilitate discussions to enable ownership of the work programme to be achieved. When organising regular meetings:

- Reinforce the need to have maximum attendance from the practice. Meeting with one or two GPs from the practice will not necessarily ensure success
- Involve all interested parties, i.e. practice nurses, practice staff responsible for managing prescribing (they often have practical answers) and practice managers
- Involve key members of the prescribing support team, e.g. prescribing support technicians. They will understand the potential barriers/solutions to any suggestions made and should understand how the practice information technology (IT) could support any initiatives agreed
- Be prepared. Ensure detailed analysis of the practice prescribing trends has been made, and that recommendations are backed up by sound evidence
- Share success stories – where methods adopted by other practices have resulted in positive outcomes, share the success:
- Use a variety of information to illustrate recommendations: graphs, trends and practice comparisons. Use IT at the meeting if necessary to provide more detailed analysis and to support visually the points being discussed
- Gain commitment at the meeting for the actions agreed and follow up the meeting with a letter detailing these actions
- Identify what resources are available to support the practice, e.g.
  - personnel – technician/pharmacists: use your skill mix wisely. It is inappropriate for clinical pharmacists to be undertaking routine simple tasks, e.g. generic changes
  - letters to support practices to implement changes; keeping patients informed at all times will aid success
  - developing medicines management/chronic disease management clinics.

CHANGE METHODOLOGIES

In supporting the prescribing support team to implement successful change, an understanding is required of the key principles that underpin successful change. There is little point in work being undertaken if, once the prescribing support team move on, the change cannot be maintained. It is important that the prescribing team:

- keep steps small
- familiarise themselves with change techniques used to facilitate acceleration of change, e.g. Plan/Do/Study/Act (PDSA) cycles
- identify successes
- identify how the successful change will be sustained and the learning from the process spread, e.g. prescribing leads forum.

The National Prescribing Centre has facilitated the Medicines Management Services Collaborative, which has supported participating sites in developing these skills within their teams. The website www. npc.co.uk has a specific area related to the collaborative and, as a result of the learning gained through the scheme, has developed service improvement guides, the first of which has now been released, with others to follow.

PRESCRIBING LEADS

Primary Care Prescribing: A bulletin for primary care trusts describes the development of a GP prescribing lead for the primary care organisation; a job description for this position is available on the National Prescribing Centre website. The concept of a GP prescribing lead at primary care organisation level can be further developed to include prescribing leads within each practice. These individuals are the key to supporting effective management of prescribing within their own practice and act as a point of contact for the prescribing support team. Offering protected time to these individuals to work on target areas has been shown to be effective in producing positive impact on prescribing issues. Primary care organisations should consider bringing these leads together on a regular basis as this provides a forum in which to share ideas, provide updates and interact with secondary care consultants in specific therapeutic areas.

In addition, the provision of comparative performance indicators often stimulates lively debate, can act as a further lever to improve prescribing performance and is best done in an open manner, naming all practices in the data. Good communication with these individuals is essential and can be supported, for example, by the development of an email group and web pages for further discussion and sharing of ideas.

Effective management of prescribing is both challenging and rewarding. The Audit Commission document (2001) summarises the requirements for good management of prescribing, i.e:

- effective strategic planning and performance management
- mechanisms to influence prescribers, based on positive, open relationships with GPs and other professionals
- appropriate direction of the efforts of the prescribing team and evaluation of their impact
- close working with other primary care organisations and secondary care.

REFERENCES

Audit Commission 2001 A spoonful of sugar: medicines management in NHS hospitals. Audit Commission, London. Available online at: http://www.audit-commission.gov.uk/reports/

Audit Commission 2003 Primary care prescribing – a bulletin for Primary Care Trusts. Audit Commission, London. Available online at: http://www.audit-commission.gov.uk/health/primaryandcommunity services/auditcommissionreports/

National Prescribing Centre 1998 GP prescribing support: a resource document and guide for the new NHS. Department of Health, London. Available online at: http://www.dh.gov.uk/assetRoot/04/11/92/11/04119211.pdf

NHS Executive and National Prescribing Centre 2000 Competencies for pharmacists working in primary care. Available online at: http://www.npc.co.uk/publications/CompPharm/competencies.htm

CHAPTER 14

Improving adherence to medication

S. Clifford, N. Barber

WHAT IS ADHERENCE?

Adherence to medication is the extent to which a patient's medication-taking behaviour coincides with the recommendations given when the patient was prescribed treatment. This behaviour is also referred to as 'compliance', but this term is becoming less frequently used because it has negative connotations that imply the patient is passive and should obey the doctor's orders. The term 'concordance' was introduced to describe a process by which a 'therapeutic alliance' is developed between doctor and patient that is conducive to discussing patients' views about their treatment (Royal Pharmaceutical Society of Great Britain 1997). The term refers to the process of communication between doctor and patient and was not introduced as a replacement for the terms 'compliance' or 'adherence'. Concordance is one of several models of prescriber–patient interactions.

NON-ADHERENCE

IS NON-ADHERENCE A PROBLEM?

Non-adherence affects approximately a third to half of patients with a chronic condition; this has wide-ranging implications. For patients, the consequences of non-adherence are unnecessary ill health, additional treatment and wasted opportunity for health gain. For the health care system, there are economic consequences from wasted medication, hospitalisations and extra treatment for the patient.

IS NON-ADHERENCE BAD?

Not necessarily so. For example, non-adherence could be a logical response to the experience of severe side effects or if the prescription is inappropriate. However, non-adherence could be a problem if patients are making the decision to behave in this way on the basis of inaccurate information and beliefs. The aim for health professionals is to ensure that patients are making adherence decisions based on informed judgements.

HOW CAN NON-ADHERENCE BE IDENTIFIED?

There is no gold standard for identifying non-adherence. This has led to much discussion over the merits of different methods and a relative impasse in the debate over which is the best method to use. The most practical way is to ask the patient. Most patients have what they consider to be a good reason for not taking their medication, and will tell you if asked in the right way.

HOW CAN WE UNDERSTAND NON-ADHERENCE?

Non-adherence is a complex behaviour that can best be understood according to whether it is intentional or unintentional (also referred to as active and passive, respectively). Intentional non-adherence is largely related to cognitive factors and unintentional non-adherence is related to circumstances or issues of ability. Table 14.1 contains some examples of reasons for the two different types of non-adherence.

Over 200 often conflicting factors thought to influence non-adherence have been reported. No demographic factors have been found to predict non-adherence consistently, so there is no such thing as an easily identifiable 'non-adherent patient'. Key influential factors are listed in Table 14.2.

Figure 14.1 illustrates the period during medication-taking when some of these factors are most likely to be relevant. As medication-taking is a dynamic process, adherence is likely to vary within the same patients over time. Patients taking more than one medication may vary in their adherence behaviour with each one.

HOW TO IMPROVE ADHERENCE

THE EVIDENCE

Compared to the volume of literature on why non-adherence occurs, there is relatively little research into how adherence can be improved.

TABLE 14.1 Examples of intentional and unintentional reasons for non-adherence

Intentional non-adherence	Unintentional non-adherence
Deciding not to get the prescription dispensed	Forgetting to get the prescription dispensed
Stopping the medication because of side effects or because feeling better	Forgetting to take the medication
Not starting the medication because of concerns about taking it	Not understanding the original treatment instructions
Fear of becoming dependent on the medication	Manual dexterity problems with opening bottles or difficulty swallowing tablets
Increasing the dose because of belief that medication is not working	Memory problems with recalling accurate treatment instructions

There has been no simple, proven effective method to improve adherence, largely because the interventions have relied solely on one method (e.g. provision of information). Given the many and varied causes of non-adherence, it is not surprising that simplistic approaches have limited success. Successful interventions have tended to be complex, so it is unclear which elements of the interventions were effective and it would be difficult to implement them in practice. However, there are some principles and insights we can give.

KEY STRATEGIES

Non-adherence is clearly complex; it can be intentional or unintentional and can arise as the result of many different factors.

> **The key to improving adherence is to identify the unique causes of non-adherence for each patient and to select the correct solutions.**

Diagnosis of the problem is crucial and this can only happen after accessing and listening to each patient's unique experience with, or 'story about', their medication. It is important also to understand how the patient perceives their illness, as this is likely to influence how they perceive their medication. The aim of exploring patients' beliefs

TABLE 14.2 Examples of key factors that influence non-adherence

Key factors	Example
Patients' beliefs about the medication	• Low perceived necessity of the medication and high level of concern about taking it • Low perceived benefits of the medication and high perceived barriers • Low perceived behavioural control and low perception of self-efficacy
Health professionals' communication with the patient	• Prescribers' overuse of a biomedical approach in the consultation and underuse of a psychosocial approach (ignoring relevant psychological and social factors) • Doctors and pharmacists giving little attention to whether patients understand or will recall the treatment instructions accurately
Depression	• Low mood, leading to decline in motivation towards taking medication
Social support	• Family or friends who have negative attitudes towards the medication or who are unsupportive
Complexity of the treatment	• Large number of medications • Dose frequency more than twice a day

is to create an opportunity to ensure that they understand the purpose and effects of their medication, to help them make an informed decision about whether to adhere.

The following recommendations for exploring adherence issues with patients are based partly on the literature and partly on our research experience; we have interviewed several hundred patients about their adherence.

1. *Start by forming some rapport* with the patient by asking a general question, such as 'How are you getting on with your medicines?'

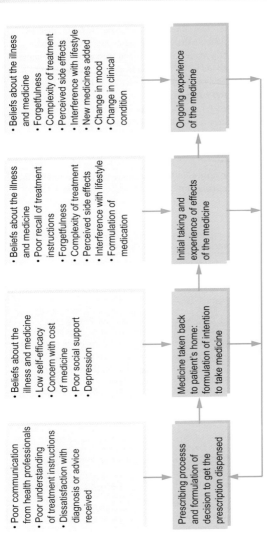

Fig. 14.1 Time that key factors are likely to influence non-adherence from the start of a new medication.

2. *Identify whether non-adherence is an issue.* A useful method is to reassure patients that many patients miss doses of their medications for a range of reasons, and then ask patients when they last missed a dose of their medication. Previous studies have shown that missing a dose in the previous 7 days is a good indication of non-adherence.

3. *Identify reasons for non-adherence.* Ask a series of questions to follow up patients' accounts of their reasons for missing a dose. You may need to explore patients' perceptions of their illness and medication, as these are likely to be salient in many explanations of non-adherence.

4. *Suggest one or more solutions.* Keep the intentional/unintentional dichotomy in mind and the different approaches that would be

---

TABLE 14.3 Examples of intentional and unintentional reasons for non-adherence and possible solutions

Intentional non-adherence	Unintentional non-adherence
Reason: Patient stops taking medication or misses doses because of perceived side effects	*Reason*: Patient misses doses because of a misunderstanding about how they should take the medication or poor recall of original treatment instructions
Solution: If appropriate, provide advice to patient to change dose frequency or time of day taken. If necessary, refer patient to their GP for a change of medication and monitoring	*Solution*: Restate the original treatment instructions. Explain why the medication was prescribed and how they should take it
Reason: Patient doesn't start or stops taking the medication because they do not feel ill (common in asymptomatic conditions such as hypertension)	*Reason*: Patient forgets their morning dose of their medication because they are in a rush to get to work
Solution: Explain to patient that their condition is asymptomatic and how the medication is necessary to prevent future health problems. Exploring patients' perceptions of their illness and its consequences will identify areas to tailor information that can promote their understanding of how the medication was intended to help their condition	*Solution*: Suggest that patient keeps a supply of their medication at work or, depending on the specific regimen, suggest that they try taking it at night instead

necessary for each type. As a general rule, unintentional non-adherence will require practical solutions, whereas intentional non-adherence will require focusing on patients' beliefs and motivations. Table 14.3 has examples of common intentional and unintentional reasons for not taking medication and possible solutions.

Some causes of non-adherence may be intractable. A patient's reason for not taking their medication may be the most logical behaviour according to their beliefs about their illness and/or medication. It is crucial not to judge as deviant patients who report non-adherence. Also, it is important to remember that medication-taking is a dynamic process, so adherence will vary over time; most of us are non-adherent some of the time. Hence, adherence needs to be monitored at frequent intervals.

Finally, monitoring adherence can form part of a regular medication review with patients. Box 14.1 is the interview guide that has been used as an effective way of discussing and resolving adherence issues, medication-related problems and information needs with patients.

Box 14.1 Interview guide for a medication review with patients

Q1 How are you getting on with your medicines?

Q2 What medicines are you taking that you get on prescription?

Q3 What illnesses are you taking your medicines to treat?

Taking each medicine in turn . . .

Q4 Do you think the medicine is helping you? Why do you think that?

Q5 Are you having any problems or concerns with it?

Q6 Do you think the medicine has made you feel worse in any way or has had any side effects?

Q7 People often miss taking doses of their medicines for a whole range of reasons. When was the last time you missed taking a dose of this medicine?

(How often missed in last week? Have any medicines have been stopped completely?)

Q8 When you have missed a dose, what have been the reasons?

Q9 Would you like any further information on how to take your medicine? (dose, times of day to take the medicine, any special instructions on how to take it, whether to take it with food or drink etc.)

Box 14.1 **Interview guide for a medication review with patients – cont'd**

Q10 Would you like any further information on the effects of your medicine? (why you are taking the medicine, how it works, how it will help your condition, etc.)

Q11 Would you like any further information on the side effects of your medicine? (types of side effects, likelihood of experiencing them and what to do if you have them)

Q12 Is there anything else about your illness or medicines I can help you with?

REFERENCE

Royal Pharmaceutical Society of Great Britain 1997 From compliance to concordance: achieving shared goals in medicine taking. Royal Pharmaceutical Society of Great Britain/Merck Sharp & Dohme, London

FURTHER READING

McDonald HP, Garg AX, Haynes RB 2002 Interventions to enhance patient adherence to medication prescriptions: scientific review. Journal of the American Medical Association 288: 2868–2879

Meichenbaum D, Turk D 1987 Factors affecting adherence. In: Meichenbaum D, Turk D (eds) Facilitating treatment adherence. Plenum Press, New York, pp 41–68

Myers L, Midence K 1998 Adherence to treatment in medical conditions. Harwood Academic Press, Amsterdam

CHAPTER 15

Informing patients about the risks of their medicines

D. K. Raynor, P. Knapp, D. C. Berry

INTRODUCTION

If patients are asked what information they want about their medicines, 'side effects' is always in the top two answers. But this is only the beginning of the story – do they just want a list, as currently provided on patient information leaflets, or do they want more?

The answer is almost certainly that they want more. If they are going to make informed decisions about taking medicines, then they need to know more about their personal risk of having those side effects. They also need to know what they can do to alleviate or reduce the consequences of them.

However, detailed information about side effect risk is no use in isolation – it needs to be balanced against information about how likely they are to benefit from the medicine. Only then can they make an informed decision. This decision will relate to their perception of:

- how important the benefits are to them
- how the negative impact of the possible side effects will affect them.

This depends on their personal values and so no one else can make these decisions for them.

This chapter is about the role of clinical pharmacists (and fellow health professionals) in answering the following questions from patients about side effects:

- What are the side effects?
- How likely are they to happen to me?
- What should I do if they happen?

and supporting them in making decisions based on this information. Essentially, this is a mixture of objective and subjective information:

- the likelihood of the side effect occurring – objective
- the patient's perceived impact of the side effects on them in particular – subjective.

WHAT ARE THE SIDE EFFECTS OF THIS MEDICINE?

This frequently asked question is often the tip of an iceberg. Underlying it is often the deeper question: 'Will this medicine do me any good and might it harm me?' If this question is asked, then you should explore the issues which prompted it.

- Has the patient had problems with side effects before?
- Does the patient already have some knowledge of the side effects of this medicine?
- Do they have doubts about the benefits of the medicine?

WHAT TERMS SHOULD I USE?

Once the context of the inquiry is clear, how do you then provide an answer to the original question? If it is a common medicine, or a more specialised medicine in your clinical specialty, then you may be in the position to be able to give summarised verbal information describing the broad advantages and/or disadvantages. You might decide to say something like 'There are a few common side effects, like x, y and z, which are mild and most people manage to cope with, and some more serious side effects, which are rare'.

However, you can see from Table 15.1 that people's interpretation of descriptive terms, such as 'common' and 'rare' (column 2) differs markedly from that of legislators (column 4); these figures are from an EU guideline on how manufacturers could express the risk of side effects using these descriptive terms. Column 3 shows that doctors also underestimate the risk, but to a lesser extent than lay people.

TABLE 15.1 Differing interpretations of vertal terms for levels of risk

Term	Lay people's interpretation	Hospital doctors' interpretation	EU guideline
Very common	65%	46%	>10%
Common	45%	–	1–10%
Uncommon	18%	–	0.1–1%
Rare	8%	2%	0.01–0.1%
Very rare	4%	–	0.001–0.01%

There are a number of other series of descriptive terms. Notably, Calman and Hine proposed a risk scale comprising high, moderate, low, very low, minimal, negligible (Calman and Hine 1995), but there is no evidence that people interpret these terms in line with the intended meaning.

It would be instructive for you to determine, in your own mind, what you mean when you yourself use terms like this. The bottom line is that, whenever such terms are used, their interpretation will vary widely between patients and the professionals who use them. Generally, people interpret such descriptive terms so as to overestimate the chance of the side effect happening compared with what was intended by the professional or regulator.

Another descriptive option is to relate the risk to the likelihood of events to which the general public can relate, such as a road accident or being struck by lighting. However, people vary widely in their judgements of the frequency of such events.

WHAT ARE THE ALTERNATIVES TO VERBAL TERMS?

If descriptive terms are open to misinterpretation, then we need to think about alternatives. These fall under the headings of *numeric* or *graphical* approaches.

The most obvious is to use the actual percentage quoted in the literature. However, problems with numerical literacy may be as common as textual literacy – not everyone understands percentages. One group of older people with ischaemic heart disease said that a 3% risk of death from surgery was a 'low' risk. You might therefore feel that using 3 in 100 rather than 3% might be preferable. This might be particularly appropriate when the numbers are very small, e.g. 1 in 10 000 rather than 0.001%. However, some people are confused by this and think that a risk of 1 in 10000 is bigger than a risk of 1 in 1000. Another suggested option is to use 'number needed to harm' (the mirror image of 'number needed to treat'). An example is saying that '*x* people would have to take the medicine for a year for one person to have side effect *y*, compared to people not taking the medicine'. However, this is a concept that the general public are unlikely to understand easily.

Giving an idea of the likelihood without using numbers at all is to relate it to the size of communities. Calman and Royston proposed the 'community risk scale', which is shown in Table 15.2. So, if a side effect occurs in 0.001% or 1 in 10000 people, then you could say that if everyone in a small town was taking the medicine, then 1 person would get the side effect. Clearly, streets, villages and towns vary in size, as do peoples' perception of their size.

So, numerical options overcome the ambiguity associated with descriptive terms, but have their own drawbacks. To overcome the problems associated with numerical illiteracy, a graphical approach can be used. There are many different types of graphical approach. An example is a diagram containing 100 'stick men', with 1 a different colour to show an incidence of 1 in 100. More research is needed to test the effectiveness of different graphical methods.

TABLE 15.2 Community risk scale

Risk	Risk description	Death rates in UK per year
1 in 1	Person	
1 in 10	Family	
1 in 100	Street	Any cause
1 in 1000	Village	Any cause age 40
1 in 10000	Small town	Road accident
1 in 100000	Large town	Murder
1 in 1000000	City	Oral contraceptives
1 in 10000000	Province/country	Lightning
1 in 100000000	Large country	Measles
1 in 1000000000	Continent	
1 in 10000000000	World	

Source: adapted with permission from Calman KC, Royston G 1997 Personal paper: risk language and dialects. British Medical Journal 315: 939–942.

OVERALL ASSESSMENT OF A MEDICINE'S RISK

A further issue when adopting any of the above approaches is that most medicines have a number of possible side effects; 10, 20 or even 30. Providing such information verbally (with effective recall) is impossible. However, a list of 20–30 percentages, graphs, etc., each linked to one of the side effects, may be equally indigestible.

WRITTEN RESOURCES

You, as a health professional, need access to reliable information to be able to inform patients. However, lack of time, and the amount of information to get across, dictate that patients also need access to such information.

The two most immediate options are the Summary of Product Characteristics (previously known as the Data Sheet), which contains the definitive list of side effects and its equivalent patient information leaflet. You can find many of these documents in the Electronic Medicines Compendium on www.medicines.org.uk. However, in most cases, the side effects are listed with little qualification. They may be divided into mild and severe, and sometimes common and rare. If you need to know the frequency of the side effect, then the *British National Formulary* (hard copy or web version) gives little further detail. This will require you to access more specialised sources of information from Medicines Information. These will include systematic reviews and specialist adverse drug reaction textbooks. This will give you a range of data, which you will need to process to make something that is meaningful for the patient. However, in many cases, drugs have not been evaluated in large trials and so the calculation of low-frequency incident rates is an inexact science. The prevalence of side effects identified in postmarketing surveillance is difficult to determine because of the uncertainties over the number of people who have taken the medicine.

WHAT SHOULD I DO IF I GET A SIDE EFFECT?

People need to know not only how likely a side effect is, but what to do if it happens. Again the terminology is important. The EU recommended the terms 'immediately' and 'as soon as possible' for the need to see a doctor urgently or less urgently, respectively. We found that there was little difference in people's interpretation of these terms. Again you need to use your professional judgement and be as specific as possible when describing the urgency.

SUPPORTING PATIENTS IN THEIR DECISION-MAKING

The need to work with patients in a partnership about their medicine-taking (concordance) has already been explored in Chapter 14. Providing people with information about side effects and their likelihood is an important part of the concordance process. However, it is difficult to separate level of risk from the 'value' attached to the side effect – what the negative effects mean for that person.

At the heart of the issue for clinical pharmacists (and all health professionals) about informing patients about the risk of side effects is that much of the general information about side effects is imprecise, and information about the individual level of risk is simply not available. Finding information about the benefits of a medicine are even less accessible. Balancing risks and benefits of medicines is complex; with medicines, there is generally one benefit but many possible risks. It is an imprecise science and a key role of the professional is to convey this to the patient. This lack of precision may be difficult for the patient to accept.

Sophisticated decision aids are available in some areas and they are increasingly available as IT-based tools. Evaluation has yielded conflicting results and further research is needed. However, such aids tend to focus on surgical choices or screening, rather than decisions about whether to take a particular medicine or medicines.

In practice, the information is rarely available at the professional's finger tips.

Until the quality and accessibility of information on side effect risk are improved, much lies on the professional's shoulders. Ideally they should be able to direct people to resources on the web or elsewhere for them to consider in their own time.

Most patients do not get information about treatment options and outcomes from the written information they receive. To support shared decision-making, information needs to be balanced about risks and benefits and honest about uncertainties and knowledge gaps.

Each side effect will have its own frequency of occurrence and each will be more or less important to individual patients, e.g. drowsiness is particularly important to someone who drives, as are aching limbs for someone sporting. You will need to ask how important the potential side effects would be to the individual patient.

You may need to use your professional judgement in advising patients about the overall risks associated with a medicine or medicine regime.

INDIVIDUAL LEVEL OF RISK

Individual level of risk is what people really want to know. How relevant is clinical trials data to the patient in front of you? Systematic reviews show that clinical risk communication is most effective if individualised calculations of risks and benefits are used. Professionals need to be able to tailor the information to needs of individual patients but often do not have the basic information. It is self-evident that trials data will relate to the individual patient only to the extent that they are using the same daily dose and length of course as in the trial. Of course, with some medicines, e.g. pain-killers, the doses taken are highly variable.

YOU'VE BEEN FRAMED

There is considerable potential for misleading patients, depending on how the information is presented. Using either relative or absolute risk is a good example. In the 1995 'pill scare', professionals, patients and the media misinterpreted the risk information by looking at the relative risk in isolation, i.e. third-generation oral contraceptives were 'twice as likely' to cause thromboembolism. The missing absolute information was that the risks were 1 in 250 000 and that the risk in pregnant women was much higher than with either type of oral contraceptive.

This is known as framing and it can be used to influence perceptions of risk – as shown in the above case, relative risk is more persuasive than absolute risk. It has been suggested that drug manufacturers attempted to enhance the apparent effectiveness of statins by emphasising the relative benefits numbers rather than the absolute benefits. So, we have to take care not to use the effect of framing to manipulate information to get the effect we want, as these different approaches lead to significantly different choices being made by patients.

As well as using relative or absolute risk, information can be framed in a positive or negative way. Edwards and Elwyn (2006) used the example of hormone replacement therapy (HRT). The risk of major fracture is 12% in women who take HRT for more than 5 years and 15% in those who do not. This can be 'framed' as:

- a 3% reduction in absolute risk
- fractures are 20% less common (relative risk reduction)
- 3% more people remain free of fractures with HRT (positive framing)
- 3% more people suffer fractures if they do not take HRT (negative framing).

In general, positive framing is more persuasive than negative framing

PRACTICAL RECOMMENDATIONS

Until the relevant data are easily accessible to clinical pharmacists, it remains difficult to meet patients' information needs. Ideally, a range of formats:

- descriptive
- numeric
- graphical

should maximise patients' understanding. However, a pragmatic approach is to combine the use of verbal and numerical terms.

Wider priorities are:

- a patient education programme to improve the consistency of understanding of whatever risk presentation methods official bodies decide to use
- risk information should be written and designed in line with professional information design specialists
- the need for regulators and policy-makers to test understanding of recommended methods of risk description before implementation.

REFERENCES

Calman K, Hine D 1995 A policy framework for commissioning cancer services. Department of Health, London
Calman KC, Royston G 1997 Personal paper: risk language and dialects. British Medical Journal 315: 939–942
Edwards A, Elwyn G 2006 Professional skills in treatment decisions. http://www.dh.gov.uk

FURTHER READING

Berry D 2004 Risk, communication and health psychology. Open University Press, Maidenhead
Berry DC, Raynor DK, Knapp P, Bersellini E 2003 Patients' understanding of risk associated with medication use. Drug Safety 26: 1–11
Edwards A 2003 Communicating risks. British Medical Journal 327: 691–692
Gigerenzer G 2002 Reckoning with risk. Penguin, Harmondsworth
Knapp P, Raynor DK, Berry DC 2004 Comparison of two methods of presenting risk information to patients about the side effects of medicines. Quality and Safety in Healthcare 13: 176–180
Paling J 2003 Strategies to help patients understand risks. British Medical Journal 327: 745–748

Substance misuse

K. Roberts, J. Sheridan, M. Walker

Substance misuse is not a new phenomenon. However, the context in which we view substance misuse today is shaped by the legal status of the drugs, the effects of drug misuse on health and social wellbeing, government and medical policy on drug misuse and the effects of substance misuse on the rest of society. In the UK, detailed frameworks for developing local systems of effective drug misuse treatment have been implemented. As a result, the numbers of misusers entering treatment continues to grow, providing greater opportunities for pharmacists to become involved on a day-to-day basis.

Although there are increasing numbers of individuals who misuse other drugs such as stimulants, this chapter will focus briefly on some clinical and practical aspects of the supply of prescribed medications to opiate-dependent clients, with a particular focus on UK practice and legal requirements. These may differ in other countries. Specific groups such as pregnant drug users, those with a dual diagnosis, young people and those in prison are not covered. The term 'client' is used throughout the chapter, and refers to patients and consumers of services.

HARM REDUCTION

Much of the service provision for drug misusers in the UK is based on the philosophy of harm reduction – i.e. enabling drug-takers who cannot or will not abstain from taking drugs in a way that causes least harm to them (and possibly to society). For many drug misusers, abstinence is not possible (at least not in the short term) and harm reduction embraces the concept of intermediate goals such as not sharing injecting equipment, reducing the frequency of injecting, reducing the amount of drug injecting, switching from injecting drugs to taking them orally (or in other ways less harmful than injecting, such as smoking, inhaling, etc.).

Personal harm, in the context of harm reduction, relates to:

- blood-borne diseases such as hepatitis B and C, human immunodeficiency virus (HIV)
- problems surrounding injecting – abscesses, deep vein thrombosis, gangrene, ulcers, septicaemia, wound botulism, tetanus
- overdose
- poor health status (for example, poor oral health and tuberculosis).

SHARED CARE AND COMMUNICATION

The UK government recommends that drug treatment focuses on service user journeys and 'flow' through drug treatment systems. This requires partnership between health and criminal justice, as well as with housing, education and employment. Where health care includes prescribed treatment, specialist support for GPs and community pharmacists is a vital part of any team approach. However, for any service to operate effectively and safely, all members must communicate regularly about agreed issues. Pharmacists providing services for drug misusers should make themselves known to their local shared care monitoring group, drug action team or local action team for advice and local protocols. More advice on practical, legal and ethical issues can be found in *Drug Misuse and Community Pharmacy*, edited by Janie Sheridan and John Strang (2003), and the *RCGP Guide to the Management of Substance Misuse in Primary Care*, edited by Clare Gerada (2005).

CONFIDENTIALITY AND PRIVACY

The Royal Pharmaceutical Society of Great Britain (RPSGB) code of ethics spells out requirements for pharmacists with regard to confidentiality. However, problem drug users often have concerns about confidentiality and are anxious about others knowing about their drug misuse, often because drug users are held in low esteem, and they may have additional worries such as children being taken into care. It is important to be clear with clients for whom you have a professional responsibility to communicate relevant information. This can be organised as part of a shared care agreement involving the pharmacist, the client and the drug clinic/prescriber. Confidentiality issues may be a problem for pharmacists when a client uses two or more services, e.g. methadone dispensing and using the needle exchange. Information should not be shared between the two services without the knowledge and agreement of the client unless there is a duty of care issue.

Pharmacists should also be cognisant of privacy issues when providing a needle exchange service or dispensing methadone and buprenorphine, especially if doses need to be consumed under the supervision of the pharmacist.

DISPENSING CONTROLLED DRUGS

Methadone is a Schedule 2 controlled drug (Misuse of Drugs Regulations 2001) and buprenorphine is a Schedule 3 controlled drug. Prescription writing requirements, record keeping and safe storage requirements all apply (see Royal Pharmaceutical Society of Great Britain 2006 and the latest version of the *British National Formulary* for details). From April 2005, pharmacist and nurse supplementary prescribers have been able to prescribe controlled drugs.

Both NHS and private prescriptions for controlled drugs are only valid for 28 days. In the case of instalment (FP10(MDA)) forms, the prescription is valid from the date of signing for 28 days or from the start date specified by the prescriber on the form (even if this is more than 28 days after the date of signing). All private prescriptions for controlled drugs are now required to be prescribed on special (pink) forms (FP10(PCD)), which the pharmacist must then forward to the Prescription Pricing Division.

While in theory the details of instalment prescriptions may not be varied, the Home Office recently confirmed that a specific form of words can be used by prescribers of controlled drugs that allows pharmacists to use their professional judgement to dispense the remainder of an instalment when a patient has missed collecting the first part. In addition, the Department of Health intends to issue guidance to support the implementation of further amendments to the Misuse of Drugs Regulations. This will include guidance on technical errors (which will allow pharmacists, in very specific circumstances, to dispense an incorrectly written controlled drug prescription without requiring the prescriber to amend the prescription prior to dispensing) and the recording of the identity of those collecting controlled drugs on behalf of patients (both public and professional).

In England, the new pharmacy contract, introduced in 2005, includes supervised administration of oral prescribed drugs (as well as pharmacy needle exchange and supplementary prescribing) as an enhanced service. Service specifications for enhanced services have been agreed with the Department of Health. Comprehensive information of the best practice guidance for commissioners and providers of pharmaceutical services for drug users can be accessed from the National Treatment Agency website, www.nta.nhs.uk (National Treatment Agency for Substance Misuse et al 2006).

METHADONE

KINETICS AND METABOLISM

Methadone is soluble in lipids and is mainly metabolised in the liver. The mean half-life of first dose is 15 hours and after repeated doses is 25 hours (Dollery 1991); however, in practice it may be much longer than this. Methadone induces its own metabolism, further confounding the issue. Furthermore there is huge interindividual variation in the clinical pharmacokinetics of methadone. An excellent reference on the implications of this for the treatment of opiate dependence can be found in a paper by Eap et al (2002). In practice, it is important that pharmacists recognise that it may take several days to achieve steady state and so they must be alert to symptoms of overdose. In addition it may take 2–3 weeks or longer before a client is stabilised on the most appropriate dose and so the client may be at risk from 'topping up' with illicit drugs in an attempt to prevent withdrawal.

DOSAGE FORMS

In the UK the majority of methadone prescriptions are for methadone mixture 1 mg in 1 ml – which should not to be confused with the 2 mg in 5 ml linctus. In the UK, although methadone mixture is available as a sugar-free preparation, this cannot be dispensed unless specifically requested by the prescriber. The sugar-free formulation has not been proved to offer any advantage over the standard and can cause gastrointestinal upset. Less frequently, 10 mg/ml ampoules (available as 1 ml, 2 ml, 3.5 ml, 5 ml) are prescribed, but clinical guidelines now recommend that these are only prescribed by specialists (e.g. specialist clinics or GPs with special interest). Stronger oral mixtures such as 10 mg in 1 ml or 20 mg in 1 ml may be used when high doses (e.g. 200 mg) are required, but require dilution if doses are not supervised and are generally restricted to use within clinics for clients on high doses where the volume of solution to be consumed can be a problem.

Although 5 mg tablets are available, doctors are advised not to prescribe them to opiate-dependent clients except in exceptional circumstances, as some drug misusers may crush and inject them, resulting in damage at the site of injecting, possibly leading to abscesses and gangrene.

TOLERANCE AND OVERDOSE

Tolerance develops within 2 weeks after repeated doses of methadone, so the same dose has less effect. Tolerance may be lost as quickly as it develops, so that taking the same dose after several days without any opioids may result in overdose. Therefore, when clients miss several consecutive days of methadone they should be referred for reassessment before being given their next dose. Death by overdose is mainly caused by respiratory depression. Naloxone (a short-acting opioid antagonist) is used to reverse opiate overdose. Repeated doses of naloxone may be required, as its effect wears off more quickly than the effects of the methadone and the client slips back into overdose. This is especially relevant when higher doses of methadone have been taken.

Signs of overdose include:

nausea and vomiting, pin-point pupils, drowsiness, cold, clammy bluish skin, reduced heart rate, breathlessness, cyanosis, pulmonary oedema.

WITHDRAWAL

This syndrome is a result of a lack of opioid combined with raised anxiety levels, due to the release of large amounts of noradrenaline (norepinephrine) (noradrenaline 'storm').

Symptoms of withdrawal include:

weakness, yawning, sneezing, sweating, goose bumps, tremors, insomnia, muscle spasms, diarrhoea.

Clients who gain a lot of weight may also find their dose does not 'hold them', as methadone is held in lipid stores, leading to symptoms of withdrawal.

DRUG INTERACTIONS

Any drugs that affect the cytochrome p450 pathway will interact with methadone, e.g. rifampicin, which increases the metabolism of methadone so that higher doses of methadone are needed. Drugs that cause central nervous system depression will cause increased sedation (e.g. alcohol, hypnotics, tricyclics and anxiolytics) and possibly increased respiratory depression. A number of drugs used in the management of HIV/AIDS interact with methadone. An excellent table of drug interactions can be found in the Department of Health's guidelines on the management of drug misuse (Department of Health 1999).

SUPERVISED CONSUMPTION OF METHADONE IN THE COMMUNITY PHARMACY

Pharmacists may be asked by the prescriber to supervise the consumption of methadone for an individual client, or there may be a scheme set up locally in conjunction with a clinic. Sometimes the request may be made by the client, to help with compliance, or possibly because they are being threatened by other drug misusers to hand over their medication. Guidelines may be obtained from the RPSGB and the National Treatment Agency's 'best practice' guidance on pharmaceutical services for drug users. Additional information may be obtained from the local Pharmaceutical Adviser, local Drug Action Team, Drug Treatment Group, Local Action Team and the RPSGB library. The Centre for Pharmacy Postgraduate Education (for England) and NHS Education Scotland: Pharmacy (for Scotland) have distance learning packs for pharmacists that cover this topic in detail, with Wales and Northern Ireland tending to use the latter.

Supervision may be requested for a number of reasons:

- **as an aid to adherence**
- **to reduce risk of overdose at start of treatment**
- **to give clients some stability**
- **to reduce outside pressures on client to sell dose**
- **to prevent diversion on to the illicit market**
- **to reduce risks of accidental overdose (particularly a problem in small children)**

Normally local protocols exist for this procedure, agreed with local drug services (including pharmacist–client agreement forms) and cover issues such as:

- dispensing to intoxicated clients
- dispensing to clients who have missed doses
- communication
- client behaviour.

To ensure methadone has been swallowed:

- **talk to clients – it's difficult to talk with a mouthful of methadone**
- **offer them a drink of water – this also helps to reduce tooth decay and offers another opportunity for some health education**

Things to remember:

- All pharmacies must have standard operating procedures (SOPs) in place to cover both the dispensing procedure and the supervised consumption procedure
- Ensure all locums understand the procedure and are willing to supervise
- Ensure that clients can be identified by locums
- Check that professional liability insurance covers such services
- All doses must be individually dispensed, i.e. the supervision procedure must be separate from the dispensing procedure. This also ensures that each dispensing is recorded on the client medication record in accordance with 'best practice'
- Pre-prepared doses must be stored in the Controlled Drugs cupboard
- Clients should be allowed to check the name, contents, label on the bottle
- After supervising consumption, retain the bottle and remove labels from used containers before disposal, to maintain client confidentiality
- Take-home doses must be supplied in a child-resistant container and clients must be frequently reminded about the risk of overdose if a dose is accidentally taken by another person – children being specifically at risk. As little as 5 ml of methadone mixture 1 mg in 1 ml can kill a child.

 Advice to new clients:

- If not being supervised, don't take the first dose of prescribed methadone while alone – have someone with you for the first 2–4 hours
- Don't mix methadone with other drugs or alcohol
- Beware of using other opioids (e.g. street heroin) as well as methadone
- All take-home doses should be stored in a cool place out of the reach of children, preferably locked up.

Discuss with prescribers/key-workers what information they would like to be fed back to them, e.g. missed doses, signs of chaotic behaviour, etc. Rules for managing intoxicated clients and clients who miss doses should be agreed with the prescribing doctor and there may be local guidelines on this (e.g. three doses missed – refer client back to prescriber for reassessment because risk of reduced tolerance could result in overdose). This information should also be conveyed to the client. Clients should be made aware that pharmacists liaise with the prescriber – this usually forms part of a shared care agreement.

BUPRENORPHINE

Buprenorphine is a partial opiate agonist and is licensed as Subutex in the UK for the management of opioid dependence as $400\,\mu g$, 2 mg and 8 mg tablets. Temgesic, which is another brand of buprenorphine, is *not* licensed for the treatment of addiction/dependence. The two products are not interchangeable; therefore it is good practice for Subutex to be prescribed by its brand name. For example, the client information leaflets are not relevant to each other. Instalment prescriptions for Subutex for the management of opiate dependence are allowed in all four UK countries. However, at the time of writing, buprenorphine prescribing is less widespread in Scotland than elsewhere in the UK. This is because of high levels of misuse of Temgesic and a high number of forged prescriptions, especially in the Glasgow area during the late 1970s and early 1980s. This history of misuse has been a major deterrent to the acceptance of Subutex in Scotland.

Buprenorphine has a long half-life and in stable opiate-dependent clients it is possible to dose on alternate days. Because buprenorphine binds very tightly to receptors, but has low intrinsic opiate agonist activity, those starting on buprenorphine who have high plasma levels of opiates (e.g. illicit heroin or methadone) will experience withdrawal-type symptoms. This is because the buprenorphine will displace the other opiate from the receptors. Therefore when transferring someone from methadone to buprenorphine, the daily methadone dose should be reduced to 30 mg or less before stopping the methadone. Buprenorphine can then be started the next day with at least 24–36 hours elapsing since the last dose of methadone has been taken. Those transferring from heroin/short-acting opioids should abstain for at least 6–8 hours prior to the first dose of buprenorphine. Ideally clients should be experiencing withdrawal symptoms before taking their first dose of buprenorphine. Excellent guidance on buprenorphine prescribing can be found in Lintzeris et al (2001) and Royal College of General Practitioners (2005).

TOLERANCE, OVERDOSE AND WITHDRAWAL

Sudden cessation of buprenorphine does not cause adverse effects because of its slow receptor dissociation. One missed dose on daily dispensing should not precipitate substantial withdrawal. Patients who have missed more than three consecutive days should be referred back to the prescribing doctor (Royal College of General Practitioners 2005). Buprenorphine is considered to be much safer in overdose than methadone, with a low risk of respiratory depression (because of its partial agonist activity). However, buprenorphine-related deaths have been reported in combination with other sedative drugs such as alcohol or benzodiazepines. High doses of naloxone (10–30 times) are needed to reverse the effects of buprenorphine and its long duration of action will also need to be taken into account.

DRUG INTERACTIONS WITH BUPRENORPHINE

Buprenorphine is metabolised via the cytochrome p450 3A4 pathway and so blood levels can be increased if it is administered at the same time as drugs such as ketoconazole, protease inhibitors or nifedipine. Precautions should be applied when prescribing buprenorphine with other central nervous system depressants.

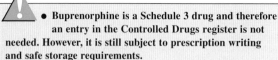

- Buprenorphine is a Schedule 3 drug and therefore an entry in the Controlled Drugs register is not needed. However, it is still subject to prescription writing and safe storage requirements.
- Instalment prescriptions should be written on blue FP10(MDA) forms. A machine-written prescription is acceptable. The prescriber's signature must be hand-written
- All doses dispensed must be documented and the RPSGB insists that each instalment must be fully labelled to ensure that a record is kept in the client medication records
- Buprenorphine is given sublingually and has the potential for diversion on to the illicit market and for injecting
- Most clients are initially dosed under supervision. This poses issues for pharmacists with regard to ensuring the dose is taken and has adequately dispersed before the client leaves the pharmacy. Other issues around supervised consumption can be found in the section above on methadone dispensing
- Pharmacists considering crushing of buprenorphine tablets need to be satisfied that this is in the patient's best interests, as there is the potential for the product's bioavailability profile to be distorted. Pharmacists who crush buprenorphine tablets may assume some liability for the supply of the product outside licensed indications. The Royal Pharmaceutical Society and the National Pharmacy Association have published advice (2005) that should be followed if a prescription requests crushing of tablets
- Local protocols should be adhered to with regard to crushing of tablets. Advice from the NPA and RPSGB should be followed in order to be covered for professional indemnity insurance purposes

Advice to new clients

Pharmacists can really help clients by explaining that, although the first 3 days' treatment may be difficult, as the dose has to be started low and rapidly increased, this quickly settles and the client will feel much better. In addition, explain to clients that taking other opioids at the same time can worsen feelings of withdrawal, as the different drugs may compete for the receptors, especially if a dose of buprenorphine has been missed. Patients should be warned that the tablets have a bitter taste.

LOFEXIDINE

Lofexidine is an alpha-2 agonist similar to clonidine. It is used in the management of opiate withdrawal as it suppresses noradrenergic neuronal hyperactivity. Although it attenuates some withdrawal symptoms, clients may need symptomatic relief from other symptoms such as diarrhoea, stomach cramps, anxiety, insomnia and pain. Side effects of lofexidine include drowsiness and dry mouth and, as it is related to clonidine, it can cause hypotension. Clients will have their blood pressure monitored while on lofexidine, although for most clients the hypotensive effect is not clinically significant. Pharmacists can provide invaluable support and encouragement to clients undergoing a detoxification.

Advice to lofexidine clients
- Lofexidine may make them drowsy
- If they feel dizzy they should consult the doctor or nurse
- Do not stand up too quickly after lying down
- Do not drive or operate machinery if feeling dizzy or drowsy

HOSPITAL PHARMACY

A number of scenarios may occur with respect to substance misusers in a hospital context. These will be dealt with briefly. Hospitals or local NHS trusts may have their own guidelines.

Particular issues relate to the management of pain in opiate-dependent clients. This is a real and mostly misunderstood issue. Clients on opiates are wrongly assumed to need less, rather than more, pain control. Buprenorphine clients will need careful handling because of the drug's antagonist properties.

Pharmacists and pharmacy technicians working in mental health trusts often work closely with drug and alcohol services, helping write policies and procedures, monitoring prescribing, providing specialist medicines information services, running patient groups, and managing in-house dispensing and supervised consumption services.

Substance misusers admitted to hospital who need prescribed Controlled Drugs for the treatment of opiate dependence

Mindful of confidentiality, the following issues should be carefully thought through:

- Before starting treatment with methadone or Subutex, a urine drug screen should be organised and a proper assessment (usually by either a specialist worker or senior registrar), otherwise there is a risk of inappropriate treatment
- Where the client states they are in receipt of a prescription for methadone (or another opioid), contact the client's prescriber to confirm this
- The community pharmacist who dispensed the methadone/ Subutex should be contacted to inform them of the situation and confirm when the last dose was dispensed or consumed
- There may be a need to prescribe drugs such as methadone to prevent the client going into withdrawal, but it is important treatment is not started until a proper assessment has been made
- Where a client is in withdrawal and there is no evidence of a pre-existing prescription, the dose should be carefully titrated in accordance with local guidelines
- If high doses are already being prescribed or demanded by clients, the dose given should be titrated up in divided doses and the client monitored for signs of overdose/withdrawal
- Always ensure that naloxone 'when required' is prescribed on the ward in case of accidental overdose
- Arrangements for discharge must be clear as there is no point starting treatment if there is no prescriber available to continue the prescription once discharged (see notes below)
- Clients on substitute opiates will need additional analgesia for pain relief – in the case of buprenorphine this may be a problem due to its partial agonist action
- Be alert to the possibility of drugs being smuggled on to wards and have procedures in place on how to manage such situations
- Be alert to the possibility of confusing strengths of methadone mixture. Always ensure that doses are expressed in milligrams not millilitres, as a ten-times error can occur as some wards in acute hospitals may have the 10 mg in 1 ml strength as stock on the ward

Clients with existing community pharmacy dispensed opiates

- Is consumption of the Controlled Drug supervised?
- How much is the client actually taking?
- Did they actually consume this last dose?
- What other drugs could they be taking?
- Is someone else collecting the client's instalment from the community pharmacy while they are in hospital?

Discharge of such clients who are currently receiving prescriptions in the community for the treatment of their drug misuse

Inform the client's prescriber and the community pharmacist as to:

- the discharge date
- whether the client received methadone/Subutex on the day of discharge
- details of any take-home doses given
- any other drugs being prescribed on discharge

Arrange for community prescription to be resumed or arrange for new prescription to be written. New clients referred for treatment are unlikely be able to get a prescription immediately until a full assessment has been made. Check procedures with local drug services/GPs.

Do not give several days' supply to a client to take home, because of the risk of overdose.

REFERENCES

Department of Health 1999 Drug misuse and dependence: guidelines on clinical management. Stationery Office, London

Dollery C 1991 Therapeutic drugs. Churchill Livingstone, Edinburgh

Eap CB, Buclin T, Baumann P 2002 Interindividual variability of the clinical pharmacokinetics of methadone. Clinical Pharmacokinetics 41: 1153–1193

Gerada C (ed.) 2005 RCGP guide to the management of substance misuse in primary care. Royal College of General Practitioners, London

Law and Ethics Bulletin 2005 Instalment dispensing of controlled drugs. Pharmaceutical Journal 275: 122

Lintzeris N, Clark N, Muhleisen P 2001 Clinical guidelines: buprenorphine treatment of heroin dependence. Turning Point Alcohol and Drug Centre, Victoria, Australia. Available online at: http://www.health.gov.au/pubhlth/nds/resources/publications/buprenorphine_guide.pdf

National Treatment Agency for Substance Misuse, Royal Pharmaceutical Society of Great Britain, Pharmaceutical Services Negotiating Committee 2006 Best practice guidance for commissioners and providers of pharmaceutical services for drug users. National Treatment Agency, London. Available online at www.nta.nhs.uk/publications/Prescribing/Pharmaceutical_services_for_drug_users.pdf

Royal College of General Practitioners 2005 Guidance for the use of buprenorphine for the treatment of opioid dependence in primary care, 2nd edn. RCGP, London.

Royal Pharmaceutical Society of Great Britain 2005 Society issues guidance on crushing buprenorphine sublingual tablets. Pharmaceutical Journal 274: 401. Available online at: http://www.pjonline.com/editorial/20050402/society/p401crushing.html

Royal Pharmaceutical Society of Great Britain 2006 Medicines, ethics and practice 30. Pharmaceutical Press, London

Sheridan J, Strang J (eds) (2003) Drug misuse and community pharmacy. Taylor & Francis, London.

USEFUL RESOURCES

Centre for Pharmacy Postgraduate Education 2006 Substance misuse, open learning pack. CPPE, University of Manchester, Manchester

Centre for Pharmacy Postgraduate Education 2002 Opiate treatment: supporting pharmacists for improved patient care. CPPE, University of Manchester, Manchester

Department of Health 2006 Safer management of controlled drugs (CDs) 2. Private CD prescriptions and other changes to the prescribing and dispensing of controlled drugs (CDs). Gateway reference 6212 March 2006) (Interim guidance – to be updated summer 2006)

Detox Handbook – available online from: http://www.exchangesupplies.org

Drugscope 0207 928 1211 http://www.drugscope.org.uk/

Gray R, Whelton J 2003 The oral health status of methadone clients in Dublin. Poster presentation. IADR 81st General Session, Gotenborg, Sweden. Journal of Dental Research (Special Issue B): 0973

Home Office (UK) 0207 273 3000

Lingford-Hughes A, Welch S, Nutt DJ; British Association for Psychopharmacology 2004. Evidence-based guidelines for the pharmacological management of substance misuse, addiction and comorbidity: recommendations from the British Association for Psychopharmacology. Journal of Psychopharmacology 18: 293–335

Methadone Handbook – available online from: http://www.exchangesupplies.org

Preston A 1996 The methadone briefing. ISDD, London. Available online at: http://www.drugtext.org/library/books/methadone/default.htm

Royal Pharmaceutical Society of Great Britain Professional Standards
    Directorate – 0207 735 9141
Royal Pharmaceutical Society of Great Britain 2006 Changes in the
    management fo CDs. Pharmaceutical Journal 277: 25
Scottish Centre for Pharmacy Postgraduate Education 2001 Pharmaceutical
    aspects of methadone prescribing. SCPPE, University of Strathclyde,
    Glasgow
Substance Misuse Management in General Practice (SMMGP) http://www.
    smmgp.demon.co.uk/
Ward J, Mattick R, Hall W 1998 Methadone maintenance treatment and other
    opioid replacement therapies. Harwood Academic, Sydney
Wills S 2005 Drugs of abuse. Pharmaceutical Press, London

CHAPTER 17

Monitoring patients with renal disease

J. G. Davies, C. Ashley, J. Harchowal

This chapter is intended to introduce clinical pharmacists to the problems associated with the use of medicines in patients with various degrees of renal impairment. While some of the material is directed at specialist renal practice, the chapter aims to support the work of individuals caring for general medical and surgical patients, with a focus on ensuring that drug use in this population is safe with respect to the degree of renal impairment present.

This chapter should help practitioners to:

- identify patients who, as a result of impaired renal function, are at risk of experiencing an adverse drug event
- review drug use in this population to resolve or prevent an adverse drug event
- orientate their practice when caring for patients with acute or chronic renal failure.

While this chapter provides a broad overview of renal impairment and a basic introduction to drug use, more detailed information can be obtained from the bibliography. The authors draw attention to the resources produced by the Renal Pharmacy Group, in particular to information contained within *The Renal Drug Handbook* (Ashley & Currie 2004) and the website of the organisation at www.renalpharmacy.org.

CHRONIC RENAL FAILURE

Chronic renal failure (CRF) is defined as either kidney damage or a glomerular filtration rate (GFR) of less than 60 ml/min for 3 months or longer. This is invariably a progressive process that results in end-stage renal failure.

END-STAGE RENAL DISEASE

End-stage renal disease (ESRD) is the irreversible deterioration of renal function to a degree that is incompatible with life (in the absence of renal replacement therapy, either by dialysis or transplantation), and is the end result of progressive chronic renal failure. In practice, a patient is usually accepted as having ESRD when their creatinine clearance is less than 10 ml/min; in many patients this corresponds to a serum creatinine of 500–700 μmol/l.

ACUTE RENAL FAILURE

Acute renal failure (ARF) is diagnosed when renal excretory function declines over hours or days. It is usually recognised when serum levels of urea and creatinine rise rapidly. There can be many causes: medical, surgical, traumatic, obstructive and obstetric. Some degree of acute impairment of renal function occurs in about 5% of hospital admissions. Two types of ARF should be distinguished: isolated failure of the kidneys, where the other organ systems function normally, and multiple organ failure. Mortality is low in those with renal failure alone (<5%), whereas it is high (>40%) in those with multiple organ failure. Most patients who develop ARF will have the condition known as *acute tubular necrosis*, so renal function usually recovers if the patient survives the causative insult. However, especially in older patients, pre-existing impairment of renal function plus multiple co-morbidities may mean that the patient achieves only partial, or even minimal, recovery of kidney function.

COMMON CAUSES OF CHRONIC RENAL FAILURE

Chronic renal failure is often a result of other disease states, some of which are listed below:

- diabetes
- hypertension
- autoimmune diseases, e.g.
  - glomerulonephritis
  - focal segmental glomerular sclerosis (FSGS)
  - multisystem vasculitis, e.g. Wegener's granulomatosuis, systemic lupus erythematosus
  - haemolytic–uraemic syndrome
  - IgA and IgM glomerulonephritis.

Other conditions can cause chronic renal damage and occasionally the patient will present with a sudden reduction in renal function, leading to a picture of ARF. This is usually reversible, but sometimes can lead to chronic renal damage and ultimately end-stage renal disease. Some examples are listed below:

- hereditary (adult polycystic kidney disease)
- ureteric obstruction/kidney stones
- chronic pyelonephritis
- drug-induced (chronic use of, e.g. analgesics, lithium)
- malignancy, e.g. multiple myeloma

COMMON CAUSES OF ACUTE RENAL FAILURE

ARF can be classified into prerenal, direct and postrenal causes depending on the precipitating factor involved, some examples of which are given below.

- *Prerenal causes* (these are the causes of ARF most commonly experienced by hospital inpatients): reduced kidney perfusion as a result of shock, major haemorrhage, volume depletion, sepsis, hypotension. Particular at-risk patients include the elderly and patients on antihypertensive medication, diuretics, non-steroidal anti-inflammatory drugs (NSAIDs), angiotensin-converting enzyme (ACE) inhibitors
- *Direct renal causes*: tubular damage caused by nephrotoxic agents (e.g. aminoglycosides, NSAIDs, cisplatin), or autoimmune diseases (see above)
- *Postrenal causes*: commonly an obstruction. This may occur in the collecting ducts of the kidneys, in the ureters or somewhere

else in the remainder of the urinary system. The obstruction can be due to crystalluria (some drugs can cause this – methotrexate, nitrofurantoin, sulphonamides), urate stone formation (following cytotoxic therapy) or direct ureteric obstruction due to conditions such as retroperitoneal fibrosis, pelvic or bladder tumours.

IDENTIFYING PATIENTS WITH RENAL IMPAIRMENT

Patients requiring close monitoring by a pharmacist can be classified into two groups:

- those patients at risk of developing renal impairment
- those patients with pre-existing renal failure.

RISK FACTORS FOR DEVELOPING RENAL IMPAIRMENT

- *Extremes of age*. An individual's renal function declines with age, and people in their 70s and 80s may have a glomerular filtration rate (GFR) of only 40–50 ml/min or even lower, despite their serum creatinine being in the normal range. Serum creatinine may only begin to rise above the upper limit of normal when more than 60–70% of nephrons are no longer functioning. In addition, elderly patients have a lower muscle mass than younger individuals so that a serum creatinine value within the normal range may accompany a degree of renal impairment.
- *Diabetes*. Both insulin-dependent and non-insulin-dependent diabetes mellitus predispose a patient to renal impairment. The rate of decline of renal function appears to be directly correlated with poor diabetic control.
- *Hypertension*. Although poor control of hypertension is a major cause of renal impairment, the damage occurs over a relatively long period of time. However, in the case of malignant hypertension, kidney damage can occur in a very short period of time.
- *Family history of renal disease*. This may include conditions such as diabetes, hypertension and hypercholesterolaemia, or inherited conditions such as adult polycystic kidney disease
- *Pre-existing renal disease*. Patients with pre-existing renal impairment are more susceptible to the effects of both prerenal failure and nephrotoxic agents, e.g. NSAIDs or a cytotoxic agent such as cisplatin. These patients are therefore more likely to experience a decline in their renal function if administered one of these agents.

- *Renal transplant.* A renal transplant recipient will only have one functioning kidney, so it is vital to avoid all nephrotoxic insults to that kidney. In addition, if the transplant is ageing, or not functioning well, then the patient will have a reasonable degree of renal insufficiency, so that all drug doses must be adjusted accordingly to avoid further kidney damage.

IDENTIFYING PATIENTS WITH PRE-EXISTING RENAL PROBLEMS

Patients with established chronic renal failure can often be identified by the drug treatment they have been prescribed. These commonly include:

- Antihypertensive therapy – patients are commonly receiving a number of different classes of drugs, e.g. ACE inhibitors, angiotensin receptor blockers, calcium antagonists, alpha-blockers or beta-blockers
- Phosphate binders, e.g. Calcichew, Titralac, Phosex, Renagel, Alu-Cap
- Vitamin D analogues, e.g. calcitriol and alfacalcidol
- High-dose loop diuretics
- Erythropoietin and iron supplements.

Box 17.1 represents the type of general patient who often develops ARF as a result of the medication prescribed.

MONITORING RENAL FUNCTION

A number of approaches can be used to monitor a patient's renal function.

COCKCROFT AND GAULT EQUATION

The Cockcroft and Gault equation is used to estimate renal function from a knowledge of the patient's serum creatinine concentration, age and body weight:

$$GFR = \frac{F \times (140 - Age\,[yrs]) \times Ideal\,body\,weight\,[kg]}{Serum\,creatinine\,[\mu mol/l]},$$

where $F = 1.23$ for males, and 1.04 for females. Ideal body weight = 50 kg + 2.3 kg for every 1 inch (2.5 cm) over 5 foot (1.50 m) in height (males); 45.5 kg + 2.3 kg for every 1 inch (2.5 cm) over 5 foot (1.50 m) in height (females).

Box 17.1 Example of a 'problem' patient

Mrs GD is a 78-year-old woman admitted for left total hip replacement. She weighs 52 kg and her serum creatinine on admission was found to be 74 μmol/l. Following surgery, she was slightly dehydrated but was only prescribed 1 litre of intravenous sodium chloride infusion (0.9%) over the next 24 hours. In addition she was prescribed diclofenac M/R 75 mg twice daily and started on intravenous gentamicin (at a dose of 120 mg twice daily) and ceftriaxone (at a dose of 1 g daily). Three days later her serum creatinine is 152 μmol/l.

The patient's problems are:

- She was volume-depleted and was not given sufficient replacement fluids, leading to reduced kidney perfusion, which contributed to her renal impairment
- She was prescribed diclofenac, which adversely affects the renal microcirculation, further reducing renal perfusion
- She was prescribed gentamicin, a known nephrotoxic agent. Given that she already had other risk factors predisposing to renal damage, the nephrotoxic effects of the gentamicin were enhanced.

According to Cockcroft and Gault, her glomerular filtration rate on admission was 45 ml/min, even though her serum creatinine concentration was at the lower end of the normal range. This often leads inexperienced junior medical staff to prescribe potentially nephrotoxic agents in the belief that the patient has 'normal' renal function. By the time her creatinine reaches 152 μmol/l, her GFR has decreased to 22 ml/min, so that she is at serious risk of developing severe renal impairment unless corrective measures are introduced.

This patient should be managed by ensuring that she receives adequate fluid replacement, stopping all nephrotoxic agents and maintaining a strict fluid balance chart. If this advice is followed her renal function should recover.

There are a number of limitations to the use of this equation:

- It is only accurate when renal function is stable, i.e. serum creatinine is not fluctuating by more than 40 μmol/l per day
- It is inaccurate when serum creatinine values are above 450 μmol/l
- It becomes inaccurate when GFR is below 20 ml/min
- It is not valid in pregnancy
- It is not valid in children
- It is not valid in the very old
- It is inaccurate in very wasted patients because they have decreased muscle mass
- It is inaccurate in amputees because of loss of muscle mass.

URINE OUTPUT

An alternative method of determining renal function is the 24-hour urine collection, to estimate the amount of creatinine cleared by the kidneys during that time period. Although often inconvenient to carry out, it does give an accurate measure of renal function. At the end of the collection period, a blood sample is taken to determine serum creatinine.

$$GFR \text{ [ml/min]} = UV/P,$$

where U = urine creatinine concentration (µmol/l), V = volume of urine collected (ml) and P = serum creatinine concentration (µmol/l).

The volume of urine should be converted into ml/min by dividing the total volume of urine collected over 24 hours by 1440 (1440 minutes in 24 hours) before entering the value into the equation. In addition, it is important to ensure that the urine concentration is entered as µmol/l rather than mmol/l, as often reported by the biochemistry laboratory.

CLASSIFICATION OF RENAL FAILURE

Once a GFR is estimated using one of the approaches described above, the degrees of renal impairment can be classified as shown in Table 17.1 (see Appendix 3 of the *British National Formulary*).

BEDSIDE MONITORING

Points to be monitored at the patient's bedside include:

- fluid balance charts (remember insensible losses)
- fluid restriction notices (watch out for the 2 litre water jug sitting by the patient on a 500 ml fluid restriction)
- patient's daily weight – if the patient gains 2 kg in 24 hours, this is equivalent to retaining 2 litres of fluid.

TABLE 17.1 Classification of degrees of renal impairment

Classification	GFR (ml/min per 1.73 m^2)	Serum creatinine (µmol/l)
Mild	20–50	150–300
Moderate	10–20	300–700
Severe	<10	>700

Oliguria = urine output <400 ml/day; anuria = urine output <50 ml/day.

DRY WEIGHT

Patients with ESRD have what is termed a 'dry' weight. Unlike ideal body weight, it is not calculated from an equation but is derived from clinical observation. The dry weight is what the patient should weigh when they have no excess fluid and they are normotensive. Each time a patient attends for dialysis, the difference between their actual weight and their dry weight determines the amount of fluid to be removed by dialysis during the visit.

BIOCHEMICAL AND HAEMATOLOGICAL PROFILE

The typical biochemistry and haematology profile of a patient with renal impairment might include:

- raised serum creatinine and urea concentrations
- raised serum potassium concentration, which should be carefully monitored for an increasing trend – some chronic renal patients often have a serum potassium at the higher end of normal with no adverse effects
- reduced serum calcium concentration
- raised serum phosphate concentration in patients with chronic renal impairment – may be lower than normal in patients in acute renal failure who are undergoing continuous renal replacement therapy (see later)
- decreased haemoglobin concentration in patients with chronic renal impairment
- reduced serum bicarbonate concentration as a result of metabolic acidosis. This occurs in both acute and chronic situations.

PHARMACEUTICAL MANAGEMENT OF PATIENTS WITH ACUTE AND CHRONIC RENAL FAILURE AND END-STAGE RENAL DISEASE

When faced with a patient who has renal impairment the following key questions should be asked:

WHAT RISK FACTORS DOES THE PATIENT EXHIBIT?

- What is the underlying cause of renal failure?
- How long has the patient had renal impairment? It is vital to gauge whether the condition is acute or chronic

- Does the patient have any risk factors for renal disease? (age, postsurgical, dehydrated)
- Check vital urea and electrolytes, particularly creatinine, urea, potassium, calcium, phosphate and haemoglobin levels
- What is the patient's blood pressure, fluid balance?
- If the condition is chronic but stable, then estimate the renal function (see above regarding measuring renal function)

WHAT DRUGS HAS THE PATIENT BEEN PRESCRIBED?

- What drugs has the patient been on long-term?
- What drugs have been started?
- Is the patient on any problem drugs? (ACE inhibitors, antihypertensives, NSAIDs, diuretics)

Drugs which can potentially cause problems can be divided into:

- those that are renally excreted, so they will accumulate in renal impairment, leading to end-organ toxicity, which is not necessarily renal toxicity – examples include opiates (increased central nervous system and respiratory depression), meropenem (seizures) and allopurinol (severe skin rash)
- those that are known to be nephrotoxic, which could potentially exacerbate the underlying renal impairment, e.g. NSAIDs, aminoglycosides, high-dose loop diuretics. This is more important in ARF, where renal function is potentially recoverable.

Boxes 17.2–17.4 provide the clinical pharmacist with a quick guide to the management of patients with acute and chronic renal failure and ESRD.

PRESCRIBING FOR PATIENTS WITH RENAL FAILURE

The pharmacokinetic properties of some drugs will change as a result of the renal impairment experienced. These changes can reflect the biochemical changes that occur in this group of patients and may additionally have pharmacodynamic consequences.

DRUG ABSORPTION

The gastrointestinal absorption of certain drugs may be impaired as a result of the uraemia and fluid retention resulting from kidney failure.

Box 17.2 Top tips for pharmaceutical management of patients in chronic renal failure

- If the patient has chronic but stable renal impairment, estimate the GFR using the Cockcroft and Gault equation (unless an accurate 24-hour urine collection is made)
- Maintain adequate fluid balance postsurgery. It is necessary to maintain kidney perfusion but, at the same time, avoid the patient becoming fluid-overloaded. Check if the patient was fluid restricted prior to admission
- Doses of antibiotics may need to be reviewed and reduced (see Ashley & Currie 2004)
- Postoperative patients: monitor postoperative pain control – avoid NSAIDs as they may precipitate acute-on-chronic renal failure. Watch out for large doses of opiates and the use of patient-controlled analgesia – reduce the dose and increase the lock-out time
- Monitor use of drugs that may decrease blood pressure, thereby decreasing kidney perfusion
- Always check the toxic effects of drugs prescribed – if in doubt – check *The Renal Drug Handbook* (Ashley & Currie 2004)
- Ensure that the patient is not given drugs that could precipitate end-stage renal failure, e.g. NSAIDs, aminoglycosides
- If the patient is on a phosphate binder, you may have to separate the timing of administration of certain antibiotics (e.g. ciprofloxacin) to avoid chelation
- Should the patient develop hyperkalaemia, calcium resonium and lactulose can effectively manage the condition for 2–3 days

---

This may cause:

- an increase in gastric ammonia, with a resulting increase in pH, so reducing the absorption of some drugs, e.g. iron and digoxin
- an oedematous gut, which may result in a decrease in local blood flow, so reducing the rate of drug absorption, e.g. chlorpropamide and frusemide.

In addition, the regular use of phosphate binders and calcium resonium may impede the absorption of some drugs and alter the absorption profile of sustained-release or enteric-coated products.

DRUG DISTRIBUTION

The protein binding of some drugs may decrease as a result of renal failure, which may increase the fraction of free drug available to exert

---

Box 17.3 Top tips for pharmaceutical management of patients in acute renal failure

- Ask yourself:
  - What is the most likely cause of the ARF?
  - How long has the patient been in ARF?
  - What is the patient's clinical condition?
  - Is the patient on any form of renal replacement therapy, e.g. dialysis or filtration? Note that if a patient is being filtered, their serum creatinine may be misleadingly low. Remember that, even if their serum creatinine is in the 150–200 mmol/l range, the patient's only renal function is the filter, so they will still only have an effective GFR of approximately 20 ml/min
- Adjust doses of all drugs according to the patient's level of renal function or mode of renal replacement therapy. Note that, in some cases, it may be necessary to prescribe larger doses of some drugs than is recommended in the standard texts for that patient's degree of renal function. An example would be a patient with life-threatening sepsis requiring large doses of antibiotics
- Avoid the use of nephrotoxic agents wherever possible
- Aim to keep the kidneys well perfused to aid recovery of renal function
- If in doubt, refer to an intensive therapy specialist

---

its effect. This is only clinically important where the drug is highly protein-bound (i.e. >80%). This decrease may be the result of:

- hypoalbuminaemia
- displacement of the drug by other compounds that compete for the binding sites, such as uraemic inhibitors or other drugs or their metabolites
- conformational changes to the albumin molecule so that the drug is unable to bind to the same extent, resulting in decreased binding.

These changes are important when phenytoin is used, as a normal (total) serum concentration may be reported, masking an increase in the free fraction. Where possible the free phenytoin concentration should be measured, or adjustments should be made to the reported total concentration using specific pharmacokinetic equations described in the standard textbooks.

Where digoxin is used, uraemic inhibitors displace it from its binding sites on skeletal muscle, thereby decreasing its apparent volume of distribution and consequently increasing the serum concentration measured.

Box 17.4 **Top tips for pharmaceutical management of patients in end-stage renal failure**

- End-stage renal failure is not reversible
- Determine the cause of the patient's renal failure
- Determine what form of dialysis the patient is on (and how long s/he has been on that form of dialysis). When is the patient's next scheduled dialysis session?
- Check the presenting complaint or the reason for the admission
- Check the patient's drug history and confirm with the patient – look for medication to treat hypertension, bone disease, anaemia, etc. Does the patient have a medication record card? If not, check with the patient's renal unit for an up-to-date medication list
- Remember to ask: Does the patient administer their erythropoietin intravenously (on dialysis) or subcutaneously? Do they receive iron and/or alfacalcidol/calcitriol intravenously on dialysis or do they take oral supplements? Does the patient usually take their antihypertensive medication before dialysis?
- Doses of all renally cleared drugs need to be checked and amended, to reduce the risk of significant accumulation, with increased incidence of side effects. The most useful reference books are those by Ashley & Currie (2004) and Aronoff et al (1999)
- The drugs that most commonly need to be amended are usually those that are normally cleared by the kidneys – e.g. antibiotics, antivirals, antifungals, painkillers – which can cause side effects and toxicity if allowed to accumulate. Note that dose reductions should always be made while taking into consideration the patient's clinical condition. In cases of life-threatening sepsis, doses greater than those recommended in the standard texts may be necessary
- If you are unsure how a drug is cleared, check the Summary of Produce Characteristics or *The Renal Drug Handbook* for information
- As patients will usually be fluid-restricted, check *The Renal Drug Handbook* to confirm minimum infusion volumes for any intravenous drugs
- Ensure that the patient does not receive large volumes of fluid in the postoperative period. Remember, the patient cannot get rid of that fluid until the next dialysis, which may be in 2–3 days time, so there is a risk of the patient becoming fluid-overloaded
- Check that the timing of drug doses around dialysis sessions is appropriate. If the patient is undergoing peritoneal dialysis, timing is not an issue, since peritoneal dialysis is usually a continuous process. However, if a patient is on intermittent haemodialysis and a drug is likely to be removed by dialysis, then the dosage regimen may need to be adjusted. If a drug is normally administered several times a day, e.g. flucloxacillin 500 mg q.d.s., then dose the patient

Box 17.4 **Top tips for pharmaceutical management of patients in end-stage renal failure – cont'd**

four times a day as usual and schedule a dialysis session for between any two doses. However, if a drug is only given once a day, e.g. meropenem 1 g o.d., schedule the dose for the same time each day. The use of supplementary doses after dialysis usually causes confusion and is to be avoided. If a drug is normally excreted via the hepatobiliary route, then elimination from the body is unlikely to be altered by renal failure, so the timing does not need to be altered

● If the patient is taking phosphate binders, remember to separate them from the dose of some antibiotics (e.g. ciprofloxacin) by approximately 2 hours

Other points:

● The use of NSAIDs is not going to cause any further reduction in renal function in patients with end-stage renal failure. It may, however, cause an increased risk of gastric irritation and potential gastrointestinal bleeding
● Hyperkalaemia may occur postoperatively, especially if the patient is not to be dialysed for 2–3 days. Calcium resonium and lactulose are effective until the patient can be dialysed again
● Occasionally, some patients will be on large doses of loop diuretics (e.g. furosemide 0.5–1 g daily) to maximise the urine output
● Try to keep the patient's sodium intake from drugs and intravenous fluids to a minimum – too much sodium will exacerbate the patient's fluid overload and hypertension

DRUG METABOLISM AND EXCRETION

Very little information is available on the impact of renal impairment on drug metabolism. Some research suggests that the metabolism of some drugs may be impaired while others suggest that an increased metabolic rate may affect others. The impact of these changes on those drugs commonly administered to patients with renal impairment is poorly understood, so the response of patients to a recently prescribed agent should always be closely monitored.

As discussed throughout this chapter, the excretion of a range of drugs and their metabolites is significantly reduced as a result of renal dysfunction. Modifications to the dosage regimens of such drugs should be guided by the texts included in the reference list at the end of the chapter.

PHARMACODYNAMIC CHANGES

Patients with renal dysfunction may demonstrate altered drug sensitivity. For example, patients with uraemia may experience gastrointestinal bleeding when administered warfarin or aspirin. Patients may also be more sensitive to the effects of sedative agents, thought to be due to an increase in the permeability of the blood–brain barrier.

When prescribing for patients with renal impairment the following guidelines should be observed:

- Prescribe a drug only if it is absolutely necessary
- Try and avoid the prolonged use of a drug
- Select a drug that has no nephrotoxic or minimal nephrotoxic properties
- Where practical, monitor the serum concentration and modify the dosage regimen on the basis of the results reported
- Monitor the patient closely for signs of toxicity.

RENAL REPLACEMENT THERAPY

When the residual renal function of the patient is insufficient to provide adequate symptom and fluid control (chronic failure) or following an acute insult where the patient's renal function rapidly declines (acute failure), artificial kidney support should be instigated. There are a number of different renal replacement therapies available to support patients with kidney failure. In ARF the processes used are continuous, as the patient requires intensive therapy and monitoring, usually on an intensive care unit. Commonly, either continuous haemofiltration or haemodialysis (also referred to as haemodiafiltration) is used.

In chronic renal failure, patients are normally managed on an outpatient basis using either continuous ambulatory peritoneal dialysis (CAPD) or intermittent haemodialysis. Brief descriptions of the common nomenclature and techniques employed are provided in Table 17.2.

PRINCIPLES OF RENAL REPLACEMENT THERAPY

The renal replacement techniques available for managing both acute and chronic renal failure employ either diffusion (dialysis), convection (ultrafiltration) or a combination of the two to effect the removal of waste products and water from the patient. For example, continuous haemofiltration removes solutes (waste products and drugs) by convective transport or ultrafiltration, i.e. the movement of fluid across a

TABLE 17.2 Nomenclature and techniques used to provide renal replacement

Renal replacement	Accepted nomenclature	Type of renal failure	Brief description of technique
Continuous arteriovenous haemofiltration	CAVH	Acute	Continuous ultrafiltration, removing a volume of between 10 and 20 litres of plasma water a day, most of which is replaced by a sterile isotonic solution. The technique employs an arterial access (usually femoral artery) to maintain the extracorporeal circuit
Continuous venovenous haemofiltration	CVVH	Acute	Similar in all aspects to CAVH except that a venous access is used and an external pump is employed to propel blood around the extracorporeal circuit. Ultrafiltration rates removing up to 50 litres of fluid a day can be achieved by increasing the speed of the blood pump
Continuous arteriovenous haemodialysis (or haemodiafiltration)	CAVHD	Acute	Both continuous ultrafiltration and diffusion are used to effect water and solute removal. CAVHD employs an arterial access to maintain the extracorporeal circuit, to which the technique of continuous dialysis is added. Dialysis fluid is introduced, usually at a rate of 1–2 l/h, into the membrane in a countercurrent direction to the blood flow. Although the ultrafiltration rate achieved by this technique is less than with CAVH, infusion of an isotonic replacement fluid is still required to maintain circulating volume

TABLE 17.2 Nomenclature and techniques used to provide renal replacement – cont'd

Renal replacement	Accepted nomenclature	Type of renal failure	Brief description of technique
Continuous venovenous haemodialysis (or haemodiafiltration)	CVVHD	Acute	Similar in all aspects to CAVHD except that a venous access is used and an external pump is employed to propel blood around the extracorporeal circuit
Continuous ambulatory peritoneal dialysis	CAPD	Chronic	Mainly diffusion to effect solute removal, with some ultrafiltration removing excess fluid. The peritoneal membrane serves as the dialysis membrane and fluid is introduced into the cavity via a catheter inserted into the abdominal wall. Once introduced, the dialysis fluid is allowed to remain for a specific period of time (the *dwell time*) before being drained out and replaced by fresh, sterile fluid. The concentration of glucose in the dialysis can be varied (from 1.36 to 6.36%) in order to control the volume of fluid removed during the process. CAPD normally employs four exchanges of fluid each day
Intermittent haemodialysis	IHD	Chronic	Mainly diffusion to effect solute removal; fluid balance is closely monitored and ultrafiltration employed to remove excess fluid. This technique requires an extracorporeal circuit to perfuse blood through the artificial kidney before returning it to the patient. Dialysis fluid is passed in a countercurrent direction to facilitate diffusion. Patients are normally connected to a haemodialysis machine (either at home or in the hospital's renal unit) for short periods of time (4–6 h) twice or three times a week

semipermeable membrane when a pressure is applied to one side of that membrane. The rate of blood flow through the membrane generates the hydrostatic pressure that forces plasma water to move across the filter, 'dragging' various solutes, including many drugs, with it. This process removes significant volumes of fluid from the patient so that accurate monitoring and replacement of fluid are essential.

Intermittent haemodialysis, on the other hand, combines the forces of convection with diffusion (the movement of solute along a concentration gradient between plasma and dialysate) to enhance the removal of these substances. The difference in flow rate that exists within the membrane, between the dialysis fluid and the blood, allows effective removal of solutes. As the solute clearance achieved by this technique is principally a result of diffusive and not convective forces, it is not necessary to generate large volumes of ultrafiltrate so that the volume of replacement fluid required is reduced compared to haemofiltration.

The renal replacement therapies available possess different clearance capabilities (usually determined in terms of urea clearance), which reflect the principles used as well as the technology that accompanies the process. In addition, the clearance achieved by any continuous technique can be varied by manipulating either the rate of ultrafiltration or the dialysis fluid. A guide to the clearance rates achieved by the various renal replacement techniques used is given in Table 17.3.

TABLE 17.3 Typical clearance values achieved by commonly used renal replacement techniques

Renal replacement technique	Mode of action	Type of renal failure used to treat	Typical clearance (ml/min)
CAPD	Dialysis and ultrafiltration	Chronic	5–8
Intermittent HD	Dialysis and ultrafiltration	Chronic	150–200
CAVH	Ultrafiltration only	Acute	10–20
CVVH	Ultrafiltration only	Acute	Up to 50
CAVHD or CVVHD	Dialysis and ultrafiltration	Acute	20–25

DOSAGE ADJUSTMENTS FOR PATIENTS RECEIVING RENAL REPLACEMENT THERAPIES

In general, it is only necessary to adjust the dosing regimen of a drug to accommodate any loss incurred as a result of renal replacement in cases where the drug is largely excreted via the kidneys. The following reference sources should be consulted when considering a specific drug:

- *Drug Prescribing in Renal Failure: Dosing guidelines for adults* (Aronoff et al 1999)
- *The Renal Drug Handbook* (Ashley & Currie 2004)
- *British National Formulary* (Appendix 3: Renal impairment)
- *Data Sheet Compendium.*

The following principles should serve to guide the clinical pharmacist:

- Dosage adjustment is only required where the drug is significantly excreted by the kidneys (i.e. >25%), as it is likely that a proportion of the dose will be removed by the renal replacement therapy employed
- Where intermittent haemodialysis is used, always administer the dose after the session is complete
- Consult recognised reference sources to guide any prescribing advice given. This includes discussing individual patient care with a renal pharmacist (where available) or an experienced practitioner
- Where the drug possesses a narrow therapeutic range, ensure that close monitoring of serum concentrations is undertaken. This information should be used to guide future dosing regimens
- No renal replacement therapy attains the same drug clearance as normal kidneys, so no dosing regimen should exceed that recommended for patients with normal renal function.

DOSAGE ADJUSTMENTS FOR PATIENTS RECEIVING CONTINUOUS RENAL REPLACEMENT THERAPIES

Many factors influence the removal of drugs by these techniques, the most important of which can be classified into either drug or system variables.

Molecular size (weight and steric hindrance) is an important factor in the clearance of a drug by haemodialysis but has less effect on clearance by haemofiltration. Convection (ultrafiltration) readily removes compounds with a molecular weight (MW) of up to 5000 (which includes most drugs; usually with an MW of between 200 and 2000) so that those factors affecting either filter blood flow or filter permeability (e.g. build-up of cells or protein on the filter surface) play a more important role in influencing drug clearance. Diffusion (dialysis) is the main driving force for drug removal during haemodialysis, so drugs with a low MW (approx. 500) are favourably cleared by such a process, while the removal of larger solutes relies more on convection. In general the following conditions favour drug removal by continuous renal replacement therapy:

- low apparent volume of distribution (<1 l/kg)
- low percentage protein binding
- low MW (<500)
- high water solubility.

In addition a number of system factors can also influence drug clearance, e.g. the type of dialysis membrane used, the blood and dialysis flow rates and the ultrafiltration rate employed.

As the majority of membranes used during continuous renal replacement therapy are synthetic co-polymers, they possess the ability to adsorb compounds on to their surface, so interactions between the membrane and drugs administered to the patient are highly complex but can have important implications for drug clearance. The degree of adsorption reflects the drug used, its concentration, the pH of the patient's blood and the type of membrane used. For example, research has shown that approximately half of the first dose of tobramycin employed in patients with ARF could bind to a polyacrylonitrile membrane. This could potentially jeopardise the management of patients with severe infection by reducing the initial aminoglycoside plasma concentration. The majority of interactions involving drug-membrane binding appear to be complete within the first few hours of filter life, so consideration should be given, when selecting a drug, to the likely consequences of this effect on the patient's clinical condition. In practice this effect is unlikely to be important for the majority of drugs commonly used on the intensive care unit. Furthermore, there is very little information available to assist the clinical pharmacist in identifying the drugs involved and the likely clinical significance.

In addition, the altered drug handling seen in critically ill patients further complicates the issue. Changes in the distribution volume of certain drugs correlates closely with the increased extracellular volume and altered protein binding reported for such patients. Such changes in pharmacokinetic parameters often result in reduced clearance and an increase in the elimination half-life, as observed for some drugs, e.g. ceftazidime and midazolam.

Displacement of drugs from their protein-binding sites by various uraemic inhibitors, bilirubin, free fatty acids or other drugs will increase the amount of unbound or active drug available for filtration, diffusion or binding to the membrane. For highly protein-bound drugs (such as phenytoin) the increase in concentration of active drug could also result in deleterious effects on the patient.

When prescribing for patients receiving continuous renal replacement therapy the following principles should be followed:

- Dosage adjustment is only clinically important when the extracorporeal elimination exceeds 25% of the total body clearance for that drug
- Consult recognised reference sources to guide any prescribing advice given. This includes discussing individual patient care with a specialist pharmacist, either a renal or critical care practitioner
- Where the drug possesses a narrow therapeutic range, ensure that close monitoring of serum concentrations is undertaken. This information should be used to guide future dosing regimens
- A dose can be selected based on an estimate of the creatinine clearance achieved by the continuous renal replacement therapy employed
- Where the drug may have an extended elimination half-life, e.g. gentamicin or digoxin, a loading dose of the drug may need to be given to ensure a more rapid response.

KIDNEY TRANSPLANTATION

Transplantation is the treatment of choice for most patients with end-stage renal failure. Although for many it can mean a return to a near-normal life, it should be remembered that transplantation is still a form of renal replacement therapy, and should be regarded as such. Transplanted kidneys are not as robust as native kidneys and so should be treated with great care. There are several key points to note.

Always check the following with transplant patients:

- When was the patient transplanted?
- Where were they transplanted? Always check the notes to see which transplant unit they are under, in case you need to contact them to clarify a drug history. Obtain the local transplant protocol if necessary.

Patients with a functioning transplant should always be receiving two or three immunosuppressants, which normally include:

- ciclosporin or tacrolimus
- azathioprine or mycophenolate mofetil (MMF)

- sirolimus
- steroids (prednisolone).

It is *vital* that the patient continues to take immunosuppressant drugs, or they will be at risk of rejecting the kidney, even if not recently transplanted.

Patients will often be on a number of supplementary treatments after a transplant. These may include:

- antihypertensive agents
- lipid-lowering agents
- aspirin
- diuretics
- prophylactic antibiotics, antifungals or antiviral agents.

Always remember to ensure that all these medications are correctly prescribed.

- Always check the patient's renal function – just because the patient has a working transplant it *does not* always mean that the patient has 'normal' renal function. Always adjust doses according to the patient's GFR or creatinine clearance, rather than the serum creatinine level. Use the Cockcroft and Gault equation with care, since the patient has only one functioning kidney. If in doubt, to obtain an accurate clearance, contact the patient's transplant unit, or ensure that a 24-hour urine collection has been done
- Most patients should be on oral immunosuppressant therapy. If a patient needs to be converted from an oral to intravenous treatment regimen, always double-check the doses in *The Renal Drug Handbook*, or seek specialist advice from a renal pharmacist, as it is rarely a one-to-one conversion
- Ciclosporin, tacrolimus and sirolimus all have a narrow therapeutic index. In addition, ciclosporin and tacrolimus are both nephrotoxic. Hence it is important to measure levels. If your hospital does not offer the required assays, liaise with the patient's transplant unit about the required monitoring. On the days that levels are monitored, the patient should not take their morning dose of immunosuppressant drugs until the blood sample has been taken, to ensure that a trough level is measured
- Most of the commonly used immunosuppressants have significant drug interactions (see below), so it is important to monitor for any

potential interactions, which could lead to either increased levels of immunosuppressants, with accompanying toxicity, or decreased levels of immunosuppression, with the risk of acute rejection
- Wherever possible avoid nephrotoxic agents (e.g. NSAIDs, aminoglycosides), as transplanted kidneys are particularly sensitive to toxic insults.

DRUG INTERACTIONS

It is important to ensure that transplanted patients do not experience any drug interactions that may compromise the function of the kidney or create other problems for the patient. There follows a brief list of the clinically important interactions that may occur.

- *Ciclosporin, tacrolimus and sirolimus* are all metabolised via the cytochrome P450 3A4 system and are therefore subject to drug interactions with many agents that affect this metabolic pathway
- Enzyme inducers – e.g. rifampicin, rifabutin, phenytoin, phenobarbital, St John's wort – will decrease plasma levels of ciclosporin, tacrolimus and sirolimus
- Enzyme inhibitors – e.g. erythromycin, clarithromycin, the imidazoles, protease inhibitors, cimetidine, grapefruit juice – will increase plasma levels of ciclosporin, tacrolimus and sirolimus
- Other drugs – e.g. NSAIDs, aminoglycosides, ciprofloxacin – will potentiate the nephrotoxicity of ciclosporin and tacrolimus
- *Mycophenolate mofetil* (MMF) has few significant interactions, but two of note are:
  – when MMF is co-prescribed with either aciclovir or ganciclovir, they will increase the plasma levels of each other
  – the absorption of MMF is decreased by antacids and cholestyramine
- *Azathioprine* has one highly significant drug interaction with potentially very serious consequences. Co-administration with allopurinol greatly enhances the effects of azathioprine, resulting in severe bone marrow suppression. It is essential that the dose of azathioprine be reduced by 50–75% if allopurinol therapy is initiated, and that the full blood count is monitored closely.

SUMMARY

This chapter has attempted to cover the range of situations in which clinical pharmacists may encounter patients with renal impairment and to offer a brief resumé of the major contributions to care that are required. We would like to direct the reader to additional information sources, in particular to *The Renal Drug Handbook* (Ashley & Currie 2004), which is the primary reference source recommended by the Renal Pharmacy Group.

REFERENCES

Aronoff GR, Berns JS, Brier ME et al 1999 Drug prescribing in renal failure, dosing guidelines for adults, 4th edn. American College of Physicians, Philadelphia, PA/RSM Press, London

Ashley C, Currie A, eds 2004 The renal drug handbook, 2nd edn. Radcliffe Medical, Oxford

USEFUL RESOURCES

Renal Association website: www.renal.org

Renal Disease and Dysfunction Module. (This is a module produced by renal pharmacists working in the South of England, accredited by the University of Brighton to provide 20 postgraduate credits)

UK Renal Pharmacy Group website: www.renalpharmacy.org

CHAPTER 18

Monitoring patients with liver disease

S. Dhillon

The liver is a key organ for elimination and is responsible for the metabolism of many drugs. It is a principal organ for drug metabolism and pharmacists need to be aware of the influence of liver disease on pharmacokinetics and drug handling.

In liver disease the capacity, i.e. ability of the liver to metabolise drugs, may be impaired. Structural or functional abnormalities will influence the ability of the liver to handle drugs effectively. Functions of the liver and their degree of impairment in liver disease will assist the pharmacist in monitoring drug therapy. The liver is the largest internal organ in the body. Pharmacists need to understand the main functions of the liver and hence any changes in these functions manifest themselves as changes in laboratory indices leading to specific clinical changes, signs and symptoms. The main functions of the liver include control of synthesis and metabolism of most proteins and coagulation factors, carbohydrate and lipids. Most importantly, the liver is the site for drug metabolism. The liver has an important role in converting excess carbohydrates and proteins into fatty acids and triglycerides. Sugars are also stored in the liver as glycogen until required by the body; the liver is responsible for glycogen breakdown and release of glucose. Finally the liver is responsible for metabolism and excretion of bilirubin and bile acids. Common causes of liver disease include alcohol, hepatitis C and hepatitis B.

COMMON SYMPTOMS OF LIVER DISEASE

- *Acute liver disease*: general symptoms of lethargy, anorexia and malaise and jaundice, but can present asymptomatically

- *Chronic liver disease* can be asymptomatic and clinically identified through abnormal biochemistry. Late presentation shows complications for liver disuse such as ascites, haematemesis, melaena, confusion and drowsiness. Other symptoms include pruritus, with or without signs of systemic disease.

DRUG-INDUCED LIVER DAMAGE

Many drugs may be implicated in drug-induced liver problems. Examples include those shown in Table 18.1.

CHANGES IN PHARMACOKINETICS IN LIVER DISEASE

These are mainly related to metabolism (Box 18.1).

INTERPRETATION OF LIVER FUNCTION TESTS

- *Bilirubin*: A raised value with other abnormal liver function tests may suggest hepatobiliary disease. Very high levels are indicative

TABLE 18.1 Drugs implicated in liver problems

Type of liver problem	Drug(s) implicated
Necrosis	Carbon tetrachloride, paracetamol, halothane
Fat	Sodium valproate
Hepatitis	Amiodarone, methyldopa, isoniazid
Hypersensitivity	Sulphonamides
Cholestasis	Sex hormones, erythromycin
Fibrosis	Methotrexate

Box 18.1 **Useful indices of liver dysfunction**

- Bilirubin
- Enzymes
- Aminotransaminases
- Alkaline phosphatase
- Gamma-glutamyl transpeptidase
- Albumin
- Coagulation factors, prothrombin time

of biliary tract obstruction. A small or moderate rise without changes in the liver enzymes will suggest problems with haemolysis or ineffective erythropoiesis

● *Aminotransferases*: Very high levels are indicative of acute hepatitis but may be raised because of myocardial damage or skeletal muscle damage. Look for alanine aminotransferase, since its more specific to the liver

● *Alkaline phosphatase*: Raised levels are seen in cholestasis but can also originate from the bone, e.g. osteomalacia

● *Gamma-glutamyl transpeptidase*: Raised levels are indicative of alcohol abuse and enzyme induction. Raised levels of this enzyme with raised levels of alkaline phosphatase will indicate cholestasis

HEPATIC BLOOD FLOW

The extent of impairment may be significant enough in cirrhosis, hepatic venous obstruction and portal vein thrombosis to affect the clearance of a number of drugs. At steady state the following equation gives the relationship between hepatic blood flow and the rate of elimination:

$$Cl_{hepatic} = Q(C_i - C_o)/C_i$$

where $Cl_{hepatic}$ is hepatic clearance, Q is hepatic blood flow, C_i is concentration of drug presented to the liver, C_o is concentration of drug leaving the liver.

Drugs that have a high extraction ratio will be affected by changes in the blood flow. The bioavailability of these drugs will be enhanced following oral administration with reduced hepatic blood flow. Clearance is hence affected by changes in hepatic blood flow. Examples include those shown in Box 18.2.

PORTAL SYSTEMIC SHUNTING

The extent or presence of porto-systemic shunts in cirrhosis or portal vein thrombosis can affect drug metabolism. Blood may be deviated

---

Box 18.2 Drugs with a high extraction ratio ($E > 0.7$)

● Propranolol
● Morphine
● Clomethiazole
● Glyceryl trinitrate

from the liver to the systemic circulation, thus increasing the bioavailability of drugs with high hepatic extraction.

HEPATOCELLULAR DAMAGE

A reduction in the functional ability of the liver to extract drugs may occur in acute liver failure. Extensive liver cell damage and necrosis and fibrosis can reduce the intrinsic clearance of a number of drugs. This will result in increased bioavailability of highly extracted drugs because of a reduction in first-pass metabolism. Low extraction ratio drugs will have reduced elimination and hence accumulation will occur. The dose may need to be reduced or the dosage interval extended. Examples include those shown in Box 18.3.

CHOLESTASIS

Cholestasis occurs when bile fails to pass from the hepatocyte to the duodenum, resulting in accumulation in the blood. Absorption of lipid-soluble drugs may be reduced in cholestasis; in addition there may be displacement of highly protein-bound drugs by competition for the binding site.

CHANGES IN PLASMA PROTEIN BINDING

Changes in protein binding will affect the clearance of those drugs that have a low extraction ratio and are binding-sensitive. Changes in protein binding for drugs with a narrow therapeutic range that are highly plasma protein-bound will have a clinical effect. In general a lower total serum concentration is measured in the presence of the same free concentration.

Box 18.3 **Drugs with a low extraction ratio ($E < 0.3$)**

- Diazepam
- Phenytoin
- Chloramphenicol
- Paracetamol
- Theophylline

PHARMACODYNAMIC CHANGES

There is an increased sensitivity to sedatives and/or hypnotics. Drugs such as benzodiazepines, hypnotics and opiates should be avoided or prescribed with caution because of the risk of encephalopathy. In addition, diuretics and drugs that result in electrolyte disturbances, e.g. hypokalaemia and hypovolaemia, may contribute to hepatic encephalopathy.

CLINICAL PHARMACY – LIVER CHECKLIST

You can assess whether you are dealing with a liver patient from the type of ward the patient is on or the consultant dealing with your patient. Other clues are below.

Prescription items
- Lactulose high-dose, e.g. 30–40 ml q.d.s.
- Neomycin
- Metronidazole
- Spironolactone
- Furosemide or metolazone
- Magnesium salts
- Vasopressin
- Octreotide
- Omeprazole
- Lamivudine
- Magnesium salts
- Chlorpheniramine
- Cholestyramine
- Vitamin K
- Multivitamins
- Ranitidine
- Bile salts
- Clomethiazole

The patient may be on the following
- Low-sodium diet
- Low-protein diet
- Sedatives restricted

The patient's physical appearance or clinical symptoms may be useful
Look for:

- Fatigue, generally run down and weight loss
- Girth measurements

- Skin sclera looks yellow
- Spider naevi
- Red palms
- Clubbing
- Dupuytren's contracture
- Confusion
- Ascites
- Oedema – lower-limb swelling.

The patient may be monitored

Look for:

- Liver function tests
- Haematology screen
- Specific markers.

Routine monitoring of laboratory tests

- Transaminases
- Gamma-glutamyl transferase
- Alkaline phosphatase
- Bilirubin
- Serum albumin.

DRUG SELECTION

Always check

- Is the drug metabolised?
- Is it high or low extraction ratio?
- Is it plasma protein-bound?
- Does it cause drug-induced liver disease?
- Is it a prodrug?
- For renally excreted drugs, does it have active metabolites that are metabolised?

Remember clinical pharmacy implications:

- Liver disease will result in impaired drug metabolism: caution and reduce dose of drugs that are metabolised
- Pharmacodynamic changes – caution with central nervous system drugs, i.e. enhanced sensitivity, caution with drugs that may precipitate encephalopathy
- Caution for drugs excreted in the bile: these will accumulate
- Hypoproteinaemia will result in reduced protein binding and toxicity if the drug is highly plasma protein-bound (>95%)
- Reduced clotting will cause increased sensitivity to oral anticoagulants
- Gastrointestinal disturbances common – watch prescribing of antacids
- Sodium and fluid retention – watch for sodium content of drugs, those causing electrolyte disturbances, watch fluid overload

Therapeutic drug level monitoring

S. Dhillon

Therapeutic drug monitoring (TDM) encompasses the measurement of serum drug levels and the application of clinical pharmacokinetics to improve patient care. The concept of clinical pharmacokinetics has developed over the last decade. TDM is defined as the use of drug levels, pharmacokinetic principles and pharmacodynamic factors to optimise drug therapy in individual patients. TDM has now developed successfully as an important area of clinical medicine. Advances in the development of sensitive and specific methods for the determination of drug and drug metabolite concentrations in biological fluids have advanced the implementation of TDM in routine clinical practice. Pharmacists should be able to apply pharmacokinetics in routine clinical practice on the wards. Pharmacists need to be able:

- to identify which drugs require TDM
- to advise when levels should be taken
- to advise as to the reasons for requesting TDM levels
- to provide an interpretation of the results
- to advise on dosage optimisation.

The interpretation of serum drug concentrations requires a knowledge of:

- applied therapeutics
- clinical pharmacokinetics
- drug handling in organ dysfunction
- drug disposition and the influence of disease states
- interpretation of biochemistry and pathology

- clinical pharmaceutics and formulations
- factors that influence patient adherence to drug regimens.

The pharmacist has a core knowledge base and skills in these subject areas and, through integrated practice and joint working with physicians, nurses and other members of the health care team, can promote the rational and cost-effective use of TDM and improve patient care.

The ward pharmacist is in a unique position of being able to identify those patients who could benefit from drug level monitoring. The pharmacist should aim to:

- advise the physician on when to sample for drug level determinations
- apply pharmacokinetic principles to help interpret the drug level
- advise on and follow-up TDM requests to ensure that appropriate action is taken.

TDM – WHICH DRUGS AND WHY?

Drugs where TDM is useful fulfil the following basic criteria:

- The intensity of the pharmacological effect is proportional to the drug concentration at the site of action
- The drugs have an established therapeutic plasma concentration range
- The relationship between plasma drug concentration and clinical effect is better than the relationship between the drug dose and its effect
- Monitoring the drug levels enhances the ability of the clinician to maximise the clinical efficacy and minimise the toxicity of the drug
- Drug toxicity and disease presentation are difficult to distinguish from clinical assessment alone
- There is a need to assess drug compliance
- There is a need to used to monitor the time course of drug interactions

THERAPEUTIC RANGE

The therapeutic range can be defined as the range of drug concentration within which the drug exhibits maximum efficacy and minimum toxicity in the majority of patients. It is important to appreciate that the therapeutic range is a statistical concept and that for some patients the levels at which they respond or exhibit toxicity may fall outside the most widely quoted ranges. Pharmacists can evaluate the drug use process to ensure that patients are on the correct medication, on the best formulation and dosage regimen and involved in monitoring and reviewing their own progress on the medication regimen. Interpretation of the therapeutic range must take into account the age of the patient, the disease state for which the drug is prescribed and any implications for altered volume of distribution or protein binding. Several examples exist where these factors will alter the therapeutic range, e.g. theophyllines in neonatal apnoea and asthma, digoxin in the treatment of heart failure or atrial fibrillation.

Drugs that are commonly monitored include:

- *aminoglycosides* – gentamicin, tobramycin, netilmicin, amikacin, vancomycin
- *anticonvulsants* – phenytoin, carbamazepine and occasionally phenobarbital
- *cardioactive agents* – digoxin, procainamide, lidocaine, disopyramide, flecainide
- *others* – theophylline, lithium, methotrexate, ciclosporin.

TDM SERVICES – WHAT YOU NEED TO KNOW

- How the service is organised, by whom? What is the level of pharmacy involvement?
- TDM service documentation e.g. request form, TDM information guide
- The role of pharmacy and clinical pharmacists on the wards
- The drugs for which the service will operate
- Types of assay techniques, sensitivity and specificity data and internal/external quality control procedures
- The days and times of assay runs
- The latest times by which the blood sample must arrive in the laboratory for inclusion in the scheduled run
- Processing and reporting method for results
- 'Out of hours' service arrangements
- How to provide dosage recommendations
- Advise on the design of appropriate assay request forms
- Ensure the TDM processes meet clinical governance requirements and minimise risk
- How the service is used in clinical situations (such as overdose)
- The availability of emergency assay techniques
- Referral arrangements to other TDM services (e.g. Poisons Unit) and their availability
- Sample collection details – the volume of blood and the type of tube

- Request form details and how the results will be reported to the physician (verbal and/or written report)
- Ensure documentation meets the clinical governance requirements.

INTERPRETATION OF SERUM DRUG LEVELS

The interpretation of results requires:

- patient's physical details
- clinical and biochemical status
- response to the medication regiment
- level of compliance and understanding of the dosage regimen
- the drug history, concurrent medication
- duration of therapy and sampling details.

All this information, together with the pharmacokinetics of the drug in question, is needed for a valid interpretation of the serum level.

Based on this information, the patient's individualised pharmacokinetic parameters can be estimated: the clearance (Cl); volume of distribution (V_d); and elimination rate constant (k).

Individualisation of the pharmacokinetic parameters requires the information above together with population pharmacokinetic data. Using population data, a set of initial pharmacokinetic parameters is calculated and a level is predicted for the time the blood sample was taken.

This value is compared with the assay result and the elimination rate constant or clearance is calculated from the measured serum level. The method of altering the elimination rate constant or clearance is done in a stepwise way, e.g. iteration can be used until the predicted level approximates the measured level. This technique can only be used if the V_d of the drug does not vary widely.

Clearance is then calculated ($k \times V_d$) and this can be compared with the population clearance. Since population parameters are mean values, it is probable that the patient's actual parameters will lie within 2 standard deviations of the mean population value. If this is the case, the individualised pharmacokinetic parameters can then be used for dosage adjustments.

If the values for the individualised clearance vary widely, then the reason for this deviation should be sought and the following factors should be checked:

- patient's concurrent drug therapy
- patient compliance
- drug interactions
- medication error

- change in patient's clinical status
- malabsorption
- incorrect assay result
- timing of sample
- site of sampling
- storage of sample (degradation or haemolysis).

If no explanation can be discovered for the deviation and all the factors above have been examined, then it is likely that the patient's data do differ significantly from the population mean data.

It is only then that the observed level is used to make future dosage recommendations and predictions. Any advice on alterations in dosage must be made in view of the patient's clinical condition and the assumptions and limitations of therapeutic ranges.

Population pharmacokinetic data monographs are summarised below. Additional sources of population pharmacokinetic data include *Avery's Drug Treatment* (Speight & Holford 1997), Appendix A.

USE OF CALCULATORS AND COMPUTER SOFTWARE PACKAGES

Pharmacokinetic interpretation of serum level data can be facilitated by using programmed calculators or computer software packages; however, this is not essential and basic clinical pharmacokinetics can be routinely applied using a calculator.

A number of aids facilitating interpretation are now available and it is advisable to assess the individual package according to the needs of the service. Some available software packages are listed in Table 19.1. Pharmacists who intend to use a software package should ensure that they understand the principles of the program, the pharmacokinetic model used and the associated assumptions and limitations of the package.

THERAPEUTIC DRUG MONITORING MONOGRAPHS

(From Evans et al 1992, Winter 2003.)

DIGOXIN

- Therapeutic range: 1–2 ng/ml
- Bioavailability (*F*)
  - for tablets: 0.63
  - for Lanoxin syrup: 0.80

TABLE 19.1 Some software packages available

Program	Hardware	Contact
Computer programs		
MWPharm Interactive curve-fitting program and patient simulations (180 drugs covered)	IBM-compatible	Mediware (MWPharm) Ltd Zenike Park 4 9747 AN Groningen Netherlands
Calculator programs		
American Society of Hospital Pharmacy	HP 41CV	ASHP 4630 Montgomery Avenue Bethesda, MD 20814 USA
Aminoglycosides Digoxin Theophylline	Texas 159	Mr D Crome Pharmacy Department Royal Liverpool Hospital Prescott St, Liverpool L7 8XP

- Salt factor (S): 1.0
- Absorption rate constant (k_a) 1.5/h

The apparent volume of distribution (adults) can be described by the following equations:

$$V_d = 3.12 \times (Cl_{cr}) + 3.84 \times (LBW) \text{ litres,}$$

or

$$V_d = 6\,l/kg.$$

LBW = lean body weight
Obesity >15% use LBW
Clearance (adults)

– without heart failure:

$$Cl\ (l/h) = 0.06 \times (Cl_{cr}) + 0.05 \times (LBW) \text{ (Age < 70 years)}$$

$$Cl\ (l/h) = 0.06 \times (Cl_{cr}) + 0.02 \times (LBW) \text{ (Age > 70 years)}$$

– with heart failure (all adults):

$$Cl\ (l/h) = 0.053 \times (Cl_{cr}) + 0.02 \times (LBW).$$

THEOPHYLLINE

- Therapeutic range: asthma 10–20 μg/ml; neonatal apnoea 5–15 μg/ml
- Bioavailability (F) is assumed to equal 1.0
- Salt factor (S):
  - 1.0 for theophylline
  - 0.79 for aminophylline
- Absorption rate constants (k_a) for sustained-release preparation (in k_a/h):
  - Phyllocontin, 0.35
  - Nuelin S-A, 0.27
  - Theo-Dur, 0.18
  - Slo-Phyllin, 0.5
  - Nuelin Liquid, 2.0

Adult data

The apparent volume of distribution (V_d) can be described by the following equations:

$$V_d = 0.5 \text{ l/kg of total body weight,}$$

$$V_d = 0.45 \times (LBW) + 0.4 \times (EBW) \text{ litres.}$$

EBW = excess body weight, EBW = total body weight − lean body weight.

Estimated clearance values from population data:

$$\text{Clearance} = 0.04 \text{ l/h/kg} \times \text{disease factor (Table 19.2).}$$

It is likely that these factors may be applied to paediatric patients. Experience is limited as most children do not suffer from concurrent diseases. Paediatric population pharmacokinetic data are given in Table 19.3.

TABLE 19.2 Disease factors for theophylline adult clearance

Disease	Factor
Non-smoker	1.0
Smoker	1.6
Congestive heart failure	0.4
Acute pulmonary oedema	0.5
Hepatic cirrhosis	0.5
Severe pulmonary obstruction	0.8

TABLE 19.3 Paediatric data for theophylline

Age	Clearance (l/h per kg)	Mean V_d (l/kg)
Neonates (premature to 6 weeks)	0.0229	0.63
Infants <6 months	0.048	0.50
Infants 6–11 months	0.12	
Children 1–4 years	0.102	0.44
Children 4–12 years	0.096	0.44

CARBAMAZEPINE

- Therapeutic range: 4–12 µg/ml
- Bioavailability: assume $F = 1$
- Absorption rate constant:
  - $k_a = 1.5/h$ (tablets)
  - $k_a = 0.33/h$ (retard)

The apparent volume of distribution (adults) can be calculated from:

$$V_d = 1.12 \text{ litres} \times (LBW)kg.$$

Clearance can be calculated from:

$$Cl = 0.056 \, l/h \text{ per kg}$$

$$Cl = 0.096 \, l/h \text{ per kg (paediatrics 4–12 years)}$$

PHENYTOIN

- Therapeutic range: 5–20 µg/ml
- Bioavailability (F): assumed to equal 1.0
- Salt factor (S): 0.92 (sodium salt).

Phenytoin shows non-linear pharmacokinetics. In practice, Michaelis–Menten pharmacokinetics are applied, and the equations are summarised below.

Population data

$$V_d = 0.65 \, l/kg$$

$$K_m = 5.7 \, mg/l \text{ (adults)}$$

$K_m = 3.2\,mg/l$ (<15 years old)

$V_m = 450 \times (wt/70)^{0.6}\,mg/day.$

To describe the relationship between the total daily dose (R [mg/day]) and the steady-state serum concentration (Cp_{ss}), where $R = D$ [dose]/τ [dosing interval]:

1. $RSF = V_m \times Cp_{ss}/K_m + Cp_{ss}$

where R = total daily dose (mg/day), V_m = maximum rate of metabolism (mg/day), K_m = plasma concentration (mg/l) at which rate of metabolism is 0.5 V_m, Cp_{ss} = steady-state serum concentration (mg/l).

2. $Cp_{ss} = K_m \times RSF/V_m - RSF$

3. $RSF = V_m - K_m \times RSF/(Cp_{ss})$

To decay a toxic plasma concentration Cp_l to a desired plasma concentration Cp:

$t_{decay} = [K_m \times \ln(Cp_l/Cp)] + (Cp1 - Cp)/V_m/V_d$

t_{decay} = time [days] to allow Cp_l to fall to Cp

where $\ln$ = natural log.

To calculate a 'corrected' Cp_{ss} for a patient with a low serum albumin:

$Cp_{adjusted} = Cp*/(1 - \alpha)(P_l/P) + \alpha$

where $Cp_{adjusted}$ = plasma concentration that would be expected if the patient had a normal serum albumin, $Cp*$ = steady-state serum level observed, P_l = serum albumin concentration observed, P = 'normal' serum albumin concentration 40 g/l, α = phenytoin free fraction (0.1).

To calculate a 'corrected' Cp_{ss} for a patient with both uraemia and hypoalbuminaemia:

$Cp_{adjusted} = Cp*(1 - \alpha)\,0.44 \times (P_l/P) + \alpha$

where 0.44 = empirical adjustment factor, $\alpha = 0.2$

Box 19.1 **Phenytoin preparations**
Injection Phenytoin sodium
Tablets Phenytoin sodium
Capsules Phenytoin sodium
Chewable tablets (Infatabs) Phenytoin
Suspension Phenytoin

REFERENCES

Dhillon S, Kostrzewski A 2006 Clinical pharmacokinetics. Pharmaceutical
    Press, London

Evans WE, Schentag JJ, Jusko WJ (eds) 1992 Applied pharmacokinetics:
    principles of therapeutic drug monitoring, 3rd edn. Applied Therapeutics,
    Vancouver

Speight TM, Holford NHG (eds) 1997 Avery's drug treatment: a guide to the
    properties, choice, therapeutic use and economic value of drugs in disease
    management, 3rd edn. Adis International, Auckland

Winter ME 2003 Basic clinical pharmacokinetics, 4th edn. Lippincott
    Williams & Wilkins, Philadelphia

REFERENCE

CHAPTER 20

Adverse reactions to drugs

SafeScript

Adverse reactions to drugs are common, so when a patient presents with a problem it is important to remember that it may be caused by a drug. When a patient is on many drugs it can be time-consuming to search through the adverse drug reaction (ADR) profile of all of them, so this chapter is constructed in reverse – the condition is listed (by Read code) and is followed by the pharmacological group of drugs that have been reported to cause that condition. Note that not all the drugs in a pharmacological group may cause the ADR. This list has been abstracted from a database package from SafeScript, which, among other functions, holds the ADR profile for around 30 000 drug products and is updated monthly.

Hospital pharmacists can now fill in yellow cards and send them to the Committee on Safety of Medicines. It is essential that they do this for *all* suspected ADRs to black-triangle drugs in the *British National Formulary* (BNF), and all serious suspected reactions to established drugs, even if the ADR is already well documented. If you are in doubt, the BNF gives examples of what constitutes a serious reaction. Community pharmacists should alert the prescriber or the patient's GP if the reaction is to an over-the-counter drug.

Adverse drug reaction	Pharmacological group
Abdomen feels bloated	Gastrointestinal agents
	Laxatives
	Somatotrophic hormones
Abdominal cramps	Anthelmintics
	Anthraquinone glycosides
	Anticholinesterase parasympathomimetics
	Antidiuretic hormones
	Antivirals
	Diagnostic agents
	Docusate

Adverse drug reaction	Pharmacological group
Abdominal cramps	Gastrointestinal agents
	Laxatives
	Monobactams
	Oestrogen antagonist antineoplastics
	Organic iodinated contrast media
	Parasympathomimetics
	Picosulphate
	Pilocarpine
	Posterior pituitary hormones
	Sweetening agents
	Typhoid vaccines
	Vasopressins
Abdominal discomfort	Anthelmintics
	Antifungals
	Antivirals
	Bile acid-binding resins
	Calcium antagonist vasodilators
	Diagnostic agents
	Ergot compounds
	Laxatives
	Lincomycins
	Lipid-regulating agents
	Macrolides
	Medicinal enzymes
	Sex hormones
	Sweetening agents
	Triazole antifungals
Abdominal distension	Bulk laxatives
	Chloral sedatives
	Hypoglycaemics
Abdominal pain	4-methanolquinoline antimalarials
	4-quinolones
	8-aminoquinoline antimalarials
	ACE inhibitors
	Amino acids
	Analgesics and anti-inflammatory drugs
	Anthelmintics
	Antiandrogens
	Antianginal vasodilators
	Anticholinesterase parasympathomimetics
	Antidepressants
	Antidiuretic hormones
	Antidotes
	Antiemetics

Adverse drug reaction	Pharmacological group
Abdominal pain	Antimalarials
	Antimuscarinics
	Antineoplastics
	Antituberculous agents
	Antiulcer agents
	Antivirals
	Aspartic acid
	Benzimidazole anthelmintics
	Bisphosphonates
	Borates
	Carbapenems
	Cardiac glycosides
	Catechol O-methyl transferase inhibitors
	Central stimulants
	Cephalosporins
	Chelating agents
	Cinchona antimalarials
	Clofibrate and analogues
	Colchicum alkaloids
	Colony-stimulating factors
	Contrast media
	Digitalis
	Dopaminergic antiparkinsonian agents
	E series prostaglandins
	Ergolines
	Ergot alkaloids
	Ergot compounds
	Essential amino acids
	Gastrointestinal agents
	Glycol and glycerol esters
	Gonad-regulating hormones
	HMG CoA-reductase inhibitors
	Hydroxyquinoline antiprotozoals
	Imidazole antifungals
	Interleukins
	Leukotriene inhibitors
	Lipid-regulating agents
	Medicinal enzymes
	Neuroleptics
	Nutritional carbohydrates
	Oestrogen antagonist antineoplastics
	Opioid antagonists
	Oral hypoglycaemics
	Oxazolidinedione antiepileptics
	Pilocarpine
	Prophylactic antiasthmatics

Adverse drug reaction	Pharmacological group
Abdominal pain	Selective serotonin reuptake-inhibiting antidepressants
	Somatotrophic hormones
	Triazole antifungals
	Vasodilator antihypertensives
	Vitamin E substances
	Vitamins
Abnormal granulation	Chlorine-releasing substances
	issue
Abnormal uterine bleeding	Anabolics
	Beta-sympathomimetic vasodilators
	Beta-2-selective stimulants
	E series prostaglandins
	Oestrogen antagonist antineoplastics
	Sex hormones
Abnormal weight gain	Aliphatic phenothiazine neuroleptics
	Alpha-blocking antihypertensives
	Anabolics
	Antiandrogens
	Antidepressants
	Antiepileptics
	Antiulcer agents
	Butyrophenone neuroleptics
	Calcium antagonist vasodilators
	Diphenylbutylpiperidine neuroleptics
	Ergot compounds
	Flupentixols
	Fluphenazine
	GABA-related antiepileptics
	Gonad-regulating hormones
	H_1-antagonist antihistamines
	Haloperidols
	Hydrazine monoamine oxidase-inhibiting antidepressants
	Immunosuppressants
	Lithium
	Monoamine oxidase-inhibiting antidepressants
	Neuroleptics
	Norgestrels
	Oestrogens
	Phenothiazine neuroleptics
	Piperazine phenothiazine neuroleptics
	Piperidine phenothiazine neuroleptics

Adverse drug reaction	Pharmacological group
Abnormal weight gain	Progestogens
	Prophylactic antiasthmatics
	Sex hormones
	Skeletal muscle relaxants
	Tetracyclic antidepressants
	Thioxanthene neuroleptics
	Tricyclic antidepressants
	Vasodilator antihypertensives
	Zuclopenthixols
Abnormal weight loss	ACE inhibitors
	Anabolics
	Antiandrogens
	Anticholinesterase parasympathomimetics
	Antidepressants
	Antiepileptics
	Antifolate antineoplastics
	Butyrophenone neuroleptics
	Fat-soluble vitamins
	Gonad-regulating hormones
	Haloperidols
	Norgestrels
	Oestrogens
	Oxazolidinedione antiepileptics
	Progestogens
	Selective serotonin reuptake-inhibiting antidepressants
	Sex hormones
	Skeletal muscle relaxants
	Tetracyclic antidepressants
	Thyroid agents
	Tricyclic antidepressants
	Vitamin D substances
	Vitamins
Abnormalities of the hair	Antiandrogens
ACE inhibitor symptom complex – collagen vascular	ACE inhibitors
Acidosis	Glycol and glycerol esters
Acne	Anabolics
	Gonad-regulating hormones
	Hydantoin antiepileptics
	Norgestrels
	Phenytoin

Adverse drug reaction	Pharmacological group
Acne	Progestogens Sex hormones
Acne-like eruption	Tars
Acquired hypothyroidism	Antithyroid agents Antituberculous agents Class III antiarrhythmics Iodides Iodine compounds Iodophors Lithium
Acquired pyloric obstruction	E series prostaglandins
Acute alcoholic intoxication	Glycols
Acute bronchitis/ bronchiolitis	Antiulcer agents
Acute chemical pulmonary oedema	Aromatics
Acute closed-angle glaucoma	Skeletal muscle relaxants
Acute confusional state	Opioid analgesics
Acute conjunctivitis	Anthelmintics Antifolate antineoplastics Antivirals Beta-2-selective stimulants Carbonic anhydrase inhibitors Organic iodinated contrast media Retinoic acid dermatological agents Sedatives
Acute coronary insufficiency	Antidiuretic hormones Posterior pituitary hormones Vasopressins
Acute cystitis	Nitrogen mustards
Acute hepatic failure	Antiepileptics Antituberculous agents Imidazole antifungals Xanthine oxidase inhibitors
Acute hepatitis	4-aminoquinoline antimalarials ACE inhibitors

Adverse drug reaction	Pharmacological group
Acute hepatitis	Aliphatic phenothiazine neuroleptics
	Analgesics and anti-inflammatory drugs
	Antiandrogens
	Antibacterial agents
	Antibiotic antituberculous agents
	Antifungals
	Antiprotozoals
	Antituberculous agents
	Beta-lactamase inhibitors
	Calcium antagonist vasodilators
	Carbazepine antiepileptics
	Chelating agents
	Class I antiarrhythmics
	Gastrointestinal agents
	Gold salts
	Histamine H_2 antagonists
	HMG CoA reductase inhibitors
	Hydantoin antiepileptics
	Hydrazine monoamine oxidase-inhibiting antidepressants
	Imidazole antifungals
	Immunosuppressants
	Indanedione anticoagulants
	Inhalation anaesthetics
	Isoxazolyl penicillins
	Macrolides
	Methadone and analogues
	Monoamine oxidase-inhibiting antidepressants
	Monoamine oxidase-inhibiting antihypertensives
	Neuroleptics
	Nitrofuran antimicrobials
	Nitrofuran antiprotozoals
	Oestrogen antagonist antineoplastics
	Oral hypoglycaemics
	Oxazolidinedione antiepileptics
	Phenytoin
	Retinoic acid dermatological agents
	Sex hormones
	Skeletal muscle relaxants
	Sulphone antileprotics
	Sulphonylurea hypoglycaemics
	Thiouracil antithyroid agents
	Thiourea antithyroid agents
	Tricyclic antidepressants

Adverse drug reaction	Pharmacological group
Acute hepatitis	Trimethoprim–sulphonamide combinations Uricosuric agents Vitamin B substances
Acute laryngitis	Medicinal enzymes
Acute myocardial infarction	ACE inhibitors Alpha-blocking vasodilators Ergot alkaloids Ergot compounds Erythropoietin Nitrogen mustards Serotonin and analogues
Acute myocarditis	Gastrointestinal agents Neuroleptics Salicylate analgesics
Acute nasopharyngitis	Analgesics and anti-inflammatory drugs
Acute necrosis of liver	Analgesics and anti-inflammatory drugs Antiepileptics Beta-blockers Centrally acting antihypertensives Ester-type anaesthetics Hydrazide antituberculous agents Inhalation anaesthetics Nitrogen mustards Salicylate analgesics Skeletal muscle relaxants Xanthine oxidase inhibitors
Acute pancreatitis	ACE inhibitors Analgesics and anti-inflammatory drugs Antiepileptics Antivirals Coumarin anticoagulants Diamidine antiprotozoals Gastrointestinal agents Histamine H_2 antagonists HMG CoA reductase inhibitors Immunosuppressants Indanedione anticoagulants Loop diuretics Nitrofuran antimicrobials Oxytetracyclines Salicylate analgesics Selective serotonin reuptake-inhibiting antidepressants

Adverse drug reaction	Pharmacological group
Acute pancreatitis	Sulphonamides
	Tetracyclines
	Thiazide diuretics
	Trimethoprim–sulphonamide combinations
Acute pericarditis	Colony-stimulating factors
	Neuroleptics
	Skeletal muscle relaxants
Acute pharyngitis	Antiulcer agents
	GABA-related antiepileptics
	H_1-antagonist antihistamines
	Medicinal enzymes
Acute renal failure	Antibacterial agents
	Antibiotic antituberculous agents
	Antineoplastics
	Antivirals
	Borates
	Carbazepine antiepileptics
	Cinchona antimalarials
	Diamidine antiprotozoals
	Immunosuppressants
	Inhalation anaesthetics
	Leech products
	Organic iodinated contrast media
	Polyene antibiotics
	Uricosuric agents
Acute renal tubular necrosis	4-quinolones
	Aminoglycosides
	Antibiotic antituberculous agents
	Antifolate antineoplastics
	Antineoplastics
	Edetates
	Immunosuppressants
	Polyene antibiotics
Acute respiratory infections	Anticholinesterase parasympathomimetics
	Lipid-regulating agents
Acute sinusitis	Antiulcer agents
	H_1-antagonist antihistamines
Acute/subacute liver necrosis	4-quinolones
	Antiandrogens
	Antidepressants
	Hydrazine monoamine oxidase-inhibiting antidepressants

Adverse drug reaction	Pharmacological group
Acute/subacute liver necrosis	Monoamine oxidase-inhibiting antidepressants Sulphonamides Trimethoprim–sulphonamide combinations Uricosuric agents
Adult respiratory distress syndrome	Blood products
Aggression	Antiepileptics Benzodiazepine sedatives Carbamate sedatives Carbazepine antiepileptics Central stimulants GABA-related antiepileptics Neuroleptics Sedatives Skeletal muscle relaxants
Agitation	4-quinolones Aliphatic phenothiazine neuroleptics Anabolics Antianginal vasodilators Anticholinesterase parasympathomimetics Antidepressants Antiepileptics Antiulcer agents Antivirals Barbiturate sedatives Benzodiazepine antagonists Beta-2-selective stimulants Butyrophenone neuroleptics Carbamate sedatives Carbazepine antiepileptics Central stimulants Chloral sedatives Corticosteroids Diphenylbutylpiperidine neuroleptics Dopaminergic antiparkinsonian agents Ergolines Flupentixols Fluphenazine GABA-related antiepileptics Haloperidols Hydrazine monoamine oxidase-inhibiting antidepressants

Adverse drug reaction	Pharmacological group
Agitation	Monoamine oxidase-inhibiting antidepressants
	Neuroleptics
	Organic iodinated contrast media
	Parasympathomimetics
	Phenothiazine neuroleptics
	Pilocarpine
	Piperazine phenothiazine neuroleptics
	Piperidine phenothiazine neuroleptics
	Sedatives
	Skeletal muscle relaxants
	Thioxanthene neuroleptics
	Thyroid agents
	Tricyclic antidepressants
	Zuclopenthixols
Agranulocytosis	4-aminoquinoline antimalarials
	4-quinolones
	ACE inhibitors
	Aliphatic phenothiazine neuroleptics
	Analgesics and anti-inflammatory drugs
	Antibacterial agents
	Antibiotic antifungals
	Antidepressants
	Antimalarials
	Antithyroid agents
	Antiulcer agents
	Antivirals
	Butyrophenone neuroleptics
	Calcium antagonist vasodilators
	Carbacephems
	Carbamate sedatives
	Carbazepine antiepileptics
	Cephalosporins
	Cephamycins
	Chelating agents
	Class I antiarrhythmics
	Diphenylbutylpiperidine neuroleptics
	Flupentixols
	Fluphenazine
	Gastrointestinal agents
	H_1-antagonist antihistamines
	Haloperidols
	Histamine H_2 antagonists
	Hydantoin antiepileptics
	Hydrazide antituberculous agents

Adverse drug reaction	*Pharmacological group*
Agranulocytosis	Indanedione anticoagulants
	Lincomycins
	Neuroleptics
	Nitrofuran antimicrobials
	Oestrogen antagonist antineoplastics
	Oral hypoglycaemics
	Phenothiazine neuroleptics
	Phenytoin
	Piperazine phenothiazine neuroleptics
	Piperidine phenothiazine neuroleptics
	Skeletal muscle relaxants
	Succinimide antiepileptics
	Sulphonamides
	Sulphone antileprotics
	Sulphonylurea hypoglycaemics
	Tetracyclic antidepressants
	Thiouracil antithyroid agents
	Thiourea antithyroid agents
	Thioxanthene neuroleptics
	Tricyclic antidepressants
	Trimethoprim–sulphonamide combinations
	Zuclopenthixols
Alcohol – toxic effect	Alcoholic disinfectants
	Antineoplastics
	Glycols
Alkaline phosphatase raised	Fat-soluble vitamins
	Vitamin A substances
	Vitamins
Alkalosis	Expectorants
Allergic alveolitis	Antineoplastics
Allergic arthritis	Chelating agents
	Tetracyclic antidepressants
Allergic dermatitis	Alcohol metabolism modifiers
	Analgesics and anti-inflammatory drugs
	Gold salts
	Sulphone antileprotics
Allergic/hypersensitivity reaction	4-quinolones
	ACE inhibitors
	Acetoglycerides
	Acridine disinfectant dyes
	Alcoholic disinfectants
	Alcoholic solvents

Adverse drug reaction	Pharmacological group
Allergic/hypersensitivity reaction	Alkali-metal soaps
	Alkyl gallates
	Alkyl sulphates
	Allantoin compounds
	Aluminium astringents
	Amide-type anaesthetics
	Amidinopenicillins
	Amino acids
	Aminobenzoate sunscreen agents
	Aminoglycosides
	Aminopenicillanic derivatives
	Aminopenicillins
	Analgesics and anti-inflammatory drugs
	Animal desensitising agents
	Anionic and ampholytic surfactants
	Anionic surfactants
	Anthelmintics
	Antibacterial agents
	Antibiotic antineoplastics
	Antibiotic antituberculous agents
	Antidiarrhoeals
	Antidiuretic hormones
	Antidotes
	Antiemetics
	Antifungals
	Antihypertensives
	Antimalarials
	Antimicrobial preservatives
	Antineoplastics
	Antioxidant preservatives
	Antipseudomonal penicillins
	Antisera
	Aromatics
	Azo colouring agents
	Barbiturate antiepileptics
	Barbiturate sedatives
	Bases
	Benzimidazole anthelmintics
	Benzoates
	Benzophenone sunscreen agents
	Benzylpenicillin and derivatives
	Beta-lactamase inhibitors
	Beta-2-selective stimulants
	Bioflavonoids
	Bismuth salts
	Bitters

Adverse drug reaction	Pharmacological group
Allergic/hypersensitivity reaction	Blood-clotting factors
	Blood products
	Bromides
	Bulk laxatives
	Carbacephems
	Carbapenems
	Carboxypenicillins
	Cardiac inotropic agents
	Catechol O-methyl transferase inhibitors
	Cellulose-derived viscosity modifiers
	Centrally acting antihypertensives
	Cephalosporins
	Cephamycins
	Chloramphenicols
	Cinchona antimalarials
	Cinnamate sunscreen agents
	Class I antiarrhythmics
	Colony-stimulating factors
	Colouring agents
	Contrast media
	Cough suppressants
	Coumarin anticoagulants
	Cyanoacrylate adhesives
	Cytoprotective agents
	Dermatological agents
	Dextrans
	Diagnostic agents
	Diagnostic dyes
	Dibenzoylmethanes
	Direct-acting anticoagulants
	Disinfectants
	Docusate
	Dopaminergic antiparkinsonian agents
	Encephalitis vaccines
	Ester-type anaesthetics
	Evening primrose oil
	Fat and vegetable oil bases
	Fatty alcohol bases
	Fixed oils
	Flavouring agents
	Fluorescein colouring agents
	Fluorescein diagnostic dyes
	Fluorocarbon blood substitutes
	Formaldehyde and related compounds
	Gastrointestinal agents
	Glucose tests

Adverse drug reaction	Pharmacological group
Allergic/hypersensitivity reaction	Glycerol
	Glycerophosphates
	Glycol and glycerol esters
	Glycols
	Gold salts
	Gonad-regulating hormones
	Grass pollens
	H_1-antagonist antihistamines
	Haemostatics
	Heparinoids
	Histamine H_2 antagonists
	HMG CoA reductase inhibitors
	Hyaluronic acid
	Hydrazide antituberculous agents
	Hydroquinone dermatological agents
	Hydroxybenzoates
	Hydroxynaphthoquinones
	Hydroxyquinoline antiprotozoals
	Hypophosphites
	Hypothalamic and pituitary hormones
	Imidazole antifungals
	Immunological agents
	Immunosuppressants
	Indanedione anticoagulants
	Influenza vaccines
	Insulin
	Interleukins
	Iodides
	Iodine compounds
	Iodophors
	Isothiazolinones
	Isoxazolyl penicillins
	Laureths
	Laxatives
	Lecithin derivatives
	Leech products
	Lincomycins
	Local anaesthetics
	Low-molecular-weight heparins
	Macrogol esters
	Macrogol ethers
	Macrolides
	Measles vaccine
	Medicinal enzymes
	Mercurial dermatological agents
	Mercurial diuretics

Adverse drug reaction	*Pharmacological group*
Allergic/hypersensitivity reaction	Metallic soaps
	Mineral acids
	Monobactams
	Monoclonal antibodies
	Mucolytics
	Natural colouring agents
	Natural penicillins
	Neuroleptics
	Nitrofuran antimicrobials
	Non-ionic surfactants
	Nonoxinols
	Nutritional agents
	Octoxinols
	Oestrogen antagonist antineoplastics
	Oral hypoglycaemics
	Organic acids
	Organic iodinated contrast media
	Organic mercurial disinfectants
	Organic solvents
	Osmotic diuretics
	Oxacephalosporins
	Oxytetracyclines
	Paraffins
	Penicillinase-resistant penicillins
	Permanganates
	Pesticides
	Petroleum distillate solvents
	Phenothiazine antihistamines
	Phenoxymethylpenicillin and derivatives
	Phenoxypenicillins
	Phenylmercuric salts
	Plastics
	Poliomyelitis vaccines
	Poloxamers
	Polyene antibiotics
	Polymyxins
	Polyoxyl stearates
	Polysorbates
	Posterior pituitary hormones
	Preservatives
	Product bases
	Promethazines
	Psoralen dermatological agents
	Pyrethroid pesticides
	Quaternary ammonium surfactants
	Retinoic acid dermatological agents

Adverse drug reaction	Pharmacological group
Allergic/hypersensitivity reaction	Salicylate analgesics
	Salicylate sunscreen agents
	Sedatives
	Selective serotonin reuptake-inhibiting antidepressants
	Serotonin and analogues
	Siliceous viscosity modifiers
	Sodium salts
	Sorbates
	Sorbitan derivatives
	Streptogramins
	Sulphated oils
	Sulphites
	Sulphonamides
	Sulphonated anionic surfactants
	Sulphonylurea hypoglycaemics
	Sunscreen agents
	Synthetic colouring agents
	Tetracyclines
	Thiazide diuretics
	Thyrotrophic hormones
	Toluidines
	Trace elements
	Tree pollens
	Triazole antifungals
	Trimethoprim and derivatives
	Trimethoprim–sulphonamide combinations .
	Triphenylmethane colouring agents
	Triphenylmethane diagnostic dyes
	Triphenylmethane disinfectant dyes
	Typhoid vaccines
	Ureido penicillins
	Uricosuric agents
	Vaccines
	Vanillas
	Vasopressins
	Vegetable gums
	Viscosity modifiers
	Vitamin B substances
	Vitamin B_1 substances
	Wax bases
Alopecia	4-aminoquinoline antimalarials
	ACE inhibitors
	Alkyl sulphonate antineoplastics
	Alkylating antineoplastics

Adverse drug reaction	Pharmacological group
Alopecia	Anabolics
	Analgesics and anti-inflammatory drugs
	Anthracycline antibiotic antineoplastics
	Antibiotic antineoplastics
	Antiepileptics
	Antifolate antineoplastics
	Antineoplastics
	Antiulcer agents
	Antivirals
	Asparaginase antineoplastics
	Benzimidazole anthelmintics
	Biguanide antimalarials
	Borates
	Carbazepine antiepileptics
	Clofibrate and analogues
	Colchicum alkaloids
	Coumarin anticoagulants
	Direct-acting anticoagulants
	Ergot compounds
	Ethyleneimine antineoplastics
	Fluorouracil
	Gold salts
	H_1-antagonist antihistamines
	Heparinoids
	Immunosuppressants
	Indanedione anticoagulants
	Low-molecular-weight heparins
	Nitrofuran antimicrobials
	Nitrogen mustards
	Nitrosoureas
	Norgestrels
	Oestrogen antagonist antineoplastics
	Progestogens
	Purine antagonist antineoplastics
	Pyrimidine antagonist antineoplastics
	Retinoic acid dermatological agents
	Selective serotonin reuptake-inhibiting antidepressants
	Sex hormones
	Sulphur mustards
	Thiouracil antithyroid agents
	Thiourea antithyroid agents
	Triazene antineoplastics
	Vinca alkaloid antineoplastics
	Xanthine oxidase inhibitors

Adverse drug reaction	Pharmacological group
Amblyopia	Antidepressants
	GABA-related antiepileptics
	Pilocarpine
Amenorrhoea	Anabolics
	Antiepileptics
	Immunosuppressants
	Oestrogen antagonist antineoplastics
	Sex hormones
Anaemia	4-quinolones
	Antibiotic antituberculous agents
	Antineoplastics
	Antivirals
	Borates
	Central stimulants
	Colony-stimulating factors
	Diamidine antiprotozoals
	Immunosuppressants
	Organic iodinated contrast media
	Polyene antibiotics
	Pyrimidine antagonist antineoplastics
	Retinoic acid dermatological agents
	Sulphone antileprotics
Anal pain	Contrast media
	Gastrointestinal agents
	Laxatives
	Medicinal enzymes
Anal/rectal ulcer	Cation exchange resins
Anaphylactic shock	4-quinolones
	Amidinopenicillins
	Aminopenicillanic derivatives
	Aminopenicillins
	Animal desensitising agents
	Antibacterial agents
	Antibiotic antituberculous agents
	Antineoplastics
	Antipseudomonal penicillins
	Antisera
	Asparaginase antineoplastics
	Bases
	Benzylpenicillin and derivatives
	Blood products
	Borates
	Carbacephems

Adverse drug reaction	Pharmacological group
Anaphylactic shock	Carbapenems
	Carboxypenicillins
	Cephalosporins
	Cephamycins
	Chelating agents
	Class III antiarrhythmics
	Colony-stimulating factors
	Contrast media
	Corticosteroids
	Corticotrophic hormones
	Dextrans
	Direct-acting anticoagulants
	Erythropoietin
	Fluorocarbon blood substitutes
	Grass pollens
	H_1-antagonist antihistamines
	Heparinoids
	Hyaluronic acid
	Immunostimulants
	Immunosuppressants
	Iron compounds
	Isoxazolyl penicillins
	Low-molecular-weight heparins
	Medicinal enzymes
	Natural penicillins
	Norgestrels
	Oestrogen antagonist antineoplastics
	Opioid analgesics
	Organic iodinated contrast media
	Parenteral anaesthetics
	Penicillinase-resistant penicillins
	Phenothiazine antihistamines
	Phenoxymethylpenicillin and derivatives
	Phenoxypenicillins
	Platelet-activating factor antagonists
	Polyene antibiotics
	Progestogens
	Promethazines
	Pyrimidine antagonist antineoplastics
	Sedatives
	Sex hormones
	Skeletal muscle relaxants
	Specific immunoglobulins
	Tree pollens
	Triazole antifungals
	Triphenylmethane diagnostic dyes
	Ureido penicillins

Adverse drug reaction	Pharmacological group
Angina pectoris	Alpha-blocking antihypertensives
	Antiandrogens
	Antidiuretic hormones
	Beta-1-selective stimulants
	Central stimulants
	Ergot compounds
	HMG CoA reductase inhibitors
	Lipid-regulating agents
	Nitrogen mustards
	Posterior pituitary hormones
	Serotonin and analogues
	Thyroid agents
	Vasopressins
Angioneurotic oedema	4-quinolones
	ACE inhibitors
	Amidinopenicillins
	Aminopenicillanic derivatives
	Aminopenicillins
	Angiotensin-inhibiting antihypertensives
	Antiepileptics
	Antipseudomonal penicillins
	Antiulcer agents
	Benzylpenicillin and derivatives
	Beta-2-selective stimulants
	Bisphosphonates
	Calcium antagonist vasodilators
	Carboxypenicillins
	Cinchona antimalarials
	Class I antiarrhythmics
	Direct-acting anticoagulants
	H_1-antagonist antihistamines
	Heparinoids
	Histamine H_2 antagonists
	HMG CoA reductase inhibitors
	Isoxazolyl penicillins
	Leukotriene inhibitors
	Lipid-regulating agents
	Low-molecular-weight heparins
	Medicinal enzymes
	Natural penicillins
	Nitrofuran antimicrobials
	Nitrofuran antiprotozoals
	Nitroimidazole antiprotozoals
	Organic iodinated contrast media
	Penicillinase-resistant penicillins
	Phenothiazine antihistamines

Adverse drug reaction	Pharmacological group
Angioneurotic oedema	Phenoxymethylpenicillin and derivatives
	Phenoxypenicillins
	Promethazines
	Skeletal muscle relaxants
	Triazole antifungals
	Ureido penicillins
Anosmia – loss of smell sense	4-quinolones
	Disinfectants
Antibody formation	Somatotrophic hormones
	Specific immunoglobulins
Anxiety	Antituberculous agents
Anxiousness	4-quinolones
	Amphetamines
	Antianginal vasodilators
	Antidepressants
	Antivirals
	Barbiturate antiepileptics
	Benzodiazepine antagonists
	Beta-2-selective stimulants
	Central stimulants
	H_1-antagonist antihistamines
	Lipid-regulating agents
	Neuroleptics
	Opioid antagonists
	Prophylactic antiasthmatics
	Selective serotonin reuptake-inhibiting antidepressants
	Skeletal muscle relaxants
	Sympathomimetics
	Tricyclic antidepressants
	Vasodilator antihypertensives
Apathy	Aliphatic phenothiazine neuroleptics
	Butyrophenone neuroleptics
	Diphenylbutylpiperidine neuroleptics
	Flupentixols
	Fluphenazine
	Haloperidols
	Neuroleptics
	Phenothiazine neuroleptics
	Piperazine phenothiazine neuroleptics
	Piperidine phenothiazine neuroleptics
	Thioxanthene neuroleptics
	Zuclopenthixols

Adverse drug reaction	Pharmacological group
Aplastic anaemia	4-aminoquinoline antimalarials
	Acetylurea antiepileptics
	Analgesics and anti-inflammatory drugs
	Antiepileptics
	Antifungals
	Antiprotozoals
	Antithyroid agents
	Carbacephems
	Carbazepine antiepileptics
	Cephalosporins
	Cephamycins
	Chelating agents
	Chloramphenicols
	Class I antiarrhythmics
	Gastrointestinal agents
	Histamine H_2 antagonists
	Hydantoin antiepileptics
	Inorganic mercury compounds
	Neuroleptics
	Nitrofuran antimicrobials
	Oral hypoglycaemics
	Organic mercurial disinfectants
	Oxazolidinedione antiepileptics
	Phenytoin
	Selective serotonin reuptake-inhibiting antidepressants
	Sulphonylurea hypoglycaemics
	Tetracyclic antidepressants
	Uricosuric agents
Apnoea	Benzodiazepine sedatives
	Carbamate sedatives
	Class III antiarrhythmics
	E series prostaglandins
	Inhalation anaesthetics
	Polymyxins
	Sedatives
	Skeletal muscle relaxants
Appetite increased	Antiandrogens
	Antidepressants
	Antiepileptics
	H_1-antagonist antihistamines
	Neuroleptics
	Skeletal muscle relaxants
	Tetracyclic antidepressants
	Tricyclic antidepressants

Adverse drug reaction	Pharmacological group
Appetite loss – anorexia	4-methanolquinoline antimalarials
	4-quinolones
	Amphetamines
	Anorectics
	Anthelmintics
	Antibiotic antituberculous agents
	Anticholinesterase parasympathomimetics
	Antidepressants
	Antiemetics
	Antiepileptics
	Antifungals
	Antimony antiprotozoals
	Antineoplastics
	Antituberculous agents
	Antiulcer agents
	Antivirals
	Benzimidazole anthelmintics
	Biguanide hypoglycaemics
	Borates
	Carbazepine antiepileptics
	Cardiac glycosides
	Catechol O-methyl transferase inhibitors
	Central stimulants
	Cephalosporins
	Chelating agents
	Clofibrate and analogues
	Colony-stimulating factors
	Digitalis
	Dopaminergic antiparkinsonian agents
	Fat-soluble vitamins
	HMG CoA reductase inhibitors
	Interleukins
	Lithium
	Nitrofuran antimicrobials
	Oestrogen antagonist antineoplastics
	Opioid antagonists
	Oxazolidinedione antiepileptics
	Polyene antibiotics
	Selective serotonin reuptake-inhibiting antidepressants
	Skeletal muscle relaxants
	Somatotrophic hormones
	Sulphone antileprotics
	Sympathomimetics
	Thiazide diuretics
	Vaccines

Adverse drug reaction	Pharmacological group
Appetite loss – anorexia	Vasodilator antihypertensives
	Vitamin D substances
	Vitamins
Arthropathy	Histamine H_2 antagonists
	Tetracyclic antidepressants
Asthenia	4-quinolones
	Anticholinesterase parasympathomimetics
	Antihypertensives
	Antineoplastics
	Antituberculous agents
	Antiulcer agents
	Antivirals
	Cephalosporins
	H_1-antagonist antihistamines
	HMG CoA reductase inhibitors
	Interleukins
	Neuroleptics
	Serotonin and analogues
Asthma	Gonad-regulating hormones
	Organic iodinated contrast media
Ataxia	4-methanolquinoline antimalarials
	4-quinolones
	Alcoholic disinfectants
	Antidepressants
	Antiemetics
	Antiepileptics
	Antineoplastics
	Antivirals
	Barbiturate antiepileptics
	Barbiturate sedatives
	Benzodiazepine sedatives
	Carbamate sedatives
	Carbazepine antiepileptics
	Class I antiarrhythmics
	Class III antiarrhythmics
	GABA-related antiepileptics
	Gastrointestinal agents
	H_1-antagonist antihistamines
	Hydantoin antiepileptics
	Lithium
	Nitroimidazole antiprotozoals
	Oxazolidinedione antiepileptics
	Phenothiazine antihistamines
	Phenytoin

Adverse drug reaction	Pharmacological group
Ataxia	Promethazines
	Sedatives
	Skeletal muscle relaxants
	Succinimide antiepileptics
Atony of bladder	Organic solvents
Atopic dermatitis and related	Antituberculous agents
	Dermatological agents
Atrophy of breast	Progestogens
	Sex hormones
Attention/concentration difficulty	Antiemetics
	Antiepileptics
	Antivirals
	Neuroleptics
Avascular necrosis, head of the femur	Corticosteroids
	Corticotrophic hormones
Backache	ACE inhibitors
	Angiotensin-inhibiting antihypertensives
	Antibacterial agents
	Antiulcer agents
	E series prostaglandins
	Gonad-regulating hormones
	Progestogens
	Sex hormones
Bacterial infection	Antiulcer agents
	Antivirals
	Corticosteroids
	Corticotrophic hormones
	Immunosuppressants
	Interleukins
	Leech products
	Medicinal enzymes
Bacterial pneumonia	Antivirals
Behavioural disturbance	Antidepressants
	Ergot compounds
	GABA-related antiepileptics
	Sedatives
	Skeletal muscle relaxants
	Tetracyclic antidepressants
	Tricyclic antidepressants
Benign neoplasm male breast	Antiandrogens

Adverse drug reaction	Pharmacological group
Biliary stasis	4-quinolones
	Beta-lactamase inhibitors
Birth trauma/asphyxia/ hypoxia	Oxytocic hormones
Bleeding time increased	Dermatological agents
	Salicylate analgesics
Blistering of skin	Retinoic acid dermatological agents
Blocked sinuses	Alpha-blocking vasodilators
Blood disorders	4-aminoquinoline antimalarials
	4-quinolones
	ACE inhibitors
	Aldosterone inhibitors
	Analgesics and anti-inflammatory drugs
	Antibacterial agents
	Antiepileptics
	Antifolate antineoplastics
	Antifungals
	Antineoplastics
	Antivirals
	Benzodiazepine sedatives
	Carbacephems
	Carbamate sedatives
	Carbapenems
	Cephalosporins
	Cephamycins
	Chelating agents
	Chloramphenicols
	Cinchona antimalarials
	Colchicum alkaloids
	Gastrointestinal agents
	Gold salts
	H_1-antagonist antihistamines
	Histamine H_2 antagonists
	Hydantoin antiepileptics
	Immunosuppressants
	Monobactams
	Nitrofuran antimicrobials
	Oxacephalosporins
	Phenothiazine antihistamines
	Phenytoin
	Polyene antibiotics
	Potassium-sparing diuretics
	Promethazines

Adverse drug reaction	Pharmacological group
Blood disorders	Retinoic acid dermatological agents
	Skeletal muscle relaxants
	Succinimide antiepileptics
	Thiazide diuretics
	Uricosuric agents
	Vasodilator antihypertensives
Blood in urine – haematuria	Alpha-blocking vasodilators
	Analgesics and anti-inflammatory drugs
	Antivirals
	Aromatics
	Chelating agents
	Colony-stimulating factors
	Gastrointestinal agents
	Haemostatics
	Salicylate analgesics
	Skeletal muscle relaxants
Blood pressure changes	Oxazolidinedione antiepileptics
Blood pressure raised	Sympathomimetics
Blood urate raised	Antivirals
	Colony-stimulating factors
	Immunosuppressants
	Loop diuretics
	Medicinal enzymes
	Nutritional carbohydrates
	Retinoic acid dermatological agents
	Thiazide diuretics
	Vasodilator antihypertensives
Blood urea raised	4-quinolones
	ACE inhibitors
	Analgesics and anti-inflammatory drugs
	Antibiotic antineoplastics
	Antivirals
	Borates
	Erythropoietin
	Immunosuppressants
	Interleukin 2
	Organic iodinated contrast media
	Vasodilator antihypertensives
Blurred vision	4-aminoquinoline antimalarials
	4-methanolquinoline antimalarials
	4-quinolones
	Aliphatic phenothiazine neuroleptics

Adverse drug reaction	Pharmacological group
Blurred vision	Anabolics
	Analgesics and anti-inflammatory drugs
	Anthelmintics
	Antiandrogens
	Antidepressants
	Antiemetics
	Antiepileptics
	Antimuscarinics
	Antineoplastics
	Antiprotozoals
	Antiulcer agents
	Barbiturate antiepileptics
	Benzodiazepine sedatives
	Butyrophenone neuroleptics
	Carbamate sedatives
	Carbazepine antiepileptics
	Carbonic anhydrase inhibitors
	Cardiac glycosides
	Central stimulants
	Centrally acting antihypertensives
	Chelating agents
	Cholinesterase reactivators
	Cinchona antimalarials
	Class I antiarrhythmics
	Clofibrate and analogues
	Corticosteroids
	Dermatological agents
	Diagnostic agents
	Digitalis
	Diphenylbutylpiperidine neuroleptics
	Dopaminergic antiparkinsonian agents
	Flupentixols
	Fluphenazine
	GABA-related antiepileptics
	Gonad-regulating hormones
	H_1-antagonist antihistamines
	Haloperidols
	Hydantoin antiepileptics
	Hydrazine monoamine oxidase-inhibiting antidepressants
	Immunosuppressants
	Interleukins
	Lithium
	Monoamine oxidase-inhibiting antidepressants
	Neuroleptics

Adverse drug reaction	Pharmacological group
Blurred vision	Oestrogen antagonist antineoplastics
	Oral hypoglycaemics
	Oxazolidinedione antiepileptics
	Oxytetracyclines
	Phenothiazine antihistamines
	Phenothiazine neuroleptics
	Phenytoin
	Piperazine phenothiazine neuroleptics
	Piperidine phenothiazine neuroleptics
	Polymyxins
	Progestogens
	Promethazines
	Retinoic acid dermatological agents
	Salicylate analgesics
	Sedatives
	Serotonin and analogues
	Sex hormones
	Skeletal muscle relaxants
	Smooth-muscle relaxants
	Tetracyclic antidepressants
	Tetracyclines
	Thioxanthene neuroleptics
	Tricyclic antidepressants
	Zuclopenthixols
Bone marrow suppression	ACE inhibitors
	Alkyl sulphonate antineoplastics
	Alkylating antineoplastics
	Anthracycline antibiotic antineoplastics
	Antibiotic antineoplastics
	Antifolate antineoplastics
	Antimalarials
	Antineoplastics
	Antivirals
	Asparaginase antineoplastics
	Ethyleneimine antineoplastics
	Fluorouracil
	Immunosuppressants
	Interleukin 2
	Loop diuretics
	Nitrogen mustards
	Nitrosoureas
	Oestrogen antagonist antineoplastics
	Purine antagonist antineoplastics
	Pyrimidine antagonist antineoplastics
	Sulphur mustards

Adverse drug reaction	Pharmacological group
Bone marrow suppression	Triazene antineoplastics
	Trimethoprim and derivatives
	Trimethoprim–sulphonamide combinations
	Vinca alkaloid antineoplastics
Bradycardia	4-methanolquinoline antimalarials
	Alpha-adrenoceptor stimulants
	Amide-type anaesthetics
	Analgesics and anti-inflammatory drugs
	Antianginal vasodilators
	Antiarrhythmics
	Anticholinesterase parasympathomimetics
	Antidotes
	Antiemetics
	Antimuscarinics
	Antineoplastics
	Benzomorphan opioid analgesics
	Beta-blockers
	Calcium antagonist vasodilators
	Calcium salts
	Cardioselective beta-blockers
	Central stimulants
	Centrally acting antihypertensives
	Class I antiarrhythmics
	Class III antiarrhythmics
	Class IV antiarrhythmics
	Diagnostic agents
	Dopaminergic antiparkinsonian agents
	E series prostaglandins
	Ergot alkaloids
	Ergot compounds
	Ester-type anaesthetics
	Gastrointestinal agents
	Histamine H_2 antagonists
	I series prostaglandins
	Inhalation anaesthetics
	Local anaesthetics
	Methadone and analogues
	Morphinan opioid analgesics
	Neuroleptics
	Nutritional fats
	Opioid analgesics
	Opioid peptides
	Opium alkaloid opioid analgesics
	Opium poppy substances
	Parasympathomimetics

Adverse drug reaction	Pharmacological group
Bradycardia	Parenteral anaesthetics
	Pethidine and analogues
	Pilocarpine
	Platelet-activating factor antagonists
	Rauwolfia antihypertensives
	Respiratory stimulants
	Selective serotonin reuptake-inhibiting antidepressants
	Serotonin and analogues
	Skeletal muscle relaxants
	Smooth-muscle relaxants
	Sympathomimetics
	Vasodilators
Breath – smell of alcohol	Alcoholic disinfectants
	Alcoholic solvents
	Glycols
Breath-holding	Inhalation anaesthetics
Breathlessness	Antiandrogens
	Antibiotic antituberculous agents
	Antineoplastics
Bronchospasm	4-quinolones
	Analgesics and anti-inflammatory drugs
	Anthelmintics
	Antiarrhythmics
	Antibacterial agents
	Antibiotic antituberculous agents
	Anticholinesterase parasympathomimetics
	Antiemetics
	Antineoplastics
	Antiulcer agents
	Beta-blockers
	Beta-2-selective stimulants
	Blood products
	Cardioselective beta-blockers
	Class III antiarrhythmics
	Competitive muscle relaxants
	Dermatological agents
	Diagnostic agents
	Diamidine antiprotozoals
	F series prostaglandins
	H_1-antagonist antihistamines
	Medicinal enzymes
	Organic iodinated contrast media

Adverse drug reaction	Pharmacological group
Bronchospasm	Parasympathomimetics
	Phenothiazine antihistamines
	Pilocarpine
	Polymyxins
	Promethazines
	Prophylactic antiasthmatics
	Pyrimidine antagonist antineoplastics
	Respiratory stimulants
	Salicylate analgesics
	Sulphites
	Sympathomimetics
	Thyrotrophic hormones
	Vasodilators
	Vinca alkaloid antineoplastics
Bullous eruption	Antiulcer agents
	Sedatives
Burning or stinging	Aluminium astringents
	Analgesics and anti-inflammatory drugs
	Antifungals
	Antivirals
	Aromatics
	Carbonic anhydrase inhibitors
	Centrally acting antihypertensives
	Chelating agents
	Corticosteroids
	Dermatological agents
	Dithranols
	Formaldehyde and related compounds
	H_1-antagonist antihistamines
	Hydroquinone dermatological agents
	Imidazole antifungals
	Immunosuppressants
	Medicinal enzymes
	Prophylactic antiasthmatics
	Psoralen dermatological agents
	Pyrethroid pesticides
	Retinoic acid dermatological agents
	Serotonin and analogues
	Triazole antifungals
	Vitamin B substances
	Vitamin D substances
Burns	Tannic acid and derivatives
Candidal vulvovaginitis	Cephalosporins

Adverse drug reaction	Pharmacological group
Candidiasis mouth/oesophagus/ gastrointestinal tract	Antiulcer agents Carbapenems
Capillary	Colony-stimulating factors hyperpermeability
Carcinoma	Triphenylmethane disinfectant dyes
Cardiac arrest	Amide-type anaesthetics Antibacterial agents Antiemetics Class IV antiarrhythmics E series prostaglandins Ester-type anaesthetics Inhalation anaesthetics Local anaesthetics Medicinal enzymes Organic iodinated contrast media Peripheral and cerebral vasodilators
Cardiac conduction disorders	4-methanolquinoline antimalarials Antiandrogens Antineoplastics Calcium antagonist vasodilators Carbazepine antiepileptics Class III antiarrhythmics
Cardiac dysrhythmias	ACE inhibitors Aliphatic phenothiazine neuroleptics Alpha-blocking antihypertensives Amphetamines Antiandrogens Antiarrhythmics Antidepressants Antiemetics Antimalarials Antimuscarinics Antineoplastics Antivirals Beta-adrenoceptor stimulants Beta-sympathomimetic vasodilators Beta-2-selective stimulants Butyrophenone neuroleptics Calcium salts Carbazepine antiepileptics Cardiac glycosides Cardiac inotropic agents

Adverse drug reaction	Pharmacological group
Cardiac dysrhythmias	Central stimulants
	Chelating agents
	Class I antiarrhythmics
	Colony-stimulating factors
	Diamidine antiprotozoals
	Digitalis
	Diphenylbutylpiperidine neuroleptics
	Dopaminergic antiparkinsonian agents
	E series prostaglandins
	Ergolines
	Ester-type anaesthetics
	Flupentixols
	Fluphenazine
	H_1-antagonist antihistamines
	Haloperidols
	Hydantoin antiepileptics
	Hydrazine monoamine oxidase-inhibiting antidepressants
	Inhalation anaesthetics
	Interleukins
	Iron compounds
	Isoprenaline
	Monoamine oxidase-inhibiting antidepressants
	Neuroleptics
	Organic iodinated contrast media
	Oxytocic hormones
	Phenothiazine antihistamines
	Phenothiazine neuroleptics
	Phenytoin
	Piperazine phenothiazine neuroleptics
	Piperidine phenothiazine neuroleptics
	Polyene antibiotics
	Potassium salts
	Promethazines
	Respiratory stimulants
	Serotonin and analogues
	Skeletal muscle relaxants
	Smooth-muscle relaxants
	Sympathomimetics
	Tetracyclic antidepressants
	Theophylline xanthines
	Thioxanthene neuroleptics
	Thyroid agents
	Tricyclic antidepressants
	Vasodilator antihypertensives

Adverse drug reaction	Pharmacological group
Cardiac dysrhythmias	Vasodilators Xanthine-containing beverages Xanthines Zuclopenthixols
Cardiac murmur	Antineoplastics
Cardiomyopathy	Amphetamines Anorectics Anthracycline antibiotic antineoplastics Central stimulants
Cardiovascular symptoms	Antianginal vasodilators Antivirals Cinchona antimalarials Competitive muscle relaxants Expectorants Hydantoin antiepileptics Immunosuppressants Inhalation anaesthetics Lithium Nitrogen mustards Phenytoin Skeletal muscle relaxants
Cataract	Aliphatic phenothiazine neuroleptics Butyrophenone neuroleptics Chelating agents Corticosteroids Corticotrophic hormones Diphenylbutylpiperidine neuroleptics Flupentixols Fluphenazine Haloperidols Neuroleptics Oestrogen antagonist antineoplastics Phenothiazine neuroleptics Piperazine phenothiazine neuroleptics Piperidine phenothiazine neuroleptics Retinoic acid dermatological agents Sex hormones Thioxanthene neuroleptics Zuclopenthixols
Cellulitis or abscess at site of injection	Aliphatic phenothiazine neuroleptics Antineoplastics Antivirals Butyrophenone neuroleptics

Adverse drug reaction	Pharmacological group
Cellulitis or abscess at site of injection	Calcitonin
	Carbapenems
	Chelating agents
	Colony-stimulating factors
	Diamidine antiprotozoals
	Diphenylbutylpiperidine neuroleptics
	Dopaminergic antiparkinsonian agents
	E series prostaglandins
	F series prostaglandins
	Flupentixols
	Fluphenazine
	Gonad-regulating hormones
	Haloperidols
	Hydantoin antiepileptics
	Imidazole antifungals
	Insulin
	Insulin zinc suspensions
	Lincomycins
	Neuroleptics
	Oestrogen antagonist antineoplastics
	Phenothiazine neuroleptics
	Phenytoin
	Piperazine phenothiazine neuroleptics
	Piperidine phenothiazine neuroleptics
	Sedatives
	Thioxanthene neuroleptics
	Vaccines
	Zuclopenthixols
Cerebellar ataxia	Fluorouracil
	Pyrimidine antagonist antineoplastics
Cerebrovascular disorders	Colony-stimulating factors
Change in bowel habit	Histamine H_2 antagonists
Change in voice	ACE inhibitors
	Anabolics
	Medicinal enzymes
	Progestogens
	Sex hormones
Changes in breast size	Gonad-regulating hormones
Chemical bronchitis/ pneumonitis	Petroleum distillate solvents
Chest pain	Alpha-blocking antihypertensives
	Antiandrogens

Adverse drug reaction	Pharmacological group
Chest pain	Antiarrhythmics
	Antibacterial agents
	Antidotes
	Antiemetics
	Antimuscarinics
	Antiulcer agents
	Beta-sympathomimetic vasodilators
	Beta-2-selective stimulants
	Calcium antagonist vasodilators
	Cardiac inotropic agents
	Central stimulants
	Chelating agents
	Class I antiarrhythmics
	Colony-stimulating factors
	Corticotrophic hormones
	E series prostaglandins
	Ergot alkaloids
	Ergot compounds
	HMG CoA reductase inhibitors
	Oestrogen antagonist antineoplastics
	Opioid antagonists
	Sedatives
	Serotonin and analogues
	Sympathomimetics
	Vasodilators
Chest tightness	Antiemetics
	Beta-sympathomimetic vasodilators
	Beta-2-selective stimulants
	Serotonin and analogues
Childhood hyperkinetic syndrome	Respiratory stimulants
Chills with fever	Alpha-blocking vasodilators
	Antineoplastics
	Antiulcer agents
	Interleukins
	Triazole antifungals
Chloasma	Norgestrels
	Oestrogens
	Progestogens
	Sex hormones
Choking sensation	Antiarrhythmics
	Vasodilators
Cholangitis	Pyrimidine antagonist antineoplastics

Adverse drug reaction	Pharmacological group
Cholesterol gall stones	Clofibrate and analogues
Cholinergic urticaria	Anticholinesterase parasympathomimetics Parasympathomimetics Pilocarpine
Choreas	Central stimulants
Choreiform movement	Ganglion-blocking antihypertensives
Chronic active hepatitis	Analgesics and anti-inflammatory drugs Centrally acting antihypertensives Hydrazide antituberculous agents Nitrofuran antimicrobials Nitrofuran antiprotozoals Retinoic acid dermatological agents Skeletal muscle relaxants Sulphonamides Tricyclic antidepressants
Chronic renal failure	Inhalation anaesthetics
Cirrhosis – non-alcoholic	Alcohol metabolism modifiers
Cold extremities	Alpha-adrenoceptor stimulants Sympathomimetics
Colicky abdominal pain	Anthelmintics Laxatives
Coma	Alcoholic disinfectants Anthelmintics Antianginal vasodilators Antivirals Aromatics Gases Lithium Organic iodinated contrast media Oxazolidinedione antiepileptics
Complete atrioventricular block	Calcium antagonist vasodilators Cardiac glycosides Class I antiarrhythmics Class IV antiarrhythmics Digitalis Histamine H_2 antagonists
Complete epiphyseal arrest	Anabolics Androgens Sex hormones Testosterones

Adverse drug reaction	Pharmacological group
Confusion	4-quinolones
	Aldosterone inhibitors
	Amide-type anaesthetics
	Analgesics and anti-inflammatory drugs
	Anthelmintics
	Antibiotic antifungals
	Anticholinesterase parasympathomimetics
	Antidepressants
	Antidotes
	Antiemetics
	Antiepileptics
	Antifungals
	Antimuscarinics
	Antineoplastics
	Antiulcer agents
	Antivirals
	Barbiturate antiepileptics
	Barbiturate sedatives
	Benzodiazepine sedatives
	Borates
	Carbacephems
	Carbamate sedatives
	Carbapenems
	Carbazepine antiepileptics
	Cardiac glycosides
	Catechol *O*-methyl transferase inhibitors
	Cephalosporins
	Cephamycins
	Cinchona antimalarials
	Class I antiarrhythmics
	Colony-stimulating factors
	Digitalis
	Dopaminergic antiparkinsonian agents
	Ergolines
	Ergot alkaloids
	Ergot compounds
	Ester-type anaesthetics
	GABA-related antiepileptics
	Ganglion-blocking antihypertensives
	Gases
	Histamine H_2 antagonists
	Hydantoin antiepileptics
	Hydrazine monoamine oxidase-inhibiting antidepressants
	Hydroxyquinoline antiprotozoals
	Immunosuppressants

Adverse drug reaction	Pharmacological group
Confusion	Local anaesthetics
	Monoamine oxidase-inhibiting antidepressants
	Opioid analgesics
	Organic iodinated contrast media
	Osmotic diuretics
	Phenytoin
	Polymyxins
	Potassium-sparing diuretics
	Respiratory stimulants
	Salicylate analgesics
	Sedatives
	Selective serotonin reuptake-inhibiting antidepressants
	Skeletal muscle relaxants
	Smooth-muscle relaxants
	Sympathomimetics
	Tetracyclic antidepressants
	Tricyclic antidepressants
Conjunctival blanching	Centrally acting antihypertensives
Conjunctival deposits	Aliphatic phenothiazine neuroleptics
	Butyrophenone neuroleptics
	Diphenylbutylpiperidine neuroleptics
	Flupentixols
	Fluphenazine
	Haloperidols
	Neuroleptics
	Phenothiazine neuroleptics
	Piperazine phenothiazine neuroleptics
	Piperidine phenothiazine neuroleptics
	Thioxanthene neuroleptics
	Zuclopenthixols
Conjunctival vascular disorders, cysts	Centrally acting antihypertensives
Constipation	ACE inhibitors
	Aliphatic phenothiazine neuroleptics
	Analgesics and anti-inflammatory drugs
	Anorectics
	Antacid gastrointestinal agents
	Antidepressants
	Antidiarrhoeals
	Antiemetics
	Antimuscarinics
	Antineoplastics

Adverse drug reaction	Pharmacological group
Constipation	Antiulcer agents
	Benzimidazole anthelmintics
	Benzomorphan opioid analgesics
	Bile acid-binding resins
	Bisphosphonates
	Butyrophenone neuroleptics
	Carbazepine antiepileptics
	Catechol O-methyl transferase inhibitors
	Centrally acting antihypertensives
	Cephalosporins
	Class I antiarrhythmics
	Class IV antiarrhythmics
	Contrast media
	Cough suppressants
	Dermatological agents
	Diphenylbutylpiperidine neuroleptics
	Dopaminergic antiparkinsonian agents
	Ergolines
	Ferric salts
	Ferrous salts
	Flupentixols
	Fluphenazine
	Ganglion-blocking antihypertensives
	Gonad-regulating hormones
	Haloperidols
	HMG CoA reductase inhibitors
	Hydrazine monoamine oxidase-inhibiting antidepressants
	Interleukins
	Iron compounds
	Methadone and analogues
	Monoamine oxidase-inhibiting antidepressants
	Morphinan cough suppressants
	Morphinan opioid analgesics
	Neuroleptics
	Oestrogen antagonist antineoplastics
	Opioid analgesics
	Opioid antagonists
	Opioid peptides
	Opium alkaloid opioid analgesics
	Opium poppy substances
	Oral hypoglycaemics
	Pethidine and analogues
	Phenothiazine neuroleptics
	Piperazine phenothiazine neuroleptics

Adverse drug reaction	Pharmacological group
Constipation	Piperidine phenothiazine neuroleptics
	Pyrimidine antagonist antineoplastics
	Selective noradrenaline reuptake-inhibiting antidepressants
	Selective serotonin reuptake-inhibiting antidepressants
	Skeletal-muscle relaxants
	Smooth-muscle relaxants
	Tetracyclic antidepressants
	Thiazide diuretics
	Thioxanthene neuroleptics
	Tricyclic antidepressants
	Vinca alkaloid antineoplastics
	Zuclopenthixols
Contact dermatitis	Aliphatic phenothiazine neuroleptics
	Anthelmintics
	Butyrophenone neuroleptics
	Chlorinated phenol disinfectants
	Dermatological agents
	Diphenylbutylpiperidine neuroleptics
	Disinfectants
	Flupentixols
	Fluphenazine
	Haloperidols
	Neuroleptics
	Phenothiazine neuroleptics
	Piperazine phenothiazine neuroleptics
	Piperidine phenothiazine neuroleptics
	Thioxanthene neuroleptics
	Vasodilator antihypertensives
	Zuclopenthixols
Contact dermatitis: dichromate	Dermatological agents
Contact dermatitis: glycol	Glycols
Contact dermatitis: mercurials	Inorganic mercury compounds
	Organic mercurial disinfectants
Contact dermatitis: solar radiation	Dermatological agents
Contact lens corneal oedema	Oestrogens
	Sex hormones
Convulsions	4-methanolquinoline antimalarials
	4-quinolones

Adverse drug reaction	Pharmacological group
Convulsions	Aliphatic phenothiazine neuroleptics
	Amide-type anaesthetics
	Analgesics and anti-inflammatory drugs
	Anthelmintics
	Antibiotic antituberculous agents
	Antidepressants
	Antidiuretic hormones
	Antifungals
	Antivirals
	Aromatics
	Benzimidazole anthelmintics
	Benzodiazepine antagonists
	Borates
	Butyrophenone neuroleptics
	Carbapenems
	Central stimulants
	Chelating agents
	Class I antiarrhythmics
	Colony-stimulating factors
	Diphenylbutylpiperidine neuroleptics
	Dopaminergic antiparkinsonian agents
	E series prostaglandins
	Erythropoietin
	Ester-type anaesthetics
	Flupentixols
	Fluphenazine
	GABA-related antiepileptics
	Ganglion-blocking antihypertensives
	Gases
	Gastrointestinal agents
	Glycols
	H_1-antagonist antihistamines
	Haloperidols
	Hydrazide antituberculous agents
	Hydrazine monoamine oxidase-inhibiting antidepressants
	Immunosuppressants
	Lithium
	Local anaesthetics
	Monoamine oxidase-inhibiting antidepressants
	Neuroleptics
	Nitroimidazole antiprotozoals
	Opioid analgesics
	Organic iodinated contrast media
	Parenteral anaesthetics

Adverse drug reaction	Pharmacological group
Convulsions	Pethidine and analogues
	Phenothiazine antihistamines
	Phenothiazine neuroleptics
	Piperazine phenothiazine neuroleptics
	Piperidine phenothiazine neuroleptics
	Polyene antibiotics
	Posterior pituitary hormones
	Promethazines
	Respiratory stimulants
	Retinoic acid dermatological agents
	Salicylate analgesics
	Selective serotonin reuptake-inhibiting antidepressants
	Skeletal muscle relaxants
	Sympathomimetics
	Tetracyclic antidepressants
	Theophylline xanthines
	Thioxanthene neuroleptics
	Tricyclic antidepressants
	Xanthine-containing beverages
	Xanthines
	Zuclopenthixols
Coordination disorders (dyspraxia)	Antibiotic antifungals
	Antiemetics
	Antiepileptics
	H_1-antagonist antihistamines
	Lithium
	Phenothiazine antihistamines
	Promethazines
	Sedatives
Corneal deposits	4-aminoquinoline antimalarials
	Analgesics and anti-inflammatory drugs
	Antiprotozoals
	Class I antiarrhythmics
	Class III antiarrhythmics
	Dermatological agents
	Salicylate analgesics
Corneal disorders	Oestrogen antagonist antineoplastics
	Sex hormones
Corneal opacity	4-aminoquinoline antimalarials
	Aliphatic phenothiazine neuroleptics
	Butyrophenone neuroleptics
	Diphenylbutylpiperidine neuroleptics
	Flupentixols

Adverse drug reaction	*Pharmacological group*
Corneal opacity	Fluphenazine
	Haloperidols
	Hydroquinone dermatological agents
	Neuroleptics
	Phenothiazine neuroleptics
	Piperazine phenothiazine neuroleptics
	Piperidine phenothiazine neuroleptics
	Retinoic acid dermatological agents
	Thioxanthene neuroleptics
	Zuclopenthixols
Coronary artery spasm	Ergot compounds
Corpus cavernosum haematoma	E series prostaglandins
	Papaverine and analogues
Corticoadrenal insufficiency	Parenteral anaesthetics
Cough	ACE inhibitors
	Anthelmintics
	Antimony antiprotozoals
	Antineoplastics
	Antiulcer agents
	Antivirals
	Aromatics
	GABA-related antiepileptics
	Gases
	Inhalation anaesthetics
	Oestrogen antagonist antineoplastics
	Organic iodinated contrast media
	Prophylactic antiasthmatics
	Pyrimidine antagonist antineoplastics
	Respiratory stimulants
Cranial nerve palsy	4-quinolones
Creatine kinase level raised	Central stimulants
	Clofibrate and analogues
	Depolarising muscle relaxants
	HMG CoA reductase inhibitors
	Neuroleptics
Crystalluria	4-quinolones
	Gastrointestinal agents
	Skeletal muscle relaxants
Cushing's syndrome	Corticosteroids
	Corticotrophic hormones

Adverse drug reaction	Pharmacological group
Cyanide – toxic effects	Vasodilator antihypertensives
Cystitis	Analgesics and anti-inflammatory drugs Antibacterial agents Antineoplastics
Darkened tongue	Antidepressants Antidiarrhoeals Antiulcer agents Bismuth salts Histamine H_2 antagonists Skeletal muscle relaxants Tetracyclic antidepressants Tricyclic antidepressants
Deafness	Antibacterial agents Antibiotic antituberculous agents Loop diuretics Macrolides Polyene antibiotics
Debility	Borates
Decreased sweating	Alpha-blocking antihypertensives
Deformity	Dermatological agents
Degenerative skin disorders	Direct-acting anticoagulants Heparinoids Low-molecular-weight heparins
Dehydration	Antifolate antineoplastics Interleukins
Delayed recovery from anaesthesia	Parenteral anaesthetics
Delirium	Cardiac glycosides Chloral sedatives Digitalis Inhalation anaesthetics Neuroleptics
Dental fluorosis	Fluorine compounds
Depression	4-quinolones Aliphatic phenothiazine neuroleptics Alpha-blocking antihypertensives Anabolics Analgesics and anti-inflammatory drugs Anorectics

Adverse drug reaction	Pharmacological group
Depression	Antibiotic antituberculous agents
	Anticholinesterase parasympathomimetics
	Antidotes
	Antiemetics
	Antiepileptics
	Antineoplastics
	Antituberculous agents
	Antiulcer agents
	Antivirals
	Barbiturate antiepileptics
	Butyrophenone neuroleptics
	Calcium antagonist vasodilators
	Carbazepine antiepileptics
	Central stimulants
	Centrally acting antihypertensives
	Diphenylbutylpiperidine neuroleptics
	Dopaminergic antiparkinsonian agents
	Flupentixols
	Fluphenazine
	GABA-related antiepileptics
	Gonad-regulating hormones
	H_1-antagonist antihistamines
	Haloperidols
	Neuroleptics
	Norgestrels
	Oestrogens
	Phenothiazine antihistamines
	Phenothiazine neuroleptics
	Piperazine phenothiazine neuroleptics
	Piperidine phenothiazine neuroleptics
	Progestogens
	Promethazines
	Rauwolfia antihypertensives
	Retinoic acid dermatological agents
	Salicylate analgesics
	Sedatives
	Sex hormones
	Skeletal muscle relaxants
	Succinimide antiepileptics
	Thioxanthene neuroleptics
	Zuclopenthixols
Dermatosis	Antiprotozoals
Desire to defecate	Anticholinesterase parasympathomimetics
	Antidiuretic hormones
	Diagnostic agents

Adverse drug reaction	Pharmacological group
Desire to defecate	Parasympathomimetics
	Pilocarpine
	Posterior pituitary hormones
	Vasopressins
Desire to micturate	Anticholinesterase parasympathomimetics
	Diagnostic agents
	Parasympathomimetics
	Pilocarpine
	Thyrotrophic hormones
Diabetes mellitus with ketoacidosis	Antivirals
Diarrhoea	4-aminoquinoline antimalarials
	4-methanolquinoline antimalarials
	4-quinolones
	ACE inhibitors
	Adrenergic neurone-blocking antihypertensives
	Alpha-blocking antihypertensives
	Alpha-blocking vasodilators
	Alpha-glucosidase inhibitors
	Amidinopenicillins
	Amino acids
	Aminopenicillanic derivatives
	Aminopenicillins
	Anabolics
	Analgesics and anti-inflammatory drugs
	Anorectics
	Antacid gastrointestinal agents
	Anthelmintics
	Antiandrogens
	Antianginal vasodilators
	Antibacterial agents
	Antibiotic antituberculous agents
	Anticholinesterase parasympathomimetics
	Antiemetics
	Antifungals
	Antihypertensives
	Antileprotics
	Antimalarials
	Antineoplastics
	Antipseudomonal penicillins
	Antituberculous agents
	Antiulcer agents
	Antivirals

Adverse drug reaction	Pharmacological group
Diarrhoea	Aspartic acid
	Benzimidazole anthelmintics
	Benzylpenicillin and derivatives
	Beta-blockers
	Biguanide antimalarials
	Biguanide hypoglycaemics
	Bile acid-binding resins
	Bile acids and salts
	Bisphosphonates
	Borates
	Carbacephems
	Carbapenems
	Carbazepine antiepileptics
	Carboxypenicillins
	Cardiac glycosides
	Cardiac inotropic agents
	Catechol *O*-methyl transferase inhibitors
	Cation exchange resins
	Central stimulants
	Centrally acting antihypertensives
	Cephalosporins
	Cephamycins
	Chloramphenicols
	Class I antiarrhythmics
	Colchicum alkaloids
	Colony-stimulating factors
	Contrast media
	Corticosteroids
	Coumarin anticoagulants
	Dermatological agents
	Diagnostic agents
	Digitalis
	E series prostaglandins
	Edetates
	Ergolines
	Essential amino acids
	Expectorants
	F series prostaglandins
	Fat-soluble vitamins
	Ferric salts
	Ferrous salts
	Fixed oils
	Gastrointestinal agents
	Glucose tests
	Glycerol
	Glycol and glycerol esters

Adverse drug reaction	Pharmacological group
Diarrhoea	Gold salts
	Gonad-regulating hormones
	H_1-antagonist antihistamines
	Haemostatics
	HMG CoA reductase inhibitors
	Hydroxynaphthoquinones
	Hydroxyquinoline antiprotozoals
	Immunosuppressants
	Indanedione anticoagulants
	Iron compounds
	Isoxazolyl penicillins
	Leukotriene inhibitors
	Lincomycins
	Lipid-regulating agents
	Lithium
	Macrolides
	Magnesium salts
	Medicinal enzymes
	Monobactams
	Natural penicillins
	Neuroleptics
	Nitrofuran antimicrobials
	Nutritional carbohydrates
	Oestrogen antagonist antineoplastics
	Opioid antagonists
	Oral hypoglycaemics
	Organic iodinated contrast media
	Oxacephalosporins
	Oxytetracyclines
	Parasympathomimetics
	Penicillinase-resistant penicillins
	Phenoxymethylpenicillin and derivatives
	Phenoxypenicillins
	Pilocarpine
	Polyene antibiotics
	Pyrimidine antagonist antineoplastics
	Salicylate analgesics
	Sedatives
	Selective serotonin reuptake-inhibiting antidepressants
	Skeletal-muscle relaxants
	Smooth-muscle relaxants
	Somatotrophic hormones
	Sulphonamides
	Tetracyclines
	Thiazide diuretics

Adverse drug reaction	Pharmacological group
Diarrhoea	Thyroid agents
	Triazole antifungals
	Trimethoprim–sulphonamide combinations
	Typhoid vaccines
	Ureido penicillins
	Vasodilators
	Vitamin D substances
	Vitamin E substances
	Vitamins
Difficulty swallowing solids	Antimuscarinics
	Smooth-muscle relaxants
Difficulty with micturition	Aliphatic phenothiazine neuroleptics
	Alkylating antineoplastics
	Antidepressants
	Antimuscarinics
	Benzomorphan opioid analgesics
	Beta-blockers
	Butyrophenone neuroleptics
	Colony-stimulating factors
	Diphenylbutylpiperidine neuroleptics
	Flupentixols
	Fluphenazine
	Haloperidols
	Hydrazine monoamine oxidase-inhibiting antidepressants
	Methadone and analogues
	Monoamine oxidase-inhibiting antidepressants
	Morphinan opioid analgesics
	Neuroleptics
	Opioid analgesics
	Opioid peptides
	Opium alkaloid opioid analgesics
	Opium poppy substances
	Organic iodinated contrast media
	Pethidine and analogues
	Phenothiazine neuroleptics
	Piperazine phenothiazine neuroleptics
	Piperidine phenothiazine neuroleptics
	Skeletal muscle relaxants
	Smooth-muscle relaxants
	Tetracyclic antidepressants
	Thioxanthene neuroleptics
	Tricyclic antidepressants
	Zuclopenthixols

Adverse drug reaction	Pharmacological group
Diplopia/double vision	Antiepileptics
	Ergolines
	GABA-related antiepileptics
	Polyene antibiotics
	Sedatives
	Skeletal muscle relaxants
Direct Coombs test positive	Carbacephems
	Carbapenems
	Centrally acting antihypertensives
	Cephalosporins
	Cephamycins
Discoloration of teeth	Antibacterial agents
	Fluorine compounds
	Oxytetracyclines
	Tetracyclines
	Trimethoprim and derivatives
	Trimethoprim–sulphonamide combinations
Disorders of calcium metabolism	Hydantoin antiepileptics
	Phenytoin
Disorders of conjunctiva	Interleukins
Disorientation	Antiemetics
Dizziness	4-methanolquinoline antimalarials
	4-quinolones
	ACE inhibitors
	Alcoholic solvents
	Aldose reductase inhibitors
	Alpha-blocking antihypertensives
	Alpha-blocking vasodilators
	Amphetamines
	Anabolics
	Analgesics and anti-inflammatory drugs
	Angiotensin-inhibiting antihypertensives
	Anorectics
	Anthelmintics
	Antiandrogens
	Antianginal vasodilators
	Antibacterial agents
	Antibiotic antifungals
	Antibiotic antituberculous agents
	Anticholinesterase parasympathomimetics
	Antidepressants
	Antidotes

Adverse drug reaction	Pharmacological group
Dizziness	Antiemetics
	Antiepileptics
	Antihypertensives
	Antineoplastics
	Antiprotozoals
	Antituberculous agents
	Antiulcer agents
	Antivirals
	Barbiturate sedatives
	Benzimidazole anthelmintics
	Beta-2-selective stimulants
	Bisphosphonates
	Calcium antagonist vasodilators
	Carbacephems
	Carbazepine antiepileptics
	Catechol O-methyl transferase inhibitors
	Central stimulants
	Centrally acting antihypertensives
	Cephalosporins
	Cephamycins
	Chelating agents
	Cholinesterase reactivators
	Class I antiarrhythmics
	Class IV antiarrhythmics
	Clofibrate and analogues
	Contrast media
	Cough suppressants
	Cytoprotective agents
	Dermatological agents
	Diagnostic agents
	Diamidine antiprotozoals
	Dopaminergic antiparkinsonian agents
	E series prostaglandins
	Ergolines
	Ergot alkaloids
	Ergot compounds
	F series prostaglandins
	GABA-related antiepileptics
	Gases
	Gonad-regulating hormones
	Haemostatics
	Histamine H_2 antagonists
	HMG CoA reductase inhibitors
	Hydantoin antiepileptics
	Hydrazine monoamine oxidase-inhibiting antidepressants

Adverse drug reaction	Pharmacological group
Dizziness	Immunosuppressants
	Monoamine oxidase-inhibiting antidepressants
	Neuroleptics
	Nitrofuran antiprotozoals
	Nitroimidazole antiprotozoals
	Oestrogen antagonist antineoplastics
	Opioid antagonists
	Organic iodinated contrast media
	Oxazolidinedione antiepileptics
	Peripheral and cerebral vasodilators
	Phenytoin
	Pilocarpine
	Progestogens
	Prophylactic antiasthmatics
	Psoralen dermatological agents
	Respiratory stimulants
	Salicylate analgesics
	Sedatives
	Selective noradrenaline reuptake-inhibiting antidepressants
	Selective serotonin reuptake-inhibiting antidepressants
	Serotonin and analogues
	Sex hormones
	Skeletal muscle relaxants
	Smooth-muscle relaxants
	Succinimide antiepileptics
	Sympathomimetics
	Tetracyclines
	Thiazide diuretics
	Thyrotrophic hormones
	Triazole antifungals
	Uricosuric agents
	Vasodilator antihypertensives
	Vitamin B substances
Drowsiness	4-quinolones
	Adrenergic neurone-blocking antihypertensives
	Alcohol metabolism modifiers
	Alcoholic disinfectants
	Alcoholic solvents
	Aliphatic phenothiazine neuroleptics
	Alpha-blocking antihypertensives
	Analgesics and anti-inflammatory drugs

Adverse drug reaction	Pharmacological group
Drowsiness	Anorectics
	Anthelmintics
	Antiandrogens
	Antibiotic antituberculous agents
	Antidepressants
	Antidiarrhoeals
	Antiemetics
	Antiepileptics
	Antineoplastics
	Antituberculous agents
	Antiulcer agents
	Antivirals
	Asparaginase antineoplastics
	Barbiturate antiepileptics
	Barbiturate sedatives
	Benzimidazole anthelmintics
	Benzodiazepine sedatives
	Benzomorphan opioid analgesics
	Butyrophenone neuroleptics
	Calcium antagonist vasodilators
	Carbamate sedatives
	Carbazepine antiepileptics
	Cardiac glycosides
	Central stimulants
	Centrally acting antihypertensives
	Cephalosporins
	Chelating agents
	Cholinesterase reactivators
	Cough suppressants
	Cytoprotective agents
	Dermatological agents
	Diagnostic agents
	Digitalis
	Diphenylbutylpiperidine neuroleptics
	Dopaminergic antiparkinsonian agents
	Ergolines
	Ergot compounds
	Flupentixols
	Fluphenazine
	GABA-related antiepileptics
	Gonad-regulating hormones
	H_1-antagonist antihistamines
	Haloperidols
	Histamine H_2 antagonists
	Hydrazine monoamine oxidase-inhibiting antidepressants

Adverse drug reaction	Pharmacological group
Drowsiness	Lithium
	Methadone and analogues
	Monoamine oxidase-inhibiting antidepressants
	Morphinan opioid analgesics
	Neuroleptics
	Nitrofuran antiprotozoals
	Nitroimidazole antiprotozoals
	Norgestrels
	Oestrogen antagonist antineoplastics
	Opioid analgesics
	Opioid peptides
	Opium alkaloid opioid analgesics
	Opium poppy substances
	Oxazolidinedione antiepileptics
	Pethidine and analogues
	Phenothiazine antihistamines
	Phenothiazine neuroleptics
	Piperazine phenothiazine neuroleptics
	Piperidine phenothiazine neuroleptics
	Progestogens
	Promethazines
	Prophylactic antiasthmatics
	Pyrimidine antagonist antineoplastics
	Retinoic acid dermatological agents
	Salicylate analgesics
	Sedatives
	Selective serotonin reuptake-inhibiting antidepressants
	Serotonin and analogues
	Sex hormones
	Skeletal muscle relaxants
	Succinimide antiepileptics
	Sympathomimetics
	Thioxanthene neuroleptics
	Xanthine oxidase inhibitors
	Zuclopenthixols
Drug dependence	Amphetamines
	Anorectics
	Benzodiazepine sedatives
	Benzomorphan opioid analgesics
	Carbamate sedatives
	Central stimulants
	Chloral sedatives
	Methadone and analogues

Adverse drug reaction	Pharmacological group
Drug dependence	Morphinan opioid analgesics
	Opioid analgesics
	Opioid peptides
	Opium alkaloid opioid analgesics
	Opium poppy substances
	Pethidine and analogues
	Sedatives
	Skeletal muscle relaxants
Drug-induced myelopathy	Hydroxyquinoline antiprotozoals
Drug psychoses	Alcohol metabolism modifiers
	Amphetamines
	Anorectics
	Antiemetics
	Antiprotozoals
	Antituberculous agents
	Antivirals
	Central stimulants
	Dopaminergic antiparkinsonian agents
	Ergolines
	Lithium
	Parenteral anaesthetics
	Sympathomimetics
Dry cough	ACE inhibitors
Dry eyes	Antimuscarinics
	Beta-blockers
	Cardiac inotropic agents
	Cardioselective beta-blockers
	Centrally acting antihypertensives
	H_1-antagonist antihistamines
	Retinoic acid dermatological agents
	Skeletal muscle relaxants
Dry hair	Fat-soluble vitamins
	Vitamin A substances
	Vitamins
Dry mouth	Aliphatic phenothiazine neuroleptics
	Alpha-blocking antihypertensives
	Alpha-blocking vasodilators
	Amphetamines
	Analgesics and anti-inflammatory drugs
	Anorectics
	Antidepressants
	Antiemetics

Adverse drug reaction	Pharmacological group
Dry mouth	Antihypertensives
	Antimuscarinics
	Antiulcer agents
	Antivirals
	Aromatics
	Benzomorphan opioid analgesics
	Butyrophenone neuroleptics
	Catechol *O*-methyl transferase inhibitors
	Central stimulants
	Centrally acting antihypertensives
	Class I antiarrhythmics
	Dermatological agents
	Diphenylbutylpiperidine neuroleptics
	Ergolines
	Flupentixols
	Fluphenazine
	H_1-antagonist antihistamines
	Haloperidols
	Hydrazine monoamine oxidase-inhibiting antidepressants
	Methadone and analogues
	Monoamine oxidase-inhibiting antidepressants
	Morphinan opioid analgesics
	Neuroleptics
	Opioid analgesics
	Opioid peptides
	Opium alkaloid opioid analgesics
	Opium poppy substances
	Pethidine and analogues
	Phenothiazine antihistamines
	Phenothiazine neuroleptics
	Piperazine phenothiazine neuroleptics
	Piperidine phenothiazine neuroleptics
	Potassium-sparing diuretics
	Promethazines
	Prophylactic antiasthmatics
	Rauwolfia antihypertensives
	Retinoic acid dermatological agents
	Sedatives
	Selective noradrenaline reuptake-inhibiting antidepressants
	Selective serotonin reuptake-inhibiting antidepressants
	Serotonin and analogues
	Skeletal muscle relaxants

Adverse drug reaction	Pharmacological group
Dry mouth	Smooth-muscle relaxants
	Sympathomimetics
	Tetracyclic antidepressants
	Thioxanthene neuroleptics
	Tricyclic antidepressants
	Zuclopenthixols
Dry skin	Antimuscarinics
	Antivirals
	Dermatological agents
	Fat-soluble vitamins
	Gonad-regulating hormones
	Retinoic acid dermatological agents
	Smooth-muscle relaxants
	Vitamin A substances
	Vitamin B substances
	Vitamins
Duodenal ulcer (DU)	Analgesics and anti-inflammatory drugs
Dysarthria	Alcoholic disinfectants
	Class I antiarrhythmics
	GABA-related antiepileptics
	Ganglion-blocking antihypertensives
	Lithium
Dyskinesia	Aliphatic phenothiazine neuroleptics
	Butyrophenone neuroleptics
	Carbazepine antiepileptics
	Catechol *O*-methyl transferase inhibitors
	Central stimulants
	Diphenylbutylpiperidine neuroleptics
	Dopaminergic antiparkinsonian agents
	Ergolines
	Flupentixols
	Fluphenazine
	Haloperidols
	Hydantoin antiepileptics
	Neuroleptics
	Phenothiazine neuroleptics
	Phenytoin
	Piperazine phenothiazine neuroleptics
	Piperidine phenothiazine neuroleptics
	Selective serotonin reuptake-inhibiting antidepressants
	Succinimide antiepileptics
	Thioxanthene neuroleptics

Adverse drug reaction	Pharmacological group
Dyskinesia	Tricyclic antidepressants
	Zuclopenthixols
Dysmenorrhoea	Immunosuppressants
Dyspepsia	4-quinolones
	ACE inhibitors
	Anabolics
	Analgesics and anti-inflammatory drugs
	Anticholinesterase parasympathomimetics
	Antidepressants
	Antimuscarinics
	Antiulcer agents
	Antivirals
	Catechol O-methyl transferase inhibitors
	Cephalosporins
	Corticosteroids
	Dermatological agents
	E series prostaglandins
	Ergolines
	Evening primrose oil
	GABA-related antiepileptics
	Gastrointestinal agents
	H_1-antagonist antihistamines
	HMG CoA reductase inhibitors
	Interleukins
	Neuroleptics
	Oestrogen antagonist antineoplastics
	Prophylactic antiasthmatics
	Salicylate analgesics
	Selective serotonin reuptake-inhibiting antidepressants
	Smooth-muscle relaxants
	Thiazide diuretics
	Triazole antifungals
Dysphagia	4-quinolones
	Skeletal muscle relaxants
Dyspnoea	4-quinolones
	Alkylating antineoplastics
	Analgesics and anti-inflammatory drugs
	Anthelmintics
	Antiarrhythmics
	Antibacterial agents
	Antidotes
	Antiemetics
	Antineoplastics

Adverse drug reaction	Pharmacological group
Dyspnoea	Antivirals
	Class I antiarrhythmics
	Colony-stimulating factors
	Corticotrophic hormones
	Diagnostic agents
	E series prostaglandins
	Ergolines
	Ergot alkaloids
	Ergot compounds
	F series prostaglandins
	Gases
	Immunosuppressants
	Interleukins
	Iron compounds
	Neuroleptics
	Oestrogen antagonist antineoplastics
	Organic iodinated contrast media
	Pyrimidine antagonist antineoplastics
	Respiratory stimulants
	Skeletal muscle relaxants
	Vasodilators
	Vinca alkaloid antineoplastics
Dysuria	Antivirals
	Gonad-regulating hormones
	Selective noradrenaline reuptake-inhibiting antidepressants
Ecchymoses	Hyaluronic acid
	Interleukins
	Selective serotonin reuptake-inhibiting antidepressants
	Skeletal muscle relaxants
Ectopic beats	Cardiac inotropic agents
	Respiratory stimulants
Ectropion	Skeletal muscle relaxants
Electrocardiogram (ECG) abnormal	4-aminoquinoline antimalarials
	Aliphatic phenothiazine neuroleptics
	Butyrophenone neuroleptics
	Calcium antagonist vasodilators
	Diphenylbutylpiperidine neuroleptics
	Edetates
	Flupentixols
	Fluphenazine
	Haloperidols

Adverse drug reaction	Pharmacological group
Electrocardiogram (ECG) abnormal	Lithium Neuroleptics Phenothiazine neuroleptics Piperazine phenothiazine neuroleptics Piperidine phenothiazine neuroleptics Thioxanthene neuroleptics Zuclopenthixols
Electroencephalogram (EEG) abnormal	Aliphatic phenothiazine neuroleptics Butyrophenone neuroleptics Diphenylbutylpiperidine neuroleptics Flupentixols Fluphenazine Haloperidols Neuroleptics Phenothiazine neuroleptics Piperazine phenothiazine neuroleptics Piperidine phenothiazine neuroleptics Pulmonary surfactants Thioxanthene neuroleptics Zuclopenthixols
Electrolytes abnormal	Antibiotic antituberculous agents Antimalarials Antineoplastics Electrolytes
Emotional instability	Antiepileptics Oestrogen antagonist antineoplastics
Encephalitis–postplague vaccination	Vaccines
Encephalopathy	Antiandrogens Antiulcer agents Interleukin 2
Endocrine, nutritional, metabolic and immunity disorders	Immunosuppressants
Enteritis/colitis	Analgesics and anti-inflammatory drugs Gold salts Immunosuppressants Retinoic acid dermatological agents
Eosinophilia	4-quinolones Antibacterial agents Antibiotic antituberculous agents

Adverse drug reaction	Pharmacological group
Eosinophilia	Antidepressants
	Antivirals
	Carbacephems
	Carbapenems
	Cephalosporins
	Cephamycins
	Dopaminergic antiparkinsonian agents
	Lincomycins
	Neuroleptics
	Oxacephalosporins
	Skeletal muscle relaxants
	Sulphonamides
	Tetracyclic antidepressants
	Tricyclic antidepressants
	Trimethoprim–sulphonamide combinations
	Xanthine oxidase inhibitors
Epididymitis	Class III antiarrhythmics
Epigastric pain	Alpha-blocking vasodilators
	Analgesics and anti-inflammatory drugs
	Beta-blockers
	Ergolines
	Ferric salts
	Ferrous salts
	Gastrointestinal agents
	Iron compounds
	Lipid-regulating agents
	Peripheral and cerebral vasodilators
	Polyene antibiotics
	Salicylate analgesics
Epileptic seizures – clonic	Anthelmintics
	Erythropoietin
Epileptic seizures – tonic	Erythropoietin
Epileptiform seizures	Organic iodinated contrast media
Epiphora – excess lacrimation	Chelating agents
	Edetates
	Opioid antagonists
	Organic iodinated contrast media
	Pilocarpine
	Prophylactic antiasthmatics
	Skeletal muscle relaxants

Adverse drug reaction	Pharmacological group
Epistaxis	Analgesics and anti-inflammatory drugs
	Angiotensin-inhibiting antihypertensives
	Antidiuretic hormones
	Colony-stimulating factors
	Corticosteroids
	Ergolines
	Gold salts
	Posterior pituitary hormones
	Retinoic acid dermatological agents
Erythema	4-methanolquinoline antimalarials
	4-quinolones
	ACE inhibitors
	Aliphatic phenothiazine neuroleptics
	Analgesics and anti-inflammatory drugs
	Antiandrogens
	Antibacterial agents
	Antibiotic antifungals
	Antifungals
	Antiulcer agents
	Benzimidazole anthelmintics
	Bisphosphonates
	Borates
	Butyrophenone neuroleptics
	Calcium antagonist vasodilators
	Carbacephems
	Carbapenems
	Carbazepine antiepileptics
	Central stimulants
	Centrally acting antihypertensives
	Cephalosporins
	Cephamycins
	Chelating agents
	Chloramphenicols
	Class I antiarrhythmics
	Class IV antiarrhythmics
	Contrast media
	Dermatological agents
	Diphenylbutylpiperidine neuroleptics
	E series prostaglandins
	F series prostaglandins
	Flupentixols
	Fluphenazine
	Gastrointestinal agents
	Haloperidols
	Hyaluronic acid

Adverse drug reaction	Pharmacological group
Erythema	Hydantoin antiepileptics
	Hydrazide antituberculous agents
	Hydroquinone dermatological agents
	Lipid-regulating agents
	Medicinal enzymes
	Neuroleptics
	Nitrofuran antimicrobials
	Oestrogens
	Oral hypoglycaemics
	Organic iodinated contrast media
	Oxytetracyclines
	Phenothiazine neuroleptics
	Phenytoin
	Piperazine phenothiazine neuroleptics
	Piperidine phenothiazine neuroleptics
	Psoralen dermatological agents
	Pyrethroid pesticides
	Pyrimidine antagonist antineoplastics
	Retinoic acid dermatological agents
	Rubefacient vasodilators
	Sex hormones
	Succinimide antiepileptics
	Sulphonamides
	Sulphonylurea hypoglycaemics
	Tetracyclines
	Thiazide diuretics
	Thiouracil antithyroid agents
	Thioxanthene neuroleptics
	Trimethoprim–sulphonamide combinations
	Vaccines
	Vasodilator antihypertensives
	Vitamin B substances
	Vitamin D substances
	Zuclopenthixols
Erythema multiforme	Antibacterial agents
	Antibiotic antifungals
	Central stimulants
	Oxazolidinedione antiepileptics
	Succinimide antiepileptics
Erythrocyte sedimentation rate raised	Fat-soluble vitamins
	Vitamin A substances
	Vitamins

Adverse drug reaction	Pharmacological group
Euphoria	Amphetamines
	Anabolics
	Analgesics and anti-inflammatory drugs
	Anorectics
	Antiemetics
	Central stimulants
	Centrally acting antihypertensives
	Corticosteroids
	Corticotrophic hormones
	Dopaminergic antiparkinsonian agents
	Prophylactic antiasthmatics
	Sedatives
	Skeletal muscle relaxants
	Succinimide antiepileptics
Exanthema	Analgesics and anti-inflammatory drugs
	Antidepressants
	Beta-2-selective stimulants
	Oestrogen antagonist antineoplastics
	Typhoid vaccines
Excessive belching	Antidiuretic hormones
	Omega-3 triglycerides
	Posterior pituitary hormones
	Vasopressins
Excessive flatulence	Lipid-regulating agents
Excessive salivation	Anticholinesterase parasympathomimetics
	Antiepileptics
	Antituberculous agents
	Benzodiazepine sedatives
	Blood products
	Calcium antagonist vasodilators
	Carbamate sedatives
	Inhalation anaesthetics
	Neuroleptics
	Parasympathomimetics
	Pilocarpine
	Respiratory stimulants
	Skeletal muscle relaxants
Excessive sweating	Amphetamines
	Analgesics and anti-inflammatory drugs
	Anorectics
	Antianginal vasodilators
	Anticholinesterase parasympathomimetics
	Antidepressants

Adverse drug reaction	Pharmacological group
Excessive sweating	Antidotes
	Benzomorphan opioid analgesics
	Beta-adrenoceptor stimulants
	Beta-sympathomimetic vasodilators
	Beta-2-selective stimulants
	Catechol O-methyl transferase inhibitors
	Central stimulants
	Chelating agents
	Colony-stimulating factors
	Diphenylbutylpiperidine neuroleptics
	Dopaminergic antiparkinsonian agents
	F series prostaglandins
	Fat-soluble vitamins
	Gonad-regulating hormones
	H_1-antagonist antihistamines
	Histamine H_2 antagonists
	Hydrazine monoamine oxidase-inhibiting antidepressants
	I series prostaglandins
	Isoprenaline
	Methadone and analogues
	Monoamine oxidase-inhibiting antidepressants
	Morphinan opioid analgesics
	Opioid analgesics
	Opioid antagonists
	Opioid peptides
	Opium alkaloid opioid analgesics
	Opium poppy substances
	Parasympathomimetics
	Pethidine and analogues
	Phenothiazine antihistamines
	Pilocarpine
	Promethazines
	Retinoic acid dermatological agents
	Sedatives
	Selective serotonin reuptake-inhibiting antidepressants
	Skeletal muscle relaxants
	Tetracyclic antidepressants
	Thyroid agents
	Tricyclic antidepressants
	Vasodilator antihypertensives
	Vitamin D substances
	Vitamins

Adverse drug reaction	Pharmacological group
Excessive thirst	Antiandrogens
	Antimuscarinics
	Fat-soluble vitamins
	Opioid antagonists
	Smooth-muscle relaxants
	Vitamin D substances
	Vitamins
Exfoliative dermatitis	Amidinopenicillins
	Aminoglycosides
	Aminopenicillanic derivatives
	Aminopenicillins
	Antibacterial agents
	Antipseudomonal penicillins
	Benzylpenicillin and derivatives
	Beta-lactamase inhibitors
	Carbapenems
	Carboxypenicillins
	Class IV antiarrhythmics
	Dithranols
	Gold salts
	Isoxazolyl penicillins
	Natural penicillins
	Oxytetracyclines
	Penicillinase-resistant penicillins
	Phenoxymethylpenicillin and derivatives
	Phenoxypenicillins
	Retinoic acid dermatological agents
	Skeletal muscle relaxants
	Sulphonamides
	Tetracyclines
	Theophylline xanthines
	Tricyclic antidepressants
	Ureido penicillins
Exfoliative erythema	Retinoic acid dermatological agents
Extrapyramidal symptoms	Aliphatic phenothiazine neuroleptics
	Alpha-blocking antihypertensives
	Antiemetics
	Antihypertensives
	Butyrophenone neuroleptics
	Centrally acting antihypertensives
	Diphenylbutylpiperidine neuroleptics
	Flupentixols
	Fluphenazine
	Gastrointestinal agents

Adverse drug reaction	*Pharmacological group*
Extrapyramidal symptoms	H₁-antagonist antihistamines
	Haloperidols
	Neuroleptics
	Phenothiazine antihistamines
	Phenothiazine neuroleptics
	Piperazine phenothiazine neuroleptics
	Piperidine phenothiazine neuroleptics
	Promethazines
	Selective serotonin reuptake-inhibiting antidepressants
	Thioxanthene neuroleptics
	Vasodilator antihypertensives
	Zuclopenthixols
Eye pain	Calcium antagonist vasodilators
Eye symptoms	Centrally acting antihypertensives
Eyelid entropion/trichiasis	Skeletal muscle relaxants
Faecal impaction	Ferric salts
	Ferrous salts
	Iron compounds
Faeces colour: dark	Antidiarrhoeals
	Antiulcer agents
	Bismuth salts
	Histamine H₂ antagonists
Falls	Dopaminergic antiparkinsonian agents
	Sedatives
Fatigue	ACE inhibitors
	Alcohol metabolism modifiers
	Alpha-blocking antihypertensives
	Analgesics and anti-inflammatory drugs
	Angiotensin-inhibiting antihypertensives
	Antiandrogens
	Antibiotic antifungals
	Antidepressants
	Antidotes
	Antiemetics
	Antiepileptics
	Antineoplastics
	Antivirals
	Beta-blockers
	Calcium antagonist vasodilators
	Cardiac glycosides
	Cardioselective beta-blockers

Adverse drug reaction	Pharmacological group
Fatigue	Central stimulants
	Class I antiarrhythmics
	Class III antiarrhythmics
	Class IV antiarrhythmics
	Clofibrate and analogues
	Colony-stimulating factors
	Digitalis
	Dopaminergic antiparkinsonian agents
	GABA-related antiepileptics
	Gonad-regulating hormones
	H_1-antagonist antihistamines
	Histamine H_2 antagonists
	HMG CoA reductase inhibitors
	Hydrazine monoamine oxidase-inhibiting antidepressants
	Immunosuppressants
	Leukotriene inhibitors
	Lipid-regulating agents
	Monoamine oxidase-inhibiting antidepressants
	Neuroleptics
	Oestrogen antagonist antineoplastics
	Opioid antagonists
	Sedatives
	Serotonin and analogues
	Skeletal muscle relaxants
	Thiazide diuretics
	Trace elements
	Vaccines
Feels hot/feverish	Antineoplastics
	Aromatics
	Serotonin and analogues
Female genital organ symptoms	Gonad-regulating hormones
Feminising effects	Oestrogens
	Sex hormones
Fertility problems	Alkyl sulphonate antineoplastics
	Alkylating antineoplastics
	Anabolics
	Carbazepine antiepileptics
	Ethyleneimine antineoplastics
	Nitrogen mustards
	Nitrosoureas

Adverse drug reaction	Pharmacological group
Fertility problems	Sulphur mustards
	Triazene antineoplastics
Fever	4-quinolones
	Anthelmintics
	Antifolate antineoplastics
	Antineoplastics
	Antithyroid agents
	Antiulcer agents
	Antivirals
	Cardiac inotropic agents
	Edetates
	Gonad-regulating hormones
	Leech products
	Platelet-activating factor antagonists
	Triazole antifungals
Fibrosing alveolitis	Class I antiarrhythmics
	Class III antiarrhythmics
	Gastrointestinal agents
Fibrosis of penis	E series prostaglandins
	Papaverine and analogues
Flatulence/wind	4-quinolones
	Alpha-glucosidase inhibitors
	Analgesics and anti-inflammatory drugs
	Antacid gastrointestinal agents
	Antimuscarinics
	Antiulcer agents
	Antivirals
	Aromatics
	Bile acid-binding resins
	Bulk laxatives
	Cephalosporins
	Chloral sedatives
	Corticosteroids
	Dichloroacetamide antiprotozoals
	E series prostaglandins
	HMG CoA reductase inhibitors
	Hypoglycaemics
	Laxatives
	Lipid-regulating agents
	Nutritional carbohydrates
	Somatotrophic hormones
	Sweetening agents
	Triazole antifungals

Adverse drug reaction	Pharmacological group
Fluid retention	Adrenergic neurone-blocking antihypertensives
	Anabolics
	Analgesics and anti-inflammatory drugs
	Androgens
	Antidiuretic hormones
	Antineoplastics
	Antiulcer agents
	Centrally acting antihypertensives
	Corticosteroids
	Corticotrophic hormones
	Liquorice
	Norgestrels
	Oestrogen antagonist antineoplastics
	Oestrogens
	Posterior pituitary hormones
	Progestogens
	Rauwolfia antihypertensives
	Salicylate analgesics
	Sex hormones
	Testosterones
	Uricosuric agents
	Vasodilator antihypertensives
Fluid/electrolyte/acid–base disorders	Neuroleptics
Flushing	ACE inhibitors
	Alpha-blocking vasodilators
	Analgesics and anti-inflammatory drugs
	Angiotensin-inhibiting antihypertensives
	Antiandrogens
	Antianginal vasodilators
	Antiarrhythmics
	Antibacterial agents
	Antibiotic antituberculous agents
	Antidepressants
	Antidotes
	Antiemetics
	Antihypertensives
	Antimuscarinics
	Antineoplastics
	Antivirals
	Benzodiazepine antagonists
	Benzomorphan opioid analgesics
	Beta-sympathomimetic vasodilators
	Beta-2-selective stimulants

Adverse drug reaction	Pharmacological group
Flushing	Calcitonin
	Calcium antagonist vasodilators
	Cinchona antimalarials
	Class IV antiarrhythmics
	Competitive muscle relaxants
	Corticotrophic hormones
	Cytoprotective agents
	Diagnostic agents
	Diamidine antiprotozoals
	Dopaminergic antiparkinsonian agents
	E series prostaglandins
	Ergolines
	Ergot compounds
	F series prostaglandins
	Gonad-regulating hormones
	Hyaluronic acid
	I series prostaglandins
	Inhalation anaesthetics
	Iron compounds
	Lipid-regulating agents
	Magnesium salts
	Methadone and analogues
	Morphinan opioid analgesics
	Oestrogen antagonist antineoplastics
	Opioid analgesics
	Opioid peptides
	Opium alkaloid opioid analgesics
	Opium poppy substances
	Organic iodinated contrast media
	Peripheral and cerebral vasodilators
	Pethidine and analogues
	Progestogens
	Rubefacient vasodilators
	Serotonin and analogues
	Sex hormones
	Smooth-muscle relaxants
	Somatotrophic hormones
	Sulphonylurea hypoglycaemics
	Thyroid agents
	Thyrotrophic hormones
	Uricosuric agents
	Vasodilators
	Vitamin B substances
Folate-deficiency anaemia	Barbiturate antiepileptics
	Gastrointestinal agents

Adverse drug reaction	Pharmacological group
Folate-deficiency anaemia	Hydantoin antiepileptics
	Phenytoin
Frostbite	Local anaesthetics
Fructose in urine	Nutritional carbohydrates
Full blood count abnormal	Analgesics and anti-inflammatory drugs
	Vasodilator antihypertensives
Galactorrhoea	Aliphatic phenothiazine neuroleptics
	Antiandrogens
	Antiemetics
	Butyrophenone neuroleptics
	Carbazepine antiepileptics
	Diphenylbutylpiperidine neuroleptics
	Flupentixols
	Fluphenazine
	Haloperidols
	Neuroleptics
	Phenothiazine neuroleptics
	Piperazine phenothiazine neuroleptics
	Piperidine phenothiazine neuroleptics
	Selective serotonin reuptake-inhibiting antidepressants
	Thioxanthene neuroleptics
	Tricyclic antidepressants
	Zuclopenthixols
Gall stones	Somatotrophic hormones
Gallbladder disorders, incl. cholestasis	ACE inhibitors
	Aliphatic phenothiazine neuroleptics
	Analgesics and anti-inflammatory drugs
	Antiandrogens
	Antibacterial agents
	Antibiotic antifungals
	Beta-lactamase inhibitors
	Chelating agents
	Coumarin anticoagulants
	Gold salts
	Histamine H_2 antagonists
	Hydantoin antiepileptics
	Immunosuppressants
	Indanedione anticoagulants
	Isoxazolyl penicillins
	Macrolides
	Methadone and analogues

Adverse drug reaction	Pharmacological group
Gallbladder disorders, incl. cholestasis	Neuroleptics Nitrofuran antimicrobials Oestrogen antagonist antineoplastics Oral hypoglycaemics Phenytoin Sex hormones Skeletal muscle relaxants Sulphonamides Sulphonylurea hypoglycaemics Thiouracil antithyroid agents Thiourea antithyroid agents Tricyclic antidepressants Trimethoprim–sulphonamide combinations
Gangrene	Ergot alkaloids Ergot compounds
Gastric ulcer	Analgesics and anti-inflammatory drugs Medicinal enzymes
Gastritis	Analgesics and anti-inflammatory drugs Antiepileptics Antiulcer agents Chloral sedatives Ergolines
Gastrointestinal disturbances	4-aminoquinoline antimalarials Alcohol metabolism modifiers Aldosterone inhibitors Alkylating antineoplastics Alpha-blocking antihypertensives Amphetamines Anabolics Anorectics Anthelmintics Antiandrogens Antibacterial agents Antibiotic antituberculous agents Anticholinesterase parasympathomimetics Antidepressants Antidotes Antiepileptics Antifolate antineoplastics Antineoplastics Antiprotozoals Antituberculous agents Antiulcer agents Antivirals

Adverse drug reaction	Pharmacological group
Gastrointestinal disturbances	Benzodiazepine sedatives
	Beta-blockers
	Biguanide antimalarials
	Bisphosphonates
	Borates
	Calcium antagonist vasodilators
	Calcium salts
	Carbamate sedatives
	Cardiac inotropic agents
	Cardioselective beta-blockers
	Central stimulants
	Centrally acting antihypertensives
	Chelating agents
	Class I antiarrhythmics
	Clofibrate and analogues
	Corticosteroids
	Cough suppressants
	Diagnostic agents
	Dopaminergic antiparkinsonian agents
	Ergot compounds
	Expectorants
	Ferric salts
	Ferrous salts
	GABA-related antiepileptics
	Gonad-regulating hormones
	H_1-antagonist antihistamines
	Haemostatics
	Hydrazine monoamine oxidase-inhibiting antidepressants
	Immunosuppressants
	Inhalation anaesthetics
	Iron compounds
	Lipid-regulating agents
	Lithium
	Loop diuretics
	Medicinal enzymes
	Mercurial diuretics
	Monoamine oxidase-inhibiting antidepressants
	Mucolytics
	Neuroleptics
	Nitroimidazole antiprotozoals
	Norgestrels
	Oestrogen antagonist antineoplastics
	Oral hypoglycaemics
	Parasympathomimetics

Adverse drug reaction	Pharmacological group
Gastrointestinal disturbances	Pesticides
	Phenothiazine antihistamines
	Pilocarpine
	Potassium-sparing diuretics
	Progestogens
	Promethazines
	Sedatives
	Sex hormones
	Skeletal muscle relaxants
	Somatotrophic hormones
	Succinimide antiepileptics
	Sulphonylurea hypoglycaemics
	Sympathomimetics
	Theophylline xanthines
	Thiazide diuretics
	Trace elements
	Uricosuric agents
	Vasodilator antihypertensives
	Vegetable astringents
	Xanthine-containing beverages
	Xanthine oxidase inhibitors
	Xanthines
Gastrointestinal haemorrhage	Alpha-blocking vasodilators
	Analgesics and anti-inflammatory drugs
	Antivirals
	Colchicum alkaloids
	Dopaminergic antiparkinsonian agents
	Selective serotonin reuptake-inhibiting antidepressants
	Uricosuric agents
Gastrojejunal ulcer	Analgesics and anti-inflammatory drugs
Giddiness	Antileprotics
	Haemostatics
	Lithium
Gilles de la Tourette's disorder	Central stimulants
Gingival hyperplasia	Calcium antagonist vasodilators
	Class IV antiarrhythmics
	Hydantoin antiepileptics
	Immunosuppressants
	Phenytoin

Adverse drug reaction	Pharmacological group
Gingivitis	Lipid-regulating agents
Glossitis	Gold salts Macrolides Sulphonamides Trimethoprim–sulphonamide combinations
Glucose tolerance test impaired	Somatotrophic hormones
Goitre	Analgesics and anti-inflammatory drugs Antithyroid agents Iodides Iodine compounds Iodine radiopharmaceuticals Iodophors Lithium
Goodpasture's syndrome	Chelating agents
Gout	Loop diuretics Thiazide diuretics
Granulomatous hepatitis	Analgesics and anti-inflammatory drugs Carbazepine antiepileptics Centrally acting antihypertensives Cinchona antimalarials Class I antiarrhythmics Hydantoin antiepileptics Oral hypoglycaemics Phenytoin Sulphonamides Sulphonylurea hypoglycaemics Vasodilator antihypertensives Xanthine oxidase inhibitors
Granulomatous lesions	Retinoic acid dermatological agents
Griping pain	Anthraquinone glycosides Docusate Laxatives Picosulphate
Growth retardation in children	Amphetamines Anorectics Central stimulants Corticosteroids Corticotrophic hormones

Adverse drug reaction	*Pharmacological group*
Guillain–Barré syndrome	Medicinal enzymes
Gynaecomastia	Aldosterone inhibitors
	Aliphatic phenothiazine neuroleptics
	Anorectics
	Antiandrogens
	Antiemetics
	Antiepileptics
	Antiulcer agents
	Butyrophenone neuroleptics
	Carbazepine antiepileptics
	Class IV antiarrhythmics
	Diphenylbutylpiperidine neuroleptics
	Flupentixols
	Fluphenazine
	Gonad-regulating hormones
	Gonadotrophic hormones
	Haloperidols
	Histamine H_2 antagonists
	Hydrazide antituberculous agents
	Imidazole antifungals
	Immunosuppressants
	Neuroleptics
	Nitrogen mustards
	Phenothiazine neuroleptics
	Piperazine phenothiazine neuroleptics
	Piperidine phenothiazine neuroleptics
	Thioxanthene neuroleptics
	Zuclopenthixols
Haematemesis	Analgesics and anti-inflammatory drugs
	Salicylate analgesics
Haematocrit – PCV – low	Antivirals
	Coumarin anticoagulants
	Indanedione anticoagulants
	Interleukins
Haematology result abnormal	Analgesics and anti-inflammatory drugs
Haemoglobin estimation	Angiotensin-inhibiting antihypertensives
Haemoglobin low	Antivirals
	GABA-related antiepileptics
	Interleukins
Haemolysis, haemoglobinuria	Antidotes
	Dermatological agents

Adverse drug reaction	Pharmacological group
Haemolytic anaemia	4-quinolones
	8-aminoquinoline antimalarials
	Aliphatic phenothiazine neuroleptics
	Analgesics and anti-inflammatory drugs
	Antiandrogens
	Antibacterial agents
	Antibiotic antituberculous agents
	Antimalarials
	Butyrophenone neuroleptics
	Carbacephems
	Centrally acting antihypertensives
	Cephalosporins
	Cephamycins
	Chelating agents
	Diphenylbutylpiperidine neuroleptics
	Dopaminergic antiparkinsonian agents
	Flupentixols
	Fluphenazine
	Haloperidols
	Neuroleptics
	Phenothiazine neuroleptics
	Piperazine phenothiazine neuroleptics
	Piperidine phenothiazine neuroleptics
	Selective serotonin reuptake-inhibiting antidepressants
	Thioxanthene neuroleptics
	Vasodilator antihypertensives
	Zuclopenthixols
Haemolytic–uraemic syndrome	Immunosuppressants
	Pyrimidine antagonist antineoplastics
Haemorrhage	Analgesics and anti-inflammatory drugs
	Antidepressants
	Coumarin anticoagulants
	Direct-acting anticoagulants
	Gold salts
	Heparinoids
	Hydrazide antituberculous agents
	Indanedione anticoagulants
	Leech products
	Low-molecular-weight heparins
	Platelet-activating factor antagonists
	Skeletal muscle relaxants
	Sulphonamides
	Tetracyclic antidepressants
	Thiouracil antithyroid agents

Adverse drug reaction	Pharmacological group
Haemorrhage	Tricyclic antidepressants
	Trimethoprim–sulphonamide combinations
Haemorrhage of rectum and anus	Analgesics and anti-inflammatory drugs
	Contrast media
	Salicylate analgesics
Haemorrhagic bullae	4-quinolones
Haemorrhagic cystitis	Antineoplastics
	Nitrogen mustards
Haemorrhagic disorder	Medicinal enzymes
Halitosis	Alcohol metabolism modifiers
Hallucinations	4-quinolones
	Analgesics and anti-inflammatory drugs
	Anorectics
	Anthelmintics
	Antidepressants
	Antiemetics
	Antifungals
	Antimuscarinics
	Antineoplastics
	Antiulcer agents
	Antivirals
	Aromatics
	Benzomorphan opioid analgesics
	Cardiac glycosides
	Catechol O-methyl transferase inhibitors
	Central stimulants
	Class I antiarrhythmics
	Digitalis
	Dopaminergic antiparkinsonian agents
	Ergolines
	Hydrazine monoamine oxidase-inhibiting antidepressants
	Methadone and analogues
	Monoamine oxidase-inhibiting antidepressants
	Morphinan opioid analgesics
	Opioid analgesics
	Opioid peptides
	Opium alkaloid opioid analgesics
	Opium poppy substances
	Parenteral anaesthetics

Adverse drug reaction	Pharmacological group
Hallucinations	Pethidine and analogues
	Respiratory stimulants
	Sedatives
	Skeletal muscle relaxants
	Smooth-muscle relaxants
Has a sore throat	Antineoplastics
Has numbness	Sedatives
Headache	4-aminoquinoline antimalarials
	4-methanolquinoline antimalarials
	4-quinolones
	ACE inhibitors
	Adrenergic-neurone-blocking antihypertensives
	Alcoholic solvents
	Aldosterone inhibitors
	Alpha-adrenoceptor stimulants
	Alpha-blocking antihypertensives
	Alpha-blocking vasodilators
	Amphetamines
	Anabolics
	Analgesics and anti-inflammatory drugs
	Angiotensin-inhibiting antihypertensives
	Anorectics
	Anthelmintics
	Antiandrogens
	Antianginal vasodilators
	Antibiotic antifungals
	Antibiotic antituberculous agents
	Anticholinesterase parasympathomimetics
	Antidepressants
	Antidiuretic hormones
	Antidotes
	Antiemetics
	Antiepileptics
	Antifolate antineoplastics
	Antifungals
	Antihypertensives
	Antileprotics
	Antimuscarinics
	Antineoplastics
	Antiprotozoals
	Antituberculous agents
	Antiulcer agents
	Antivirals

Adverse drug reaction	Pharmacological group
Headache	Barbiturate sedatives
	Benzimidazole anthelmintics
	Benzodiazepine sedatives
	Benzomorphan opioid analgesics
	Beta-adrenoceptor stimulants
	Beta-blockers
	Beta-2-selective stimulants
	Bisphosphonates
	Calcium antagonist vasodilators
	Carbacephems
	Carbamate sedatives
	Carbapenems
	Carbazepine antiepileptics
	Carbonic anhydrase inhibitors
	Cardiac glycosides
	Cardiac inotropic agents
	Catechol O-methyl transferase inhibitors
	Central stimulants
	Centrally acting antihypertensives
	Cephalosporins
	Cephamycins
	Chelating agents
	Chloral sedatives
	Cholinesterase reactivators
	Cinchona antimalarials
	Class I antiarrhythmics
	Class III antiarrhythmics
	Class IV antiarrhythmics
	Clofibrate and analogues
	Colony-stimulating factors
	Contrast media
	Corticosteroids
	Cough suppressants
	Dermatological agents
	Diagnostic agents
	Digitalis
	Dopaminergic antiparkinsonian agents
	E series prostaglandins
	Edetates
	Ergolines
	Ergot alkaloids
	Ergot compounds
	Evening primrose oil
	F series prostaglandins
	Fat-soluble vitamins
	GABA-related antiepileptics

Adverse drug reaction	Pharmacological group
Headache	Gases
	Gastrointestinal agents
	Gonad-regulating hormones
	Gonadotrophic hormones
	H_1-antagonist antihistamines
	Haemostatics
	Histamine H_2 antagonists
	HMG CoA reductase inhibitors
	Hyaluronic acid
	Hydantoin antiepileptics
	Hydrazine monoamine oxidase-inhibiting antidepressants
	Hydroxynaphthoquinones
	I series prostaglandins
	Imidazole antifungals
	Immunosuppressants
	Inhalation anaesthetics
	Isoprenaline
	Leukotriene inhibitors
	Lipid-regulating agents
	Macrolides
	Methadone and analogues
	Monoamine oxidase-inhibiting antidepressants
	Morphinan opioid analgesics
	Mucolytics
	Neuroleptics
	Nitrofuran antiprotozoals
	Nitroimidazole antiprotozoals
	Oestrogen antagonist antineoplastics
	Oestrogens
	Opioid analgesics
	Opioid antagonists
	Opioid peptides
	Opium alkaloid opioid analgesics
	Opium poppy substances
	Oral hypoglycaemics
	Organic iodinated contrast media
	Osmotic diuretics
	Oxazolidinedione antiepileptics
	Oxytetracyclines
	Pethidine and analogues
	Phenothiazine antihistamines
	Phenytoin
	Polyene antibiotics
	Posterior pituitary hormones

Adverse drug reaction	Pharmacological group
Headache	Progestogens
	Promethazines
	Prophylactic antiasthmatics
	Psoralen dermatological agents
	Retinoic acid dermatological agents
	Salicylate analgesics
	Sedatives
	Selective serotonin reuptake-inhibiting antidepressants
	Sex hormones
	Skeletal muscle relaxants
	Smooth-muscle relaxants
	Succinimide antiepileptics
	Sulphone antileprotics
	Sulphonylurea hypoglycaemics
	Sympathomimetics
	Tetracyclines
	Theophylline xanthines
	Thiazide diuretics
	Thiouracil antithyroid agents
	Thiourea antithyroid agents
	Thyroid agents
	Triazole antifungals
	Uricosuric agents
	Vaccines
	Vasodilator antihypertensives
	Vasodilators
	Vitamin B substances
	Vitamin D substances
	Vitamins
	Xanthine-containing beverages
	Xanthine oxidase inhibitors
	Xanthines
Hearing difficulty	Chelating agents
	Retinoic acid dermatological agents
Hearing symptoms	4-quinolones
Heart failure	Anabolics
	Anthelmintics
	Antiandrogens
	Antiulcer agents
	Beta-blockers
	Cardioselective beta-blockers
	Class I antiarrhythmics
	Colony-stimulating factors
	Liquorice

Adverse drug reaction	Pharmacological group
Heartburn	Antibacterial agents Bile acid-binding resins Ergot compounds Gastrointestinal agents Lipid-regulating agents
Heinz-body anaemia	Gastrointestinal agents
Hemianopia	Ergolines
Hepatic coma	Anabolics
Hepatomegaly	Antituberculous agents Antivirals Fat-soluble vitamins Vitamin A substances Vitamins
Hiccough	Barbiturate anaesthetics Cytoprotective agents Oxazolidinedione antiepileptics Succinimide antiepileptics
Hirsutism	Anabolics Corticosteroids Corticotrophic hormones Hydantoin antiepileptics Immunosuppressants Norgestrels Oestrogen antagonist antineoplastics Phenytoin Progestogens Sex hormones Vasodilator antihypertensives
Hoarseness	Retinoic acid dermatological agents
Hyperactivity	Carbacephems Cephalosporins Cephamycins
Hyperaemia of conjunctiva	Alpha-blocking vasodilators Centrally acting antihypertensives F series prostaglandins H_1-antagonist antihistamines
Hyperaesthesia	Antivirals
Hyperammonaemia	Antiepileptics Expectorants

Adverse drug reaction	Pharmacological group
Hypercalcaemia	Anabolics
	Androgens
	Antacid gastrointestinal agents
	Calcium salts
	Fat-soluble vitamins
	Gonad-regulating hormones
	Sex hormones
	Testosterones
	Thiazide diuretics
	Vitamin A substances
	Vitamin D substances
	Vitamins
Hypercalciuria	Fat-soluble vitamins
	Vitamin D substances
	Vitamins
Hyperfibrinogenaemia	Blood-clotting factors
Hyperglycaemia	Analgesics and anti-inflammatory drugs
	Antidepressants
	Antivirals
	Asparaginase antineoplastics
	Diamidine antiprotozoals
	Glucose tests
	HMG CoA reductase inhibitors
	Hydrazide antituberculous agents
	Immunosuppressants
	Loop diuretics
	Neuroleptics
	Progestogens
	Sex hormones
	Skeletal muscle relaxants
	Somatotrophic hormones
	Tetracyclic antidepressants
	Thiazide diuretics
	Tricyclic antidepressants
	Vasodilator antihypertensives
Hyperkalaemia	ACE inhibitors
	Aldosterone inhibitors
	Analgesics and anti-inflammatory drugs
	Angiotensin-inhibiting antihypertensives
	Depolarising muscle relaxants
	Diamidine antiprotozoals
	Erythropoietin
	Immunosuppressants

Adverse drug reaction	Pharmacological group
Hyperkalaemia	Potassium salts
	Potassium-sparing diuretics
Hyperkinesia	Barbiturate antiepileptics
	Ergolines
	Neuroleptics
Hyperphosphataemia	Electrolyte anions
	Erythropoietin
	Fat-soluble vitamins
	Vitamin D substances
	Vitamins
Hyperpigmentation	Antineoplastics
	Tetracyclines
Hyperpyrexia	Borates
Hyperreflexia	Lithium
Hypertension	Alpha-adrenoceptor stimulants
	Amphetamines
	Analgesics and anti-inflammatory drugs
	Anorectics
	Antidepressants
	Antineoplastics
	Antiulcer agents
	Antivirals
	Benzodiazepine antagonists
	Beta-adrenoceptor stimulants
	Beta-1-selective stimulants
	Central stimulants
	Chelating agents
	Corticosteroids
	Corticotrophic hormones
	Dopaminergic antiparkinsonian agents
	Ergot alkaloids
	Ergot compounds
	Erythropoietin
	F series prostaglandins
	Gases
	Gonad-regulating hormones
	Immunosuppressants
	Inhalation anaesthetics
	Liquorice
	Neuroleptics
	Opioid analgesics
	Oxytocic hormones

Adverse drug reaction	Pharmacological group
Hypertension	Parenteral anaesthetics
	Pilocarpine
	Platelet-activating factor antagonists
	Respiratory stimulants
	Salicylate analgesics
	Serotonin and analogues
	Skeletal muscle relaxants
	Sympathomimetics
	Thyrotrophic hormones
	Xanthine oxidase inhibitors
Hypertensive encephalopathy	Erythropoietin
Hypertonic uterus	E series prostaglandins
	F series prostaglandins
Hypertrophic cardiomyopathy	Immunosuppressants
Hypertrophy of breast	Oestrogens
	Sex hormones
	Tricyclic antidepressants
Hypertrophy of clitoris	Progestogens
	Sex hormones
Hypertrophy of salivary gland	Beta-sympathomimetic vasodilators
	Beta-2-selective stimulants
Hyperventilation	Cholinesterase reactivators
Hypervitaminosis A	Retinoic acid dermatological agents
Hypocalcaemia	Antineoplastics
	Antivirals
	Bisphosphonates
	Cytoprotective agents
	Diamidine antiprotozoals
	Loop diuretics
Hypochloraemia	Loop diuretics
	Thiazide diuretics
Hypoglycaemia	4-quinolones
	Alcoholic disinfectants
	Antidepressants
	Antituberculous agents
	Antivirals
	Cinchona antimalarials
	Class I antiarrhythmics

Adverse drug reaction	Pharmacological group
Hypoglycaemia	Diamidine antiprotozoals
	HMG CoA reductase inhibitors
	Insulin
	Insulin zinc suspensions
	Oral hypoglycaemics
	Skeletal muscle relaxants
	Tetracyclic antidepressants
	Tricyclic antidepressants
Hypokalaemia	Antineoplastics
	Antiulcer agents
	Beta-blockers
	Beta-2-selective stimulants
	Carbonic anhydrase inhibitors
	Carboxypenicillins
	Corticosteroids
	Corticotrophic hormones
	Diphenylbutylpiperidine neuroleptics
	E series prostaglandins
	Glucose tests
	Interleukins
	Liquorice
	Lithium
	Loop diuretics
	Penicillinase-resistant penicillins
	Polyene antibiotics
	Thiazide diuretics
Hypomagnesaemia	Aminoglycosides
	Antibacterial agents
	Antineoplastics
	Bisphosphonates
	Cation exchange resins
	Immunosuppressants
	Loop diuretics
	Polyene antibiotics
	Thiazide diuretics
Hypomania	Antidepressants
	Barbiturate antiepileptics
	Dopaminergic antiparkinsonian agents
	Hydrazine monoamine oxidase-inhibiting antidepressants
	Monoamine oxidase-inhibiting antidepressants
	Selective serotonin reuptake-inhibiting antidepressants

Adverse drug reaction	Pharmacological group
Hypomania	Skeletal muscle relaxants
	Tetracyclic antidepressants
	Tricyclic antidepressants
Hypoparathyroidism	Iodine radiopharmaceuticals
Hypophosphataemia	Antineoplastics
Hyposmolality/ hyponatraemia	ACE inhibitors
	Aldosterone inhibitors
	Analgesics and anti-inflammatory drugs
	Antidepressants
	Antidiuretic hormones
	Carbazepine antiepileptics
	Hydrazine monoamine oxidase-inhibiting antidepressants
	Loop diuretics
	Monoamine oxidase-inhibiting antidepressants
	Posterior pituitary hormones
	Potassium-sparing diuretics
	Selective serotonin reuptake-inhibiting antidepressants
	Skeletal muscle relaxants
	Sulphonylurea hypoglycaemics
	Tetracyclic antidepressants
	Thiazide diuretics
	Tricyclic antidepressants
	Vinca alkaloid antineoplastics
Hypotension	4-quinolones
	ACE inhibitors
	Alcoholic disinfectants
	Aliphatic phenothiazine neuroleptics
	Alpha-blocking antihypertensives
	Amide-type anaesthetics
	Anorectics
	Antianginal vasodilators
	Antibacterial agents
	Anticholinesterase parasympathomimetics
	Antidiarrhoeals
	Antidotes
	Antiemetics
	Antineoplastics
	Antivirals
	Benzodiazepine sedatives
	Benzomorphan opioid analgesics
	Beta-adrenoceptor stimulants

Adverse drug reaction	Pharmacological group
Hypotension	Beta-sympathomimetic vasodilators
	Beta-2-selective stimulants
	Butyrophenone neuroleptics
	Calcium antagonist vasodilators
	Carbamate sedatives
	Cardiac inotropic agents
	Central stimulants
	Centrally acting antihypertensives
	Chelating agents
	Class I antiarrhythmics
	Class II antiarrhythmics
	Class IV antiarrhythmics
	Colony-stimulating factors
	Competitive muscle relaxants
	Corticotrophic hormones
	Cytoprotective agents
	Diagnostic agents
	Diamidine antiprotozoals
	Diphenylbutylpiperidine neuroleptics
	Dopaminergic antiparkinsonian agents
	E series prostaglandins
	Edetates
	Ergolines
	Ester-type anaesthetics
	Flupentixols
	Fluphenazine
	H_1-antagonist antihistamines
	Haloperidols
	Hydantoin antiepileptics
	I series prostaglandins
	Immunosuppressants
	Inhalation anaesthetics
	Interleukin 2
	Isoprenaline
	Local anaesthetics
	Loop diuretics
	Medicinal enzymes
	Mercurial diuretics
	Methadone and analogues
	Morphinan opioid analgesics
	Neuroleptics
	Opioid analgesics
	Opioid peptides
	Opium alkaloid opioid analgesics
	Opium poppy substances
	Organic iodinated contrast media

Adverse drug reaction	Pharmacological group
Hypotension	Parasympathomimetics
	Peripheral and cerebral vasodilators
	Pethidine and analogues
	Phenothiazine antihistamines
	Phenothiazine neuroleptics
	Phenytoin
	Pilocarpine
	Piperazine phenothiazine neuroleptics
	Piperidine phenothiazine neuroleptics
	Potassium-sparing diuretics
	Promethazines
	Pyrimidine antagonist antineoplastics
	Sedatives
	Selective noradrenaline reuptake-inhibiting antidepressants
	Selective serotonin reuptake-inhibiting antidepressants
	Skeletal muscle relaxants
	Sympathomimetics
	Thioxanthene neuroleptics
	Triazole antifungals
	Vasodilator antihypertensives
	Vasodilators
	Zuclopenthixols
Hypothermia	Aliphatic phenothiazine neuroleptics
	Benzomorphan opioid analgesics
	Butyrophenone neuroleptics
	Diphenylbutylpiperidine neuroleptics
	Flupentixols
	Fluphenazine
	Haloperidols
	Methadone and analogues
	Morphinan opioid analgesics
	Neuroleptics
	Opioid analgesics
	Opioid peptides
	Opium alkaloid opioid analgesics
	Opium poppy substances
	Pethidine and analogues
	Phenothiazine neuroleptics
	Piperazine phenothiazine neuroleptics
	Piperidine phenothiazine neuroleptics
	Thioxanthene neuroleptics
	Zuclopenthixols

Adverse drug reaction	Pharmacological group
Impotence	ACE inhibitors
	Aldosterone inhibitors
	Aliphatic phenothiazine neuroleptics
	Anorectics
	Antiandrogens
	Antidepressants
	Antiulcer agents
	Butyrophenone neuroleptics
	Carbazepine antiepileptics
	Centrally acting antihypertensives
	Clofibrate and analogues
	Diphenylbutylpiperidine neuroleptics
	Flupentixols
	Fluphenazine
	Gonad-regulating hormones
	Haloperidols
	Histamine H_2 antagonists
	HMG CoA reductase inhibitors
	Neuroleptics
	Opioid antagonists
	Phenothiazine neuroleptics
	Piperazine phenothiazine neuroleptics
	Piperidine phenothiazine neuroleptics
	Selective noradrenaline reuptake-inhibiting antidepressants
	Thiazide diuretics
	Thioxanthene neuroleptics
	Zuclopenthixols
Inappropriate ADH secretion syndrome	Antidepressants
	Carbazepine antiepileptics
	Lithium
	Skeletal muscle relaxants
	Sulphonylurea hypoglycaemics
	Tetracyclic antidepressants
	Tricyclic antidepressants
	Vinca alkaloid antineoplastics
Incontinence of urine	Alpha-blocking antihypertensives
	Neuroleptics
	Skeletal muscle relaxants
Incontinent of faeces	Lipid-regulating agents
Increased growth	Androgens
	Sex hormones
	Testosterones

Adverse drug reaction	Pharmacological group
Increased menstrual loss	Gonad-regulating hormones
Indirect Coombs test positive	Carbapenems Centrally acting antihypertensives
Induration of skin at site of injection	Aliphatic phenothiazine neuroleptics Butyrophenone neuroleptics Carbapenems Diphenylbutylpiperidine neuroleptics Flupentixols Fluphenazine Haloperidols Lincomycins Neuroleptics Phenothiazine neuroleptics Piperazine phenothiazine neuroleptics Piperidine phenothiazine neuroleptics Thioxanthene neuroleptics Vaccines Vinca alkaloid antineoplastics Zuclopenthixols
Infection	Antifolate antineoplastics Antineoplastics Immunosuppressants
Inflammation of eyelids	Beta-2-selective stimulants H_1-antagonist antihistamines Skeletal muscle relaxants
Influenza-like syndrome	Antibiotic antituberculous agents Antiepileptics Antiulcer agents Antivirals Chelating agents Erythropoietin Leukotriene inhibitors Lipid-regulating agents Tetracyclic antidepressants
Inhibited female orgasm	Antidepressants
Inhibited male orgasm	Adrenergic neurone-blocking antihypertensives Alpha-blocking antihypertensives Antidepressants Centrally acting antihypertensives Opioid antagonists

Adverse drug reaction	Pharmacological group
Insomnia	4-quinolones
	ACE inhibitors
	Aliphatic phenothiazine neuroleptics
	Amphetamines
	Anabolics
	Analgesics and anti-inflammatory drugs
	Anorectics
	Anthelmintics
	Antiandrogens
	Anticholinesterase parasympathomimetics
	Antidepressants
	Antiemetics
	Antiepileptics
	Antihypertensives
	Antimalarials
	Antiulcer agents
	Antivirals
	Beta-blockers
	Beta-2-selective stimulants
	Butyrophenone neuroleptics
	Calcium antagonist vasodilators
	Carbacephems
	Cardiac inotropic agents
	Cardioselective beta-blockers
	Catechol O-methyl transferase inhibitors
	Central stimulants
	Centrally acting antihypertensives
	Cephalosporins
	Cephamycins
	Class III antiarrhythmics
	Corticosteroids
	Diphenylbutylpiperidine neuroleptics
	Dopaminergic antiparkinsonian agents
	Ergolines
	Ergot compounds
	Flupentixols
	Fluphenazine
	Ganglion-blocking antihypertensives
	Gonad-regulating hormones
	H_1-antagonist antihistamines
	Haloperidols
	HMG CoA reductase inhibitors
	Hydantoin antiepileptics
	Hydroxynaphthoquinones
	Monoamine oxidase-inhibiting antidepressants

Adverse drug reaction	Pharmacological group
Insomnia	Neuroleptics
	Norgestrels
	Opioid antagonists
	Oxazolidinedione antiepileptics
	Phenothiazine antihistamines
	Phenothiazine neuroleptics
	Phenytoin
	Piperazine phenothiazine neuroleptics
	Piperidine phenothiazine neuroleptics
	Progestogens
	Promethazines
	Pyrimidine antagonist antineoplastics
	Salicylate analgesics
	Selective noradrenaline reuptake-inhibiting antidepressants
	Selective serotonin reuptake-inhibiting antidepressants
	Sex hormones
	Skeletal muscle relaxants
	Sulphone antileprotics
	Sympathomimetics
	Theophylline xanthines
	Thioxanthene neuroleptics
	Xanthine-containing beverages
	Xanthines
	Zuclopenthixols
Interstitial lung disease	Antiandrogens
Interstitial nephritis	4-quinolones
	ACE inhibitors
	Amidinopenicillins
	Aminopenicillanic derivatives
	Aminopenicillins
	Antibacterial agents
	Antibiotic antituberculous agents
	Antipseudomonal penicillins
	Antituberculous agents
	Antiulcer agents
	Barbiturate antiepileptics
	Benzylpenicillin and derivatives
	Beta-lactamase inhibitors
	Carbacephems
	Carboxypenicillins
	Centrally acting antihypertensives
	Cephalosporins
	Cephamycins

Adverse drug reaction	Pharmacological group
Interstitial nephritis	Gastrointestinal agents
	Histamine H_2 antagonists
	Hydantoin antiepileptics
	Hydrazide antituberculous agents
	Immunosuppressants
	Isoxazolyl penicillins
	Loop diuretics
	Macrolides
	Natural penicillins
	Penicillinase-resistant penicillins
	Phenoxymethylpenicillin and derivatives
	Phenoxypenicillins
	Phenytoin
	Sulphonamides
	Tetracyclines
	Thiazide diuretics
	Ureido penicillins
	Xanthine oxidase inhibitors
Interstitial pneumonia	Antifolate antineoplastics
	Chelating agents
	Class III antiarrhythmics
	Gastrointestinal agents
	Gold salts
	Nitrofuran antimicrobials
	Nitrofuran antiprotozoals
Intestinal obstruction	Bulk laxatives
	Hypoglycaemics
Intracerebral haemorrhage	Sympathomimetics
Intravascular coagulation	Cinchona antimalarials
Involuntary movements	Barbiturate anaesthetics
	Dopaminergic antiparkinsonian agents
	Parenteral anaesthetics
	Selective serotonin reuptake-inhibiting antidepressants
Iritis	Analgesics and anti-inflammatory drugs
	F series prostaglandins
Irritability	Amphetamines
	Anorectics
	Antidotes
	Antiepileptics
	Aromatics

Adverse drug reaction	Pharmacological group
Irritability	Central stimulants
	GABA-related antiepileptics
	Opioid antagonists
	Respiratory stimulants
	Sedatives
Ischaemic heart disease	Serotonin and analogues
Itching	4-quinolones
	Analgesics and anti-inflammatory drugs
	Anthelmintics
	Antifungals
	Antineoplastics
	Antiulcer agents
	Antivirals
	Calcium antagonist vasodilators
	Central stimulants
	Cephalosporins
	Cough suppressants
	Dermatological agents
	Hyaluronic acid
	Imidazole antifungals
	Leukotriene inhibitors
	Lipid-regulating agents
	Oestrogens
	Oral hypoglycaemics
	Prophylactic antiasthmatics
	Psoralen dermatological agents
	Retinoic acid dermatological agents
	Sex hormones
	Triazole antifungals
	Vitamin D substances
Itchy eyes	H_1-antagonist antihistamines
	Organic iodinated contrast media
Jaundice	4-quinolones
	ACE inhibitors
	Aliphatic phenothiazine neuroleptics
	Anabolics
	Androgens
	Antiandrogens
	Antibacterial agents
	Antibiotic antituberculous agents
	Antidepressants
	Antiepileptics
	Antifungals
	Antituberculous agents

Adverse drug reaction	Pharmacological group
Jaundice	Benzodiazepine sedatives
	Beta-lactamase inhibitors
	Borates
	Butyrophenone neuroleptics
	Carbamate sedatives
	Carbazepine antiepileptics
	Carbonic anhydrase inhibitors
	Chelating agents
	Class I antiarrhythmics
	Diphenylbutylpiperidine neuroleptics
	Flupentixols
	Fluphenazine
	Haloperidols
	HMG CoA reductase inhibitors
	Hydrazine monoamine oxidase-inhibiting antidepressants
	Inhalation anaesthetics
	Leukotriene inhibitors
	Lincomycins
	Macrolides
	Monoamine oxidase-inhibiting antidepressants
	Neuroleptics
	Nitrofuran antimicrobials
	Nitrofuran antiprotozoals
	Norgestrels
	Oestrogen antagonist antineoplastics
	Oestrogens
	Oral hypoglycaemics
	Phenothiazine neuroleptics
	Piperazine phenothiazine neuroleptics
	Piperidine phenothiazine neuroleptics
	Progestogens
	Retinoic acid dermatological agents
	Sedatives
	Sex hormones
	Skeletal muscle relaxants
	Sulphonamides
	Sulphonylurea hypoglycaemics
	Tetracyclic antidepressants
	Thiazide diuretics
	Thiouracil antithyroid agents
	Thiourea antithyroid agents
	Thioxanthene neuroleptics
	Tricyclic antidepressants
	Trimethoprim–sulphonamide combinations

Adverse drug reaction	Pharmacological group
Jaundice	Uricosuric agents
	Zuclopenthixols
Keratitis	Skeletal muscle relaxants
Ketonuria	Chloral sedatives
L-eye completely blind	Hydroxyquinoline antiprotozoals
Lactic acidosis	Antivirals
	Biguanide hypoglycaemics
	Nutritional carbohydrates
Lactose intolerance	Nutritional carbohydrates
Lagophthalmos	Skeletal muscle relaxants
Laryngeal oedema	Medicinal enzymes
	Organic iodinated contrast media
Laryngospasm	Inhalation anaesthetics
	Respiratory stimulants
Lens opacity	Antineoplastics
Leukocytosis	Aliphatic phenothiazine neuroleptics
	Antibiotic antituberculous agents
	Antiulcer agents
	Butyrophenone neuroleptics
	Diphenylbutylpiperidine neuroleptics
	E series prostaglandins
	F series prostaglandins
	Flupentixols
	Fluphenazine
	Haloperidols
	Neuroleptics
	Phenothiazine neuroleptics
	Piperazine phenothiazine neuroleptics
	Piperidine phenothiazine neuroleptics
	Thioxanthene neuroleptics
	Zuclopenthixols
Leukopenia	4-methanolquinoline antimalarials
	4-quinolones
	Aliphatic phenothiazine neuroleptics
	Amidinopenicillins
	Aminopenicillanic derivatives
	Aminopenicillins
	Analgesics and anti-inflammatory drugs
	Antibacterial agents

Adverse drug reaction	Pharmacological group
Leukopenia	Antibiotic antifungals
	Antibiotic antituberculous agents
	Antidepressants
	Antiepileptics
	Antifungals
	Antipseudomonal penicillins
	Antithyroid agents
	Antiulcer agents
	Antivirals
	Benzimidazole anthelmintics
	Benzylpenicillin and derivatives
	Beta-sympathomimetic vasodilators
	Beta-2-selective stimulants
	Butyrophenone neuroleptics
	Carbazepine antiepileptics
	Carboxypenicillins
	Central stimulants
	Chelating agents
	Diamidine antiprotozoals
	Diphenylbutylpiperidine neuroleptics
	Dopaminergic antiparkinsonian agents
	Flupentixols
	Fluphenazine
	Gastrointestinal agents
	H_1-antagonist antihistamines
	Haloperidols
	Hydantoin antiepileptics
	Hydrazine monoamine oxidase-inhibiting antidepressants
	Immunosuppressants
	Indanedione anticoagulants
	Inhalation anaesthetics
	Isoxazolyl penicillins
	Monoamine oxidase-inhibiting antidepressants
	Natural penicillins
	Neuroleptics
	Nitroimidazole antiprotozoals
	Organic iodinated contrast media
	Oxacephalosporins
	Penicillinase-resistant penicillins
	Phenothiazine neuroleptics
	Phenoxymethylpenicillin and derivatives
	Phenoxypenicillins
	Phenytoin
	Piperazine phenothiazine neuroleptics

Adverse drug reaction	Pharmacological group
Leukopenia	Piperidine phenothiazine neuroleptics
	Progestogens
	Pyrimidine antagonist antineoplastics
	Sex hormones
	Skeletal muscle relaxants
	Succinimide antiepileptics
	Sulphonamides
	Tetracyclic antidepressants
	Thioxanthene neuroleptics
	Tricyclic antidepressants
	Trimethoprim–sulphonamide combinations
	Ureido penicillins
	Zuclopenthixols
Leukorrhoea	Cephalosporins
Lichenified skin	Beta-blockers
Lid retraction or lag	Centrally acting antihypertensives
Light-headedness	Analgesics and anti-inflammatory drugs
	Anthelmintics
	Antiarrhythmics
	Antidepressants
	Antivirals
	Benzodiazepine sedatives
	Calcium antagonist vasodilators
	Carbamate sedatives
	Dopaminergic antiparkinsonian agents
	Gastrointestinal agents
	Oestrogen antagonist antineoplastics
	Sedatives
	Sex hormones
	Skeletal muscle relaxants
	Vasodilators
Liver enzymes abnormal	4-quinolones
	Angiotensin-inhibiting antihypertensives
	Anthelmintics
	Antiandrogens
	Antibiotic antituberculous agents
	Antidepressants
	Antiemetics
	Antifolate antineoplastics
	Antimalarials
	Antineoplastics
	Antiulcer agents
	Antivirals

Adverse drug reaction	Pharmacological group
Liver enzymes abnormal	Bile acids and salts
	Calcium antagonist vasodilators
	Carbapenems
	Central stimulants
	Cephalosporins
	Chelating agents
	Colony-stimulating factors
	Dopaminergic antiparkinsonian agents
	H_1-antagonist antihistamines
	Leukotriene inhibitors
	Low-molecular-weight heparins
	Mucolytics
	Oestrogen antagonist antineoplastics
	Oral hypoglycaemics
	Parasympathomimetics
	Pyrimidine antagonist antineoplastics
	Retinoic acid dermatological agents
	Sedatives
	Sex hormones
	Skeletal muscle relaxants
	Sulphonylurea hypoglycaemics
	Uricosuric agents
Liver function tests abnormal	4-methanolquinoline antimalarials
	Acetylurea antiepileptics
	Aldosterone inhibitors
	Aliphatic phenothiazine neuroleptics
	Alkylating antineoplastics
	Alpha-blocking vasodilators
	Anabolics
	Analgesics and anti-inflammatory drugs
	Angiotensin-inhibiting antihypertensives
	Anthelmintics
	Antiandrogens
	Antibacterial agents
	Antibiotic antituberculous agents
	Antiepileptics
	Antifungals
	Antineoplastics
	Antituberculous agents
	Antiulcer agents
	Antivirals
	Aromatics
	Asparaginase antineoplastics
	Beta-blockers
	Bile acids and salts

Adverse drug reaction	Pharmacological group
Liver function tests abnormal	Borates
	Butyrophenone neuroleptics
	Calcium antagonist vasodilators
	Cardiac inotropic agents
	Catechol O-methyl transferase inhibitors
	Central stimulants
	Centrally acting antihypertensives
	Cephalosporins
	Coumarin anticoagulants
	Diamidine antiprotozoals
	Diphenylbutylpiperidine neuroleptics
	Flupentixols
	Fluphenazine
	GABA-related antiepileptics
	H_1-antagonist antihistamines
	Haloperidols
	Histamine H_2 antagonists
	HMG CoA reductase inhibitors
	Immunosuppressants
	Indanedione anticoagulants
	Inhalation anaesthetics
	Interleukin 2
	Laxatives
	Methadone and analogues
	Neuroleptics
	Nitrogen mustards
	Oestrogens
	Opioid antagonists
	Parasympathomimetics
	Peripheral and cerebral vasodilators
	Phenothiazine antihistamines
	Phenothiazine neuroleptics
	Piperazine phenothiazine neuroleptics
	Piperidine phenothiazine neuroleptics
	Polyene antibiotics
	Promethazines
	Pyrimidine antagonist antineoplastics
	Selective noradrenaline reuptake-inhibiting antidepressants
	Selective serotonin reuptake-inhibiting antidepressants
	Serotonin and analogues
	Sex hormones
	Skeletal muscle relaxants
	Somatotrophic hormones
	Succinimide antiepileptics

Adverse drug reaction	Pharmacological group
Liver function tests abnormal	Tannic acid and derivatives
	Tetracyclines
	Thioxanthene neuroleptics
	Triazole antifungals
	Uricosuric agents
	Vitamin B substances
	Xanthine oxidase inhibitors
	Zuclopenthixols
Liver moderately enlarged	Leukotriene inhibitors
Local irritation	4-quinolones
	Aldehyde disinfectants
	Aluminium astringents
	Antifungals
	Aromatic solvents
	Aromatics
	Biguanide disinfectants
	Carbamate pesticides
	Carbonic anhydrase inhibitors
	Cellulose-derived viscosity modifiers
	Chlorinated pesticides
	Chlorine-releasing substances
	Dermatological agents
	Disinfectants
	Dithranols
	F series prostaglandins
	Formaldehyde and related compounds
	Glycols
	H_1-antagonist antihistamines
	Hydroquinone dermatological agents
	Hydroxyquinoline antiprotozoals
	Magnesium salts
	Medicinal enzymes
	Organic solvents
	Organophosphate pesticides
	Pesticides
	Phenol disinfectants
	Podophyllums
	Prophylactic antiasthmatics
	Pyrethroid pesticides
	Retinoic acid dermatological agents
	Rubefacient vasodilators
	Tars
	Triphenylmethane disinfectant dyes
	Vitamin B substances

Adverse drug reaction	Pharmacological group
Locomotor impairment	H_1-antagonist antihistamines
	Organic iodinated contrast media
	Phenothiazine antihistamines
	Promethazines
Loss of libido	Alcohol metabolism modifiers
	Anorectics
	Antiandrogens
	Antidepressants
	Antiemetics
	Benzodiazepine sedatives
	Carbamate sedatives
	Gonad-regulating hormones
	Hydrazine monoamine oxidase-inhibiting antidepressants
	Monoamine oxidase-inhibiting antidepressants
	Norgestrels
	Progestogens
	Selective serotonin reuptake-inhibiting antidepressants
	Sex hormones
	Skeletal muscle relaxants
	Tetracyclic antidepressants
	Tricyclic antidepressants
Lung disease	Nitrofuran antimicrobials
	Nitrofuran antiprotozoals
Lupus erythematosus	Hydrazide antituberculous agents
Lymphadenopathy	Anthelmintics
	Antiepileptics
	Carbazepine antiepileptics
	Hydantoin antiepileptics
	Oxazolidinedione antiepileptics
	Phenytoin
	Xanthine oxidase inhibitors
Lymphoedema	Antiandrogens
	Somatotrophic hormones
Lymphopenia	Bisphosphonates
	Immunosuppressants
Malaise/lethargy	4-aminoquinoline antimalarials
	Aldosterone inhibitors
	Alpha-blocking antihypertensives
	Anorectics

Adverse drug reaction	Pharmacological group
Malaise/lethargy	Anthelmintics
	Antiandrogens
	Anticholinesterase parasympathomimetics
	Antidotes
	Antiepileptics
	Antifolate antineoplastics
	Antineoplastics
	Antiulcer agents
	Antivirals
	Barbiturate antiepileptics
	Calcium antagonist vasodilators
	Central stimulants
	Chelating agents
	Edetates
	Encephalitis vaccines
	Ergolines
	Fat-soluble vitamins
	Influenza vaccines
	Leukotriene inhibitors
	Lipid-regulating agents
	Measles vaccine
	Oestrogen antagonist antineoplastics
	Opioid antagonists
	Oxazolidinedione antiepileptics
	Pesticides
	Poliomyelitis vaccines
	Pyrimidine antagonist antineoplastics
	Retinoic acid dermatological agents
	Sedatives
	Skeletal muscle relaxants
	Specific immunoglobulins
	Typhoid vaccines
	Vaccines
	Vitamin D substances
	Vitamins
	Xanthine oxidase inhibitors
Malignant hyperpyrexia	Aliphatic phenothiazine neuroleptics
	Butyrophenone neuroleptics
	Competitive muscle relaxants
	Depolarising muscle relaxants
	Diphenylbutylpiperidine neuroleptics
	Flupentixols
	Fluphenazine
	Haloperidols
	Inhalation anaesthetics
	Neuroleptics

Adverse drug reaction	Pharmacological group
Malignant hyperpyrexia	Parenteral anaesthetics Phenothiazine neuroleptics Piperazine phenothiazine neuroleptics Piperidine phenothiazine neuroleptics Thioxanthene neuroleptics Zuclopenthixols
Malignant neoplasm of thyroid gland	Iodine radiopharmaceuticals
Mastodynia – pain in breast	Antiandrogens Gonad-regulating hormones Norgestrels Oestrogens Progestogens Sex hormones Vasodilator antihypertensives
Megaloblastic anaemia	Antibiotic antituberculous agents Trimethoprim and derivatives Trimethoprim–sulphonamide combinations
Melaena	Analgesics and anti-inflammatory drugs Salicylate analgesics
Memory loss – amnesia	Antimuscarinics Benzodiazepine sedatives Carbamate sedatives GABA-related antiepileptics Hydroxyquinoline antiprotozoals Sedatives Skeletal muscle relaxants Smooth-muscle relaxants
Meningism	Benzimidazole anthelmintics Organic iodinated contrast media
Meningitis – aseptic	Analgesics and anti-inflammatory drugs Salicylate analgesics
Menopause	Gonad-regulating hormones
Menorrhagia	E series prostaglandins Gold salts
Menstrual disorders	Aldosterone inhibitors Aliphatic phenothiazine neuroleptics Antibiotic antituberculous agents Borates Butyrophenone neuroleptics

Adverse drug reaction	Pharmacological group
Menstrual disorders	Corticosteroids
	Diphenylbutylpiperidine neuroleptics
	Flupentixols
	Fluphenazine
	Gonad-regulating hormones
	Haloperidols
	Lipid-regulating agents
	Neuroleptics
	Norgestrels
	Phenothiazine neuroleptics
	Piperazine phenothiazine neuroleptics
	Piperidine phenothiazine neuroleptics
	Progestogens
	Retinoic acid dermatological agents
	Sex hormones
	Thioxanthene neuroleptics
	Tricyclic antidepressants
	Zuclopenthixols
Mercury – toxic effect	Inorganic mercury compounds
	Mercurial dermatological agents
	Organic mercurial disinfectants
Metabolic acidosis	4-quinolones
	Alcoholic disinfectants
	Nutritional carbohydrates
Metabolic alkalosis	Electrolyte anions
	Loop diuretics
	Thiazide diuretics
Methaemoglobinaemia	8-aminoquinoline antimalarials
	Amide-type anaesthetics
	Antianginal vasodilators
	Antidotes
	Dermatological agents
	Disinfectants
Microangiopathic haemolytic anaemia	Pyrimidine antagonist antineoplastics
Micturition frequency	Pilocarpine
Migraine	Anabolics
	Gonad-regulating hormones
Mild memory disturbance	GABA-related antiepileptics
	Sedatives

Adverse drug reaction	Pharmacological group
Mood changes	ACE inhibitors
	Benzomorphan opioid analgesics
	Gases
	Gonad-regulating hormones
	Gonadotrophic hormones
	Methadone and analogues
	Morphinan opioid analgesics
	Opioid analgesics
	Opioid peptides
	Opium alkaloid opioid analgesics
	Opium poppy substances
	Pethidine and analogues
	Retinoic acid dermatological agents
	Sedatives
Multiple pregnancy	Gonadotrophic hormones
Muscle cramps	ACE inhibitors
	Aldosterone inhibitors
	Anabolics
	Antiulcer agents
	Beta-2-selective stimulants
	Calcium antagonist vasodilators
	Carbonic anhydrase inhibitors
	Central stimulants
	Corticosteroids
	Diagnostic agents
	Diuretics
	Edetates
	Ergolines
	Ergot compounds
	Histamine H_2 antagonists
	HMG CoA reductase inhibitors
	Immunosuppressants
	Loop diuretics
	Mercurial diuretics
	Oestrogen antagonist antineoplastics
	Osmotic diuretics
	Potassium-sparing diuretics
	Sympathomimetics
	Thiazide diuretics
	Thyroid agents
Muscle hypertonia	Carbacephems
	Cephalosporins
	Cephamycins
	Parenteral anaesthetics

Adverse drug reaction	Pharmacological group
Muscle hypotonia	Antiepileptics
Muscle spasm	Progestogens
	Sex hormones
Muscle weakness	4-methanolquinoline antimalarials
	4-quinolones
	Alpha-blocking antihypertensives
	Antibiotic antituberculous agents
	Anticholinesterase parasympathomimetics
	Antidepressants
	Antiulcer agents
	Beta-blockers
	Carbamate sedatives
	Cholinesterase reactivators
	E series prostaglandins
	Hydrazine monoamine oxidase-inhibiting antidepressants
	Immunosuppressants
	Liquorice
	Lithium
	Monoamine oxidase-inhibiting antidepressants
	Parasympathomimetics
	Pilocarpine
	Polymyxins
	Sedatives
	Serotonin and analogues
	Skeletal muscle relaxants
Muscular fasciculation	Antianginal vasodilators
	Anticholinesterase parasympathomimetics
	Depolarising muscle relaxants
	Gases
	Parasympathomimetics
	Pilocarpine
	Respiratory stimulants
	Skeletal muscle relaxants
Muscular incoordination	Anthelmintics
Musculoskeletal pain	Antibiotic antituberculous agents
	Antifolate antineoplastics
	Antineoplastics
	Antivirals
	Bisphosphonates
	Colony-stimulating factors
	Depolarising muscle relaxants

Adverse drug reaction	Pharmacological group
Musculoskeletal pain	Gonad-regulating hormones
	Immunosuppressants
	Oestrogen antagonist antineoplastics
	Opioid antagonists
	Polyene antibiotics
	Skeletal muscle relaxants
Myalgia	4-methanolquinoline antimalarials
	4-quinolones
	Analgesics and anti-inflammatory drugs
	Anthelmintics
	Antidepressants
	Antifungals
	Antineoplastics
	Antiulcer agents
	Antivirals
	Beta-2-selective stimulants
	Clofibrate and analogues
	Colony-stimulating factors
	Depolarising muscle relaxants
	Edetates
	Gonad-regulating hormones
	H_1-antagonist antihistamines
	Histamine H_2 antagonists
	Interleukins
	Loop diuretics
	Phenothiazine antihistamines
	Promethazines
	Retinoic acid dermatological agents
	Sex hormones
	Thiourea antithyroid agents
Myalgia/myositis	Cardiac inotropic agents
	Clofibrate and analogues
	HMG CoA reductase inhibitors
Myasthenia gravis	Oxazolidinedione antiepileptics
Myasthenic syndrome	Aminoglycosides
	Antibacterial agents
	Chelating agents
	Clofibrate and analogues
Mycoses	Antivirals
	Corticosteroids
	Corticotrophic hormones
	Immunosuppressants

Adverse drug reaction	Pharmacological group
Myoclonus	Carbapenems
	Class I antiarrhythmics
Myoglobinuria	Clofibrate and analogues
	HMG CoA reductase inhibitors
Myopathy	Antibiotic antituberculous agents
	Antivirals
	Class III antiarrhythmics
	Clofibrate and analogues
	Expectorants
	Haemostatics
	HMG CoA reductase inhibitors
	Immunosuppressants
Myopia	Thiazide diuretics
Nail disorders	Antineoplastics
Nasal congestion	Adrenergic neurone-blocking antihypertensives
	Aliphatic phenothiazine neuroleptics
	Alpha-adrenoceptor stimulants
	Alpha-blocking antihypertensives
	Butyrophenone neuroleptics
	Centrally acting antihypertensives
	Cough suppressants
	Diphenylbutylpiperidine neuroleptics
	Dopaminergic antiparkinsonian agents
	Edetates
	Ergot compounds
	Flupentixols
	Fluphenazine
	Haemostatics
	Haloperidols
	Neuroleptics
	Phenothiazine neuroleptics
	Piperazine phenothiazine neuroleptics
	Piperidine phenothiazine neuroleptics
	Rauwolfia antihypertensives
	Sedatives
	Smooth-muscle relaxants
	Thioxanthene neuroleptics
	Zuclopenthixols
Nasal symptoms	Antivirals
Nausea	4-aminoquinoline antimalarials
	4-methanolquinoline antimalarials

Adverse drug reaction	Pharmacological group
Nausea	4-quinolones
	8-aminoquinoline antimalarials
	ACE inhibitors
	Alcohol metabolism modifiers
	Aldosterone inhibitors
	Alkyl sulphonate antineoplastics
	Alkylating antineoplastics
	Alpha-blocking antihypertensives
	Alpha-blocking vasodilators
	Amino acids
	Aminopenicillins
	Anabolics
	Analgesics and anti-inflammatory drugs
	Angiotensin-inhibiting antihypertensives
	Anthelmintics
	Anthracycline antibiotic antineoplastics
	Antiandrogens
	Antianginal vasodilators
	Antiarrhythmics
	Antibacterial agents
	Antibiotic antifungals
	Antibiotic antineoplastics
	Antibiotic antituberculous agents
	Anticholinesterase parasympathomimetics
	Antidepressants
	Antidiarrhoeals
	Antidiuretic hormones
	Antidotes
	Antiemetics
	Antiepileptics
	Antifolate antineoplastics
	Antifungals
	Antihypertensives
	Antileprotics
	Antimalarials
	Antineoplastics
	Antiprotozoals
	Antithyroid agents
	Antituberculous agents
	Antiulcer agents
	Antivirals
	Aromatics
	Asparaginase antineoplastics
	Aspartic acid
	Barbiturate antiepileptics
	Benzimidazole anthelmintics

Adverse drug reaction	Pharmacological group
Nausea	Benzodiazepine antagonists
	Benzomorphan opioid analgesics
	Beta-blockers
	Beta-sympathomimetic vasodilators
	Beta-1-selective stimulants
	Beta-2-selective stimulants
	Biguanide hypoglycaemics
	Bile acid-binding resins
	Bismuth salts
	Bisphosphonates
	Blood products
	Calcitonin
	Calcium antagonist vasodilators
	Carbacephems
	Carbapenems
	Carbazepine antiepileptics
	Cardiac glycosides
	Cardiac inotropic agents
	Catechol O-methyl transferase inhibitors
	Central stimulants
	Centrally acting antihypertensives
	Cephalosporins
	Cephamycins
	Chelating agents
	Chloramphenicols
	Cholinesterase reactivators
	Cinchona antimalarials
	Class I antiarrhythmics
	Class II antiarrhythmics
	Class III antiarrhythmics
	Class IV antiarrhythmics
	Clofibrate and analogues
	Colchicum alkaloids
	Colony-stimulating factors
	Contrast media
	Corticosteroids
	Cough suppressants
	Coumarin anticoagulants
	Cytoprotective agents
	Dermatological agents
	Diagnostic agents
	Diamidine antiprotozoals
	Digitalis
	Dopaminergic antiparkinsonian agents
	E series prostaglandins
	Edetates

Adverse drug reaction	Pharmacological group
Nausea	Ergolines
	Ergot alkaloids
	Ergot compounds
	Essential amino acids
	Ethyleneimine antineoplastics
	Evening primrose oil
	Expectorants
	F series prostaglandins
	Fat-soluble vitamins
	Ferric salts
	Ferrous salts
	Fluorouracil
	GABA-related antiepileptics
	Gases
	Gastrointestinal agents
	Glucose tests
	Glycol and glycerol esters
	Glycols
	Gonad-regulating hormones
	H_1-antagonist antihistamines
	Haemostatics
	Histamine H_2 antagonists
	HMG CoA reductase inhibitors
	Hydantoin antiepileptics
	Hydrazide antituberculous agents
	Hydroxynaphthoquinones
	Imidazole antifungals
	Immunosuppressants
	Indanedione anticoagulants
	Inhalation anaesthetics
	Iron compounds
	Laxatives
	Leukotriene inhibitors
	Lincomycins
	Lipid-regulating agents
	Loop diuretics
	Macrolides
	Medicinal enzymes
	Methadone and analogues
	Monoamine oxidase-inhibiting antidepressants
	Monobactams
	Morphinan opioid analgesics
	Neuroleptics
	Nitrofuran antimicrobials
	Nitrofuran antiprotozoals

Adverse drug reaction	Pharmacological group
Nausea	Nitrogen mustards
	Nitroimidazole antiprotozoals
	Nitrosoureas
	Oestrogen antagonist antineoplastics
	Oestrogens
	Omega-3 triglycerides
	Opioid analgesics
	Opioid antagonists
	Opioid peptides
	Opium alkaloid opioid analgesics
	Opium poppy substances
	Oral hypoglycaemics
	Organic iodinated contrast media
	Oxazolidinedione antiepileptics
	Oxytetracyclines
	Parasympathomimetics
	Peripheral and cerebral vasodilators
	Pethidine and analogues
	Phenytoin
	Pilocarpine
	Platelet-activating factor antagonists
	Polyene antibiotics
	Posterior pituitary hormones
	Progestogens
	Prophylactic antiasthmatics
	Purine antagonist antineoplastics
	Pyrimidine antagonist antineoplastics
	Respiratory stimulants
	Retinoic acid dermatological agents
	Salicylate analgesics
	Sedatives
	Selective serotonin reuptake-inhibiting antidepressants
	Serotonin and analogues
	Sex hormones
	Skeletal muscle relaxants
	Somatotrophic hormones
	Sulphonamides
	Sulphone antileprotics
	Sulphur mustards
	Sympathomimetics
	Tetracyclic antidepressants
	Tetracyclines
	Theophylline xanthines
	Thiazide diuretics
	Thiouracil antithyroid agents

Adverse drug reaction	Pharmacological group
Nausea	Thiourea antithyroid agents
	Thyrotrophic hormones
	Triazene antineoplastics
	Triazole antifungals
	Tricyclic antidepressants
	Trimethoprim and derivatives
	Trimethoprim–sulphonamide combinations
	Triphenylmethane diagnostic dyes
	Typhoid vaccines
	Uricosuric agents
	Vaccines
	Vasodilator antihypertensives
	Vasodilators
	Vasopressins
	Vinca alkaloid antineoplastics
	Vitamin B substances
	Vitamin D substances
	Vitamins
	Xanthine-containing beverages
	Xanthines
Neoplasms	Immunosuppressants
Nephritis, nephrosis	Organic iodinated contrast media
Nephrotic syndrome	Antithyroid agents
	Chelating agents
	Gastrointestinal agents
	Mercurial dermatological agents
	Oxazolidinedione antiepileptics
	Uricosuric agents
Nerves – nervousness	4-quinolones
	ACE inhibitors
	Amphetamines
	Analgesics and anti-inflammatory drugs
	Anorectics
	Antidepressants
	Antimuscarinics
	Antiulcer agents
	Antivirals
	Beta-2-selective stimulants
	Carbacephems
	Central stimulants
	Cephalosporins
	Cephamycins
	Dopaminergic antiparkinsonian agents
	GABA-related antiepileptics

Adverse drug reaction	Pharmacological group
Nerves – nervousness	Gonad-regulating hormones
	Hydantoin antiepileptics
	Hydrazine monoamine oxidase-inhibiting antidepressants
	Interleukins
	Monoamine oxidase-inhibiting antidepressants
	Neuroleptics
	Opioid antagonists
	Phenytoin
	Progestogens
	Sedatives
	Selective serotonin reuptake-inhibiting antidepressants
	Sex hormones
	Skeletal muscle relaxants
Neurological symptoms	Antiepileptics
	Antivirals
	Gastrointestinal agents
	Glycols
	Immunosuppressants
	Organic iodinated contrast media
Neutropenia	8-aminoquinoline antimalarials
	ACE inhibitors
	Angiotensin-inhibiting antihypertensives
	Antibacterial agents
	Antineoplastics
	Antivirals
	Carbapenems
	Central stimulants
	Chelating agents
	Gastrointestinal agents
	H_1-antagonist antihistamines
	Lincomycins
	Macrolides
	Monobactams
	Neuroleptics
	Oxazolidinedione antiepileptics
	Retinoic acid dermatological agents
	Thiazide diuretics
	Thiourea antithyroid agents
Newborn disseminated intravascular coagulation	E series prostaglandins

Adverse drug reaction	Pharmacological group
Night blindness	Retinoic acid dermatological agents
Night terrors	Amphetamines Anorectics Central stimulants
Nightmares	Aliphatic phenothiazine neuroleptics Antivirals Butyrophenone neuroleptics Calcium antagonist vasodilators Class III antiarrhythmics Diphenylbutylpiperidine neuroleptics Flupentixols Fluphenazine Haloperidols Neuroleptics Phenothiazine neuroleptics Piperazine phenothiazine neuroleptics Piperidine phenothiazine neuroleptics Sedatives Thioxanthene neuroleptics Zuclopenthixols
Non-alcoholic fatty liver	Antivirals Oestrogen antagonist antineoplastics Sex hormones
Numbness	Analgesics and anti-inflammatory drugs Organic iodinated contrast media
Nystagmus	Alcoholic disinfectants Anticholinesterase parasympathomimetics Class I antiarrhythmics GABA-related antiepileptics Hydantoin antiepileptics Parasympathomimetics Phenytoin Pilocarpine Skeletal muscle relaxants
Obstetric trauma	Oxytocic hormones
Oedema	4-quinolones Alpha-blocking antihypertensives Anabolics Analgesics and anti-inflammatory drugs Androgens Anthelmintics Antiandrogens

Adverse drug reaction	Pharmacological group
Oedema	Antibiotic antituberculous agents
	Antidepressants
	Antiepileptics
	Antifolate antineoplastics
	Antineoplastics
	Antiulcer agents
	Antivirals
	Calcium antagonist vasodilators
	Carbazepine antiepileptics
	Class IV antiarrhythmics
	Colony-stimulating factors
	Dermatological agents
	Dopaminergic antiparkinsonian agents
	E series prostaglandins
	Ergot compounds
	Gonad-regulating hormones
	Gonadotrophic hormones
	Hydrazine monoamine oxidase-inhibiting antidepressants
	Immunosuppressants
	Interleukins
	Lithium
	Monoamine oxidase-inhibiting antidepressants
	Neuroleptics
	Oestrogen antagonist antineoplastics
	Organic iodinated contrast media
	Progestogens
	Pyrethroid pesticides
	Pyrimidine antagonist antineoplastics
	Salicylate analgesics
	Sex hormones
	Testosterones
	Vasodilator antihypertensives
Oedema of eyelid	Centrally acting antihypertensives
	Erythropoietin
Oedema of glottis	Phenol disinfectants
Oedema of larynx	Phenol disinfectants
Oesophagitis	Amidinopenicillins
	Analgesics and anti-inflammatory drugs
	Antimuscarinics
	Bisphosphonates
	Salicylate analgesics
	Tetracyclines

Adverse drug reaction	Pharmacological group
Oligospermia	Gastrointestinal agents
Oliguria	Alpha-blocking vasodilators Cardiac inotropic agents Lithium
Onycholysis	ACE inhibitors
Optic neuritis	Antituberculous agents Chloramphenicols Class III antiarrhythmics Hydrazide antituberculous agents Retinoic acid dermatological agents
Oral aphthae	Analgesics and anti-inflammatory drugs Antibiotic antineoplastics Antifolate antineoplastics Antivirals Biguanide antimalarials Fluorouracil Gold salts Monobactams Pyrimidine antagonist antineoplastics
Organic psychotic conditions	Aromatics
Orofacial dyskinesia	Central stimulants Dopaminergic antiparkinsonian agents H_1-antagonist antihistamines
Osteomalacia	Aldosterone inhibitors Antacid gastrointestinal agents Barbiturate sedatives Bisphosphonates Hydantoin antiepileptics Phenytoin
Osteoporosis	Antiandrogens Bisphosphonates Corticosteroids Corticotrophic hormones Direct-acting anticoagulants Gonad-regulating hormones Heparinoids Low-molecular-weight heparins Thyroid agents
Other penile inflammatory disorders	E series prostaglandins

Adverse drug reaction	Pharmacological group
Ototoxicity – deafness	Aminoglycosides Antibacterial agents Antineoplastics
Ovarian cysts	Gonad-regulating hormones
Ovarian hyperstimulation	Sex hormones
Pain	Antifolate antineoplastics Antivirals Central stimulants Interleukins Medicinal enzymes
Pain at injection site	Alpha-blocking vasodilators Antidotes Antivirals Cardiac inotropic agents Contrast media H_1-antagonist antihistamines Hyaluronic acid Leech products Medicinal enzymes Penicillinase-resistant penicillins Phenothiazine antihistamines Vinca alkaloid antineoplastics
Pain in joints – arthralgia	4-quinolones Amidinopenicillins Aminopenicillanic derivatives Aminopenicillins Anthelmintics Antidotes Antifungals Antineoplastics Antipseudomonal penicillins Antituberculous agents Antiulcer agents Antivirals Benzylpenicillin and derivatives Carbacephems Carbazepine antiepileptics Carboxypenicillins Central stimulants Cephalosporins Cephamycins Class I antiarrhythmics Gastrointestinal agents

Adverse drug reaction	Pharmacological group
Pain in joints – arthralgia	Histamine H_2 antagonists
	Hydrazide antituberculous agents
	Isoxazolyl penicillins
	Natural penicillins
	Nitrofuran antimicrobials
	Oestrogen antagonist antineoplastics
	Penicillinase-resistant penicillins
	Phenoxymethylpenicillin and derivatives
	Phenoxypenicillins
	Polyene antibiotics
	Prophylactic antiasthmatics
	Retinoic acid dermatological agents
	Tetracyclic antidepressants
	Thiouracil antithyroid agents
	Thiourea antithyroid agents
	Ureido penicillins
	Vaccines
	Xanthine oxidase inhibitors
Pain in testicle	E series prostaglandins
Painful extremities	Antidotes
	Cardiac inotropic agents
	Clofibrate and analogues
Painful swallowing	Antineoplastics
Painful urination	Analgesics and anti-inflammatory drugs
	Organic iodinated contrast media
Pallor	Aliphatic phenothiazine neuroleptics
	Analgesics and anti-inflammatory drugs
	Antidiuretic hormones
	Butyrophenone neuroleptics
	Diphenylbutylpiperidine neuroleptics
	Dopaminergic antiparkinsonian agents
	Flupentixols
	Fluphenazine
	Haloperidols
	I series prostaglandins
	Neuroleptics
	Phenothiazine neuroleptics
	Piperazine phenothiazine neuroleptics
	Piperidine phenothiazine neuroleptics
	Posterior pituitary hormones
	Thioxanthene neuroleptics
	Vasopressins
	Zuclopenthixols

Adverse drug reaction	*Pharmacological group*
Palpitations	ACE inhibitors
	Alpha-adrenoceptor stimulants
	Alpha-blocking antihypertensives
	Amphetamines
	Analgesics and anti-inflammatory drugs
	Anorectics
	Antianginal vasodilators
	Antidepressants
	Antimuscarinics
	Benzomorphan opioid analgesics
	Beta-sympathomimetic vasodilators
	Beta-2-selective stimulants
	Calcium antagonist vasodilators
	Central stimulants
	Centrally acting antihypertensives
	Class I antiarrhythmics
	Corticosteroids
	E series prostaglandins
	Ergolines
	Ergot alkaloids
	Ergot compounds
	Gases
	Gonad-regulating hormones
	H_1-antagonist antihistamines
	Methadone and analogues
	Morphinan opioid analgesics
	Opioid analgesics
	Opioid peptides
	Opium alkaloid opioid analgesics
	Opium poppy substances
	Pethidine and analogues
	Phenothiazine antihistamines
	Promethazines
	Sedatives
	Selective serotonin reuptake-inhibiting antidepressants
	Serotonin and analogues
	Smooth-muscle relaxants
	Sympathomimetics
	Theophylline xanthines
	Vasodilator antihypertensives
	Vitamin B substances
	Xanthine-containing beverages
	Xanthines
Pancreatic steatorrhoea	Somatotrophic hormones

Adverse drug reaction	Pharmacological group
Pancytopenia	4-quinolones
	Antibacterial agents
	Antithyroid agents
	Antivirals
	Benzimidazole anthelmintics
	Oxazolidinedione antiepileptics
	Selective serotonin reuptake-inhibiting antidepressants
Papilloedema	Interleukins
	Retinoic acid dermatological agents
Paraesthesia	4-methanolquinoline antimalarials
	4-quinolones
	ACE inhibitors
	Antidepressants
	Antiepileptics
	Antimuscarinics
	Antiulcer agents
	Antivirals
	Carbamate sedatives
	Carbapenems
	Carbazepine antiepileptics
	Carbonic anhydrase inhibitors
	Central stimulants
	Class I antiarrhythmics
	Colony-stimulating factors
	Ergot compounds
	Gonad-regulating hormones
	H_1-antagonist antihistamines
	HMG CoA reductase inhibitors
	Hydroxyquinoline antiprotozoals
	Immunosuppressants
	Interleukins
	Neuroleptics
	Organic iodinated contrast media
	Oxazolidinedione antiepileptics
	Phenothiazine antihistamines
	Polymyxins
	Promethazines
	Selective noradrenaline reuptake-inhibiting antidepressants
	Serotonin and analogues
	Skeletal muscle relaxants
	Thiazide diuretics
	Vitamin D substances
	Xanthine oxidase inhibitors

Adverse drug reaction	Pharmacological group
Paralysis	Antianginal vasodilators
	Antibiotic antituberculous agents
	Anticholinesterase parasympathomimetics
	Chelating agents
	Organic iodinated contrast media
	Parasympathomimetics
	Pilocarpine
	Skeletal muscle relaxants
Paralytic ileus	Antidepressants
	Calcium antagonist vasodilators
	Skeletal muscle relaxants
	Tetracyclic antidepressants
	Tricyclic antidepressants
	Vinca alkaloid antineoplastics
Paronychia of finger	Retinoic acid dermatological agents
Paronychia of toe	Retinoic acid dermatological agents
Parotid swelling	Encephalitis vaccines
	Influenza vaccines
	Measles vaccine
	Organic iodinated contrast media
	Poliomyelitis vaccines
	Typhoid vaccines
	Vaccines
Parotitis	Analgesics and anti-inflammatory drugs
Paroxysmal choreo-athetosis	Central stimulants
Paroxysmal nocturnal haemoglobinuria	Chloramphenicols
Paroxysmal supraventricular tachycardia	Anthracycline antibiotic antineoplastics
	H_1-antagonist antihistamines
Paroxysmal ventricular tachycardia	Antimalarials
	Beta-blockers
	Inhalation anaesthetics
	Lipid-regulating agents
Partial atrioventricular block	Calcium antagonist vasodilators
	Cardiac glycosides
	Class I antiarrhythmics
	Class IV antiarrhythmics
	Digitalis
	Histamine H_2 antagonists

Adverse drug reaction	Pharmacological group
Patches of alopecia	Alkylating antineoplastics
	Analgesics and anti-inflammatory drugs
	Antibacterial agents
	Antifolate antineoplastics
	Antineoplastics
	Antituberculous agents
	Gonad-regulating hormones
	HMG CoA reductase inhibitors
	Interleukins
	Oestrogen antagonist antineoplastics
	Oxazolidinedione antiepileptics
	Pyrimidine antagonist antineoplastics
Peeling skin	Retinoic acid dermatological agents
Pellagra	Antituberculous agents
	Hydrazide antituberculous agents
Pemphigus	Chelating agents
Peptic ulcer	Analgesics and anti-inflammatory drugs
	Antineoplastics
	Corticosteroids
	Corticotrophic hormones
	Salicylate analgesics
	Uricosuric agents
Peptic ulcer symptoms	Central stimulants
Perioperative haemorrhage/ haematoma	Analgesics and anti-inflammatory drugs
Perineal pain	4-quinolones
	Corticosteroids
	E series prostaglandins
	Oestrogens
	Respiratory stimulants
Peripheral autonomic neuropathy	Antineoplastics
	Antivirals
	HMG CoA reductase inhibitors
	Vinca alkaloid antineoplastics
Peripheral enthesopathies	4-quinolones
	Interleukins
Peripheral neuritis or neuropathy	4-aminoquinoline antimalarials
	4-quinolones
	Alcohol metabolism modifiers

Adverse drug reaction	Pharmacological group
Peripheral neuritis or neuropathy	Analgesics and anti-inflammatory drugs
	Antibiotic antifungals
	Antidepressants
	Antineoplastics
	Antituberculous agents
	Antivirals
	Chloramphenicols
	Class I antiarrhythmics
	Class III antiarrhythmics
	Colchicum alkaloids
	Dermatological agents
	Dopaminergic antiparkinsonian agents
	Gold salts
	Hydantoin antiepileptics
	Hydrazide antituberculous agents
	Hydrazine monoamine oxidase-inhibiting antidepressants
	Immunosuppressants
	Monoamine oxidase-inhibiting antidepressants
	Nitrofuran antimicrobials
	Nitroimidazole antiprotozoals
	Phenytoin
	Polyene antibiotics
	Salicylate analgesics
	Sulphone antileprotics
	Vasodilator antihypertensives
	Vinca alkaloid antineoplastics
	Xanthine oxidase inhibitors
Peripheral neuropathy	Antituberculous agents
	Dermatological agents
	Vitamin B_6 substances
Peripheral vascular symptoms	Beta-blockers
	Cardioselective beta-blockers
	Platelet-activating factor antagonists
	Respiratory stimulants
Persistent miosis	Alpha-blocking antihypertensives
	Anticholinesterase parasympathomimetics
	Aromatics
	Benzomorphan opioid analgesics
	Methadone and analogues
	Morphinan opioid analgesics
	Opioid analgesics
	Opioid peptides

Adverse drug reaction	Pharmacological group
Persistent miosis	Opium alkaloid opioid analgesics
	Opium poppy substances
	Parasympathomimetics
	Pethidine and analogues
	Pilocarpine
Persistent mydriasis	Antimuscarinics
	Aromatics
	Centrally acting antihypertensives
	Ganglion-blocking antihypertensives
	Neuroleptics
	Smooth-muscle relaxants
Personality disorders	Acetylurea antiepileptics
	Central stimulants
	Dopaminergic antiparkinsonian agents
	Oxazolidinedione antiepileptics
Petechiae	4-quinolones
	Organic iodinated contrast media
	Skeletal muscle relaxants
Phlebitis and thrombophlebitis	4-quinolones
	Antibacterial agents
	Antibiotic antituberculous agents
	Antivirals
	Benzodiazepine sedatives
	Carbamate sedatives
	Carbapenems
	Gonad-regulating hormones
	Haemostatics
	Immunosuppressants
	Lincomycins
	Macrolides
	Oestrogen antagonist antineoplastics
	Osmotic diuretics
	Penicillinase-resistant penicillins
	Sedatives
	Skeletal muscle relaxants
	Vasodilator antihypertensives
Phocomelia limb unspecified	Dermatological agents
Phocomelia upper limb NOS	Dermatological agents
Photophobia	Centrally acting antihypertensives
	Neuroleptics

Adverse drug reaction	Pharmacological group
Photophobia	Oxazolidinedione antiepileptics
	Retinoic acid dermatological agents
	Skeletal muscle relaxants
	Succinimide antiepileptics
Photosensitivity	4-quinolones
	Aliphatic phenothiazine neuroleptics
	Aminobenzoate sunscreen agents
	Analgesics and anti-inflammatory drugs
	Anthelmintics
	Antibiotic antifungals
	Antiepileptics
	Antifungals
	Antineoplastics
	Antituberculous agents
	Antiulcer agents
	Aromatics
	Benzophenone sunscreen agents
	Carbazepine antiepileptics
	Chlorinated phenol disinfectants
	Cinnamate sunscreen agents
	Class I antiarrhythmics
	Class III antiarrhythmics
	Dibenzoylmethanes
	Diphenylbutylpiperidine neuroleptics
	Disinfectants
	Flupentixols
	Fluphenazine
	Gastrointestinal agents
	H_1-antagonist antihistamines
	Loop diuretics
	Neuroleptics
	Oxytetracyclines
	Phenothiazine antihistamines
	Phenothiazine neuroleptics
	Piperazine phenothiazine neuroleptics
	Piperidine phenothiazine neuroleptics
	Potassium-sparing diuretics
	Promethazines
	Retinoic acid dermatological agents
	Salicylate sunscreen agents
	Sulphonylurea hypoglycaemics
	Sunscreen agents
	Tars
	Tetracyclines
	Thiazide diuretics

Adverse drug reaction	Pharmacological group
Photosensitivity	Thioxanthene neuroleptics Tricyclic antidepressants Vegetable astringents Zuclopenthixols
Pleural effusion	Colony-stimulating factors Ergolines Skeletal muscle relaxants
Pneumonitis	Antifolate antineoplastics Antivirals Class I antiarrhythmics Thiazide diuretics
Pneumothorax	Antivirals
Polyarteritis nodosa	Hydantoin antiepileptics Phenytoin
Polydipsia	Lithium
Polyuria	Alkylating antineoplastics Alpha-blocking antihypertensives Calcium antagonist vasodilators Fat-soluble vitamins Lithium Skeletal muscle relaxants Uricosuric agents Vitamin D substances Vitamins
Postoperative urinary tract infection	Haemostatics
Postoperative haematoma formation	Analgesics and anti-inflammatory drugs Platelet-activating factor antagonists
Postmenopausal bleeding	E series prostaglandins
Postural hypotension	Adrenergic neurone-blocking antihypertensives Aliphatic phenothiazine neuroleptics Alpha-blocking antihypertensives Alpha-blocking vasodilators Angiotensin-inhibiting antihypertensives Anthelmintics Antianginal vasodilators Antidepressants Antineoplastics Antituberculous agents

Adverse drug reaction	Pharmacological group
Postural hypotension	Benzomorphan opioid analgesics
	Beta-blockers
	Centrally acting antihypertensives
	Class I antiarrhythmics
	Dopaminergic antiparkinsonian agents
	Ergolines
	Ergot compounds
	Hydrazine monoamine oxidase-inhibiting antidepressants
	Methadone and analogues
	Monoamine oxidase-inhibiting antidepressants
	Morphinan opioid analgesics
	Neuroleptics
	Opioid analgesics
	Opioid peptides
	Opium alkaloid opioid analgesics
	Opium poppy substances
	Peripheral and cerebral vasodilators
	Pethidine and analogues
	Potassium-sparing diuretics
	Rauwolfia antihypertensives
	Skeletal muscle relaxants
	Tetracyclic antidepressants
	Thiazide diuretics
	Tricyclic antidepressants
	Vasodilator antihypertensives
Premature ejaculation	Antidepressants
Premenstrual tension syndrome	Norgestrels
	Oestrogens
	Progestogens
	Sex hormones
Priapism	Alpha-blocking vasodilators
	Androgens
	Antidepressants
	E series prostaglandins
	Neuroleptics
	Papaverine and analogues
	Testosterones
Primary malignant neoplasm of liver	Anabolics
Primary pulmonary hypertension	Anorectics

Adverse drug reaction	Pharmacological group
Prolactin level increased	Antiemetics
	Neuroleptics
Proteinuria	Analgesics and anti-inflammatory drugs
	Antineoplastics
	Antivirals
	Carbazepine antiepileptics
	Chelating agents
	Colony-stimulating factors
	Gastrointestinal agents
	Gold salts
Prothrombin time increased	4-quinolones
	Class III antiarrhythmics
	Oxacephalosporins
Proximal myopathy	Corticosteroids
	Corticotrophic hormones
Pruritus	4-methanolquinoline antimalarials
	4-quinolones
	Anabolics
	Anthelmintics
	Antiandrogens
	Antibacterial agents
	Antifungals
	Antimalarials
	Antineoplastics
	Antiulcer agents
	Antivirals
	Benzimidazole anthelmintics
	Benzomorphan opioid analgesics
	Beta-2-selective stimulants
	Bile acids and salts
	Blood products
	Calcium antagonist vasodilators
	Carbacephems
	Carbapenems
	Central stimulants
	Cephalosporins
	Cephamycins
	Class IV antiarrhythmics
	Clofibrate and analogues
	Colony-stimulating factors
	Dichloroacetamide antiprotozoals
	Fluorocarbon blood substitutes
	Gold salts
	Gonad-regulating hormones

Adverse drug reaction	Pharmacological group
Pruritus	HMG CoA reductase inhibitors
	Imidazole antifungals
	Immunosuppressants
	Methadone and analogues
	Morphinan opioid analgesics
	Nitrofuran antimicrobials
	Oestrogen antagonist antineoplastics
	Opioid analgesics
	Opioid peptides
	Opium alkaloid opioid analgesics
	Opium poppy substances
	Organic iodinated contrast media
	Pethidine and analogues
	Pyrethroid pesticides
	Pyrimidine antagonist antineoplastics
	Retinoic acid dermatological agents
	Skeletal muscle relaxants
	Thiouracil antithyroid agents
	Thiourea antithyroid agents
	Triazole antifungals
	Trimethoprim and derivatives
	Trimethoprim–sulphonamide combinations
	Vitamin B substances
Pruritus ani	Analgesics and anti-inflammatory drugs
	Salicylate analgesics
Pruritus of genital organs	Oestrogen antagonist antineoplastics
	Sex hormones
Pseudomembranous colitis – *Clostridium difficile*	4-quinolones
	Aminoglycosides
	Antibacterial agents
	Antibiotic antituberculous agents
	Carbacephems
	Carbapenems
	Cephalosporins
	Cephamycins
	Lincomycins
	Macrolides
	Oxytetracyclines
	Sulphonamides
	Tetracyclines
	Trimethoprim–sulphonamide combinations
Psoriasiform rash	Antivirals
	Lithium

Adverse drug reaction	Pharmacological group
Psychiatric disturbances	4-aminoquinoline antimalarials
	4-methanolquinoline antimalarials
	4-quinolones
	Acetylurea antiepileptics
	Analgesics and anti-inflammatory drugs
	Anorectics
	Antibiotic antituberculous agents
	Antidepressants
	Antiepileptics
	Antimuscarinics
	Carbapenems
	Carbazepine antiepileptics
	Class I antiarrhythmics
	Corticosteroids
	Corticotrophic hormones
	Dopaminergic antiparkinsonian agents
	Ergot compounds
	GABA-related antiepileptics
	Hydrazide antituberculous agents
	Opioid analgesics
	Polymyxins
	Salicylate analgesics
	Smooth-muscle relaxants
	Succinimide antiepileptics
Ptosis	Alpha-blocking vasodilators
	Skeletal muscle relaxants
Pulmonary eosinophilia	Selective serotonin reuptake-inhibiting antidepressants
Pulmonary fibrosis	Alkyl sulphonate antineoplastics
	Analgesics and anti-inflammatory drugs
	Antibiotic antineoplastics
	Class I antiarrhythmics
	Class III antiarrhythmics
	Gastrointestinal agents
	Gold salts
	Nitrofuran antimicrobials
	Nitrofuran antiprotozoals
	Nitrogen mustards
	Nitrosoureas
Pulmonary haemorrhage	Pulmonary surfactants
Pulmonary oedema	Analgesics and anti-inflammatory drugs
	Beta-sympathomimetic vasodilators
	Beta-2-selective stimulants

Adverse drug reaction	Pharmacological group
Pulmonary oedema	Colony-stimulating factors
	Ergot alkaloids
	Ergot compounds
	F series prostaglandins
	Glycols
	Haloperidols
	Interleukin 2
	Morphinan opioid analgesics
	Nitrofuran antiprotozoals
	Opioid antagonists
	Organic iodinated contrast media
	Oxytocic hormones
	Polyene antibiotics
	Sympathomimetics
	Thiazide diuretics
Punctate keratitis	Anthelmintics
Pyrexia	4-quinolones
	Aliphatic phenothiazine neuroleptics
	Amidinopenicillins
	Aminopenicillanic derivatives
	Aminopenicillins
	Anthelmintics
	Antibacterial agents
	Antibiotic antituberculous agents
	Antiepileptics
	Antimuscarinics
	Antineoplastics
	Antipseudomonal penicillins
	Antituberculous agents
	Antiulcer agents
	Antivirals
	Benzimidazole anthelmintics
	Benzylpenicillin and derivatives
	Bisphosphonates
	Butyrophenone neuroleptics
	Carbacephems
	Carbapenems
	Carbazepine antiepileptics
	Carboxypenicillins
	Central stimulants
	Cephalosporins
	Cephamycins
	Chelating agents
	Class I antiarrhythmics
	Colony-stimulating factors

Adverse drug reaction	Pharmacological group
Pyrexia	Diphenylbutylpiperidine neuroleptics
	E series prostaglandins
	Encephalitis vaccines
	F series prostaglandins
	Flupentixols
	Fluphenazine
	Gastrointestinal agents
	Gold salts
	Haloperidols
	Hydantoin antiepileptics
	Hydrazide antituberculous agents
	Hydroxynaphthoquinones
	Indanedione anticoagulants
	Influenza vaccines
	Inhalation anaesthetics
	Isoxazolyl penicillins
	Macrogol ethers
	Measles vaccine
	Natural penicillins
	Neuroleptics
	Norgestrels
	Oral hypoglycaemics
	Penicillinase-resistant penicillins
	Phenothiazine neuroleptics
	Phenoxymethylpenicillin and derivatives
	Phenoxypenicillins
	Phenytoin
	Piperazine phenothiazine neuroleptics
	Piperidine phenothiazine neuroleptics
	Poliomyelitis vaccines
	Polyene antibiotics
	Progestogens
	Selective serotonin reuptake-inhibiting antidepressants
	Sex hormones
	Smooth-muscle relaxants
	Sulphonylurea hypoglycaemics
	Thioxanthene neuroleptics
	Typhoid vaccines
	Ureido penicillins
	Vaccines
	Vasodilator antihypertensives
	Vitamin B substances
	Xanthine oxidase inhibitors
	Zuclopenthixols

Adverse drug reaction	Pharmacological group
R-eye completely blind	Hydroxyquinoline antiprotozoals
Raised intracranial pressure	4-quinolones Anthelmintics Class III antiarrhythmics Colony-stimulating factors Oxytetracyclines Progestogens Retinoic acid dermatological agents Sex hormones Tetracyclines
Raised intraocular pressure	Antianginal vasodilators Antimuscarinics Ganglion-blocking antihypertensives Hyaluronic acid Smooth-muscle relaxants
Rash	4-methanolquinoline antimalarials 4-quinolones ACE inhibitors Aldosterone inhibitors Aliphatic phenothiazine neuroleptics Alkylating antineoplastics Aminopenicillins Anabolics Analgesics and anti-inflammatory drugs Angiotensin-inhibiting antihypertensives Anorectics Anthelmintics Antiandrogens Antibacterial agents Antibiotic antifungals Antibiotic antituberculous agents Antidepressants Antidotes Antiemetics Antiepileptics Antifolate antineoplastics Antifungals Antimalarials Antineoplastics Antithyroid agents Antiulcer agents Antivirals Aromatics Barbiturate antiepileptics

Adverse drug reaction	Pharmacological group
Rash	Benzimidazole anthelmintics
	Benzodiazepine sedatives
	Beta-blockers
	Bisphosphonates
	Butyrophenone neuroleptics
	Calcium antagonist vasodilators
	Carbacephems
	Carbamate sedatives
	Carbapenems
	Carbonic anhydrase inhibitors
	Cardioselective beta-blockers
	Central stimulants
	Centrally acting antihypertensives
	Cephalosporins
	Cephamycins
	Chelating agents
	Chloral sedatives
	Cinchona antimalarials
	Class I antiarrhythmics
	Class III antiarrhythmics
	Clofibrate and analogues
	Colchicum alkaloids
	Colony-stimulating factors
	Competitive muscle relaxants
	Corticosteroids
	Cough suppressants
	Coumarin anticoagulants
	Dermatological agents
	Diamidine antiprotozoals
	Diphenylbutylpiperidine neuroleptics
	Dopaminergic antiparkinsonian agents
	E series prostaglandins
	Edetates
	Encephalitis vaccines
	Ergolines
	Ergot compounds
	F series prostaglandins
	Flupentixols
	Fluphenazine
	Gastrointestinal agents
	Gonad-regulating hormones
	H_1-antagonist antihistamines
	Haemostatics
	Haloperidols
	Histamine H_2 antagonists
	HMG CoA reductase inhibitors

Adverse drug reaction	Pharmacological group
Rash	Hyaluronic acid
	Hydantoin antiepileptics
	Hydrazine monoamine oxidase-inhibiting antidepressants
	Hydroxynaphthoquinones
	Imidazole antifungals
	Immunosuppressants
	Indanedione anticoagulants
	Influenza vaccines
	Inorganic mercury compounds
	Interleukins
	Leukotriene inhibitors
	Lincomycins
	Lipid-regulating agents
	Loop diuretics
	Macrolides
	Measles vaccine
	Medicinal enzymes
	Monoamine oxidase-inhibiting antidepressants
	Monobactams
	Mucolytics
	Neuroleptics
	Nitrofuran antimicrobials
	Nitrofuran antiprotozoals
	Nitroimidazole antiprotozoals
	Oestrogen antagonist antineoplastics
	Oestrogens
	Opioid antagonists
	Oral hypoglycaemics
	Organic iodinated contrast media
	Organic mercurial disinfectants
	Oxazolidinedione antiepileptics
	Pesticides
	Phenothiazine antihistamines
	Phenothiazine neuroleptics
	Phenytoin
	Piperazine phenothiazine neuroleptics
	Piperidine phenothiazine neuroleptics
	Poliomyelitis vaccines
	Polyene antibiotics
	Potassium-sparing diuretics
	Progestogens
	Promethazines
	Prophylactic antiasthmatics
	Pyrethroid pesticides

Adverse drug reaction	Pharmacological group
Rash	Pyrimidine antagonist antineoplastics
	Retinoic acid dermatological agents
	Salicylate analgesics
	Sedatives
	Sex hormones
	Skeletal muscle relaxants
	Smooth-muscle relaxants
	Succinimide antiepileptics
	Sulphonamides
	Sulphonylurea hypoglycaemics
	Sympathomimetics
	Tetracyclic antidepressants
	Tetracyclines
	Thiazide diuretics
	Thiouracil antithyroid agents
	Thiourea antithyroid agents
	Thioxanthene neuroleptics
	Triazole antifungals
	Tricyclic antidepressants
	Trimethoprim and derivatives
	Trimethoprim–sulphonamide combinations
	Typhoid vaccines
	Uricosuric agents
	Vaccines
	Vasodilator antihypertensives
	Vasodilators
	Vitamin B substances
	Xanthine oxidase inhibitors
	Zuclopenthixols
Rate of respiration changes	Gases
Raynaud's phenomenon	Antibiotic antineoplastics
	Centrally acting antihypertensives
	Ergolines
RBCs – reticulocytes present	Antivirals
Reactive confusion	Opioid analgesics
Rectal discharge	Lipid-regulating agents
Rectal pain	Analgesics and anti-inflammatory drugs
	Lipid-regulating agents
	Salicylate analgesics
	Sedatives

Adverse drug reaction	Pharmacological group
Recurrent erosion of cornea	Centrally acting antihypertensives F series prostaglandins
Recurrent manic episodes	Central stimulants Selective serotonin reuptake-inhibiting antidepressants
Recurrent upper respiratory tract infection	Angiotensin-inhibiting antihypertensives
Red blood cell aplasia and hypoplasia	Antiepileptics Carbonic anhydrase inhibitors
Red/green colour blindness	Antituberculous agents
Redness of eye	Sympathomimetics
Reduced sebum production	Antiandrogens
Reflux oesophagitis	Antivirals
Renal function tests abnormal	ACE inhibitors Acetylurea antiepileptics Alkylating antineoplastics Antibacterial agents Antibiotic antituberculous agents Antiepileptics Antineoplastics Antiulcer agents Beta-2-selective stimulants Borates Chloral sedatives Clofibrate and analogues Colchicum alkaloids HMG CoA reductase inhibitors Immunosuppressants Liquorice Lithium Oxytetracyclines Polyene antibiotics Pyrimidine antagonist antineoplastics Selective noradrenaline reuptake-inhibiting antidepressants Somatotrophic hormones Tetracyclines Thiazide diuretics

Adverse drug reaction	Pharmacological group
Renal function tests abnormal	Trimethoprim and derivatives Trimethoprim–sulphonamide combinations
Renal stones	Antiepileptics Antivirals
Repeated rapid eye movement sleep interruptions	Anticholinesterase parasympathomimetics Parasympathomimetics Pilocarpine
Resorcinol hypothyroidism	Dermatological agents
Respiratory arrest	Organic iodinated contrast media
Respiratory depression	Amide-type anaesthetics Anthelmintics Antidiarrhoeals Antiepileptics Antivirals Barbiturate anaesthetics Barbiturate antiepileptics Barbiturate sedatives Benzomorphan opioid analgesics Competitive muscle relaxants Cough suppressants Depolarising muscle relaxants Ester-type anaesthetics Ganglion-blocking antihypertensives Inhalation anaesthetics Local anaesthetics Methadone and analogues Morphinan cough suppressants Morphinan opioid analgesics Opioid analgesics Opioid peptides Opium alkaloid opioid analgesics Opium poppy substances Pethidine and analogues Sedatives Skeletal muscle relaxants
Respiratory distress	Hydantoin antiepileptics Phenytoin
Respiratory symptoms	ACE inhibitors Antibiotic antituberculous agents Hydantoin antiepileptics Phenytoin

Adverse drug reaction	Pharmacological group
Restlessness	4-quinolones
	Amphetamines
	Anorectics
	Antianginal vasodilators
	Antiemetics
	Antivirals
	Barbiturate antiepileptics
	Central stimulants
	Diphenylbutylpiperidine neuroleptics
	Dopaminergic antiparkinsonian agents
	Monoamine oxidase-inhibiting antidepressants
	Respiratory stimulants
	Sedatives
	Skeletal muscle relaxants
	Sympathomimetics
	Thyroid agents
Retinal damage	4-aminoquinoline antimalarials
Retinal detachments and defects	Antivirals
Retinal exudate or deposits	Aliphatic phenothiazine neuroleptics
	Butyrophenone neuroleptics
	Diphenylbutylpiperidine neuroleptics
	Flupentixols
	Fluphenazine
	Haloperidols
	Neuroleptics
	Phenothiazine neuroleptics
	Piperazine phenothiazine neuroleptics
	Piperidine phenothiazine neuroleptics
	Thioxanthene neuroleptics
	Zuclopenthixols
Retinopathy	Antineoplastics
	Chelating agents
	Gases
	Oestrogen antagonist antineoplastics
	Sex hormones
Retroperitoneal fibrosis	Beta-blockers
	Cardioselective beta-blockers
	Ergolines
	Ergot alkaloids
	Ergot compounds
	Haloperidols

Adverse drug reaction	Pharmacological group
Retroperitoneal fibrosis	Morphinan opioid analgesics
	Salicylate analgesics
Retrosternal pain	Antianginal vasodilators
	Antimony antiprotozoals
	Vasodilator antihypertensives
Rhabdomyolysis	4-quinolones
	Aliphatic phenothiazine neuroleptics
	Barbiturate anaesthetics
	Barbiturate antiepileptics
	Barbiturate sedatives
	Benzodiazepine sedatives
	Benzomorphan opioid analgesics
	Clofibrate and analogues
	Colchicum alkaloids
	Dopaminergic antiparkinsonian agents
	Fluphenazine
	Histamine H_2 antagonists
	HMG CoA reductase inhibitors
	Hydrazine monoamine oxidase-inhibiting antidepressants
	Lithium
	Methadone and analogues
	Monoamine oxidase-inhibiting antidepressants
	Monoamine oxidase-inhibiting antihypertensives
	Morphinan opioid analgesics
	Neuroleptics
	Opioid analgesics
	Opioid peptides
	Opium alkaloid opioid analgesics
	Opium poppy substances
	Pethidine and analogues
	Phenothiazine antihistamines
	Phenothiazine neuroleptics
	Piperazine phenothiazine neuroleptics
	Piperidine phenothiazine neuroleptics
	Polyene antibiotics
	Promethazines
	Retinoic acid dermatological agents
	Theophylline xanthines
	Trimethoprim–sulphonamide combinations
Rhinitis	Antineoplastics
	Antiulcer agents

Adverse drug reaction	Pharmacological group
Rhinitis	Ergolines
	GABA-related antiepileptics
	H₁-antagonist antihistamines
	Neuroleptics
	Organic iodinated contrast media
	Pilocarpine
	Pyrimidine antagonist antineoplastics
Rhinorrhoea	Alpha-blocking vasodilators
	Oestrogen antagonist antineoplastics
Rickets	Hydantoin antiepileptics
	Phenytoin
Right upper quadrant pain	Leukotriene inhibitors
Rigors	Colony-stimulating factors
Ruptured uterus	E series prostaglandins
	Oxytocic hormones
Saliva – abnormal coloration	Antibiotic antituberculous agents
	Antiprotozoals
	Dopaminergic antiparkinsonian agents
Seborrhoea	Progestogens
	Sex hormones
Seborrhoeic dermatitis	Anabolics
Sedation	Aliphatic phenothiazine neuroleptics
	Alpha-blocking antihypertensives
	Antidepressants
	Antifungals
	Antihypertensives
	Antineoplastics
	Butyrophenone neuroleptics
	Centrally acting antihypertensives
	Diphenylbutylpiperidine neuroleptics
	Dopaminergic antiparkinsonian agents
	Flupentixols
	Fluphenazine
	GABA-related antiepileptics
	Ganglion-blocking antihypertensives
	Haloperidols
	Neuroleptics
	Pesticides
	Phenothiazine neuroleptics
	Piperazine phenothiazine neuroleptics

Adverse drug reaction	Pharmacological group
Sedation	Piperidine phenothiazine neuroleptics
	Rauwolfia antihypertensives
	Skeletal muscle relaxants
	Tetracyclic antidepressants
	Thioxanthene neuroleptics
	Tricyclic antidepressants
	Zuclopenthixols
Semen sample volume	Neuroleptics
Sensory symptoms	Diagnostic agents
	Organic iodinated contrast media
	Serotonin and analogues
Serum bicarbonate abnormal	Antivirals
Serum bilirubin raised	Angiotensin-inhibiting antihypertensives
	Anthelmintics
	Antibacterial agents
	Antivirals
	Carbapenems
Serum cholesterol raised	Anabolics
	Antidepressants
	Antivirals
	Loop diuretics
	Retinoic acid dermatological agents
	Thiazide diuretics
Serum creatinine abnormal	Cephalosporins
Serum creatinine raised	4-quinolones
	ACE inhibitors
	Analgesics and anti-inflammatory drugs
	Angiotensin-inhibiting antihypertensives
	Antibacterial agents
	Antibiotic antineoplastics
	Antivirals
	Borates
	Erythropoietin
	Immunosuppressants
	Interleukin 2
	Organic iodinated contrast media
	Vasodilator antihypertensives
Serum lipids high	Asparaginase antineoplastics

Adverse drug reaction	Pharmacological group
Serum sickness	Carbacephems Cephalosporins Cephamycins
Serum sodium level abnormal	Sulphonylurea hypoglycaemics
Serum triglycerides raised	Anabolics Antivirals Loop diuretics Retinoic acid dermatological agents Thiazide diuretics
Severe uterine contractions	Anthelmintics E series prostaglandins F series prostaglandins
Sexual dysfunction	Adrenergic neurone-blocking antihypertensives Alpha-blocking antihypertensives Antidepressants Centrally acting antihypertensives Opioid antagonists Piperidine phenothiazine neuroleptics
Sexual precocity	Androgens Gonadotrophic hormones Testosterones
Shivering	Alpha-blocking vasodilators Anabolics Antibacterial agents Antibiotic antineoplastics Antibiotic antituberculous agents Antidepressants Antivirals Blood-clotting factors Blood products Cardiac inotropic agents Contrast media Cytoprotective agents E series prostaglandins F series prostaglandins Immunosuppressants Opioid antagonists Osmotic diuretics Pilocarpine

Adverse drug reaction	*Pharmacological group*
Shivering	Skeletal muscle relaxants
	Specific immunoglobulins
Sideroblastic anaemia	Antituberculous agents
Sinoatrial block	Calcium antagonist vasodilators
	Class I antiarrhythmics
Sinus tachycardia	Respiratory stimulants
Skeletal hyperostosis	Interleukins
	Retinoic acid dermatological agents
Skin and finger nail pigmentation	4-aminoquinoline antimalarials
	Aliphatic phenothiazine neuroleptics
	Antibiotic antineoplastics
	Antileprotics
	Antiprotozoals
	Antivirals
	Butyrophenone neuroleptics
	Cardiac inotropic agents
	Dermatological agents
	Diphenylbutylpiperidine neuroleptics
	F series prostaglandins
	Flupentixols
	Fluphenazine
	Haloperidols
	Hydroquinone dermatological agents
	Hydroxyquinoline antiprotozoals
	Neuroleptics
	Phenothiazine neuroleptics
	Piperazine phenothiazine neuroleptics
	Piperidine phenothiazine neuroleptics
	Retinoic acid dermatological agents
	Sulphonamides
	Thioxanthene neuroleptics
	Zuclopenthixols
Skin disorders/reactions	4-aminoquinoline antimalarials
	Alcohol metabolism modifiers
	Analgesics and anti-inflammatory drugs
	Antibiotic antineoplastics
	Antineoplastics
	Biguanide antimalarials
	Bisphosphonates
	Borates
	Chelating agents
	Erythropoietin
	Thiazide diuretics

Adverse drug reaction	Pharmacological group
Skin nodules	Dopaminergic antiparkinsonian agents
Skin pigmented over lesions	Antileprotics
Skin scaling	Retinoic acid dermatological agents
Skin ulceration	Dopaminergic antiparkinsonian agents Pyrimidine antagonist antineoplastics
Slurred speech	Hydantoin antiepileptics Phenytoin Polymyxins
Sneezing	Cytoprotective agents Edetates
Soiling – encopresis	Lipid-regulating agents
Somnolence	Anticholinesterase parasympathomimetics Antiepileptics Antimuscarinics Antiulcer agents Antivirals Central stimulants Dermatological agents Dopaminergic antiparkinsonian agents Inhalation anaesthetics Neuroleptics Serotonin and analogues
Sore gums	Gold salts
Sore mouth	Antineoplastics Antivirals Oestrogen antagonist antineoplastics Phenol disinfectants
Sore throat	ACE inhibitors Anthelmintics Antiulcer agents Antivirals Centrally acting antihypertensives Corticosteroids Gold salts Oestrogen antagonist antineoplastics Prophylactic antiasthmatics
Spasm of sphincter of Oddi	Benzomorphan opioid analgesics Methadone and analogues

Adverse drug reaction	Pharmacological group
Spasm of sphincter of Oddi	Morphinan opioid analgesics
	Opioid analgesics
	Opioid peptides
	Opium alkaloid opioid analgesics
	Opium poppy substances
	Pethidine and analogues
Spasmodic torticollis	Skeletal muscle relaxants
Speech problems	Dopaminergic antiparkinsonian agents
	Skeletal muscle relaxants
Sperm absent – azoospermia	Anabolics
	Androgens
	Antiandrogens
	Antivirals
	Testosterones
Sperm morphology affected	Antibiotic antifungals
Sperm no./ml very low: 0–10 million	Antivirals
Splenomegaly	Colony-stimulating factors
Spontaneous bruising	Gold salts
	Low-molecular-weight heparins
	Skeletal muscle relaxants
Steroid acne	Corticosteroids
	Corticotrophic hormones
Steroid facies	Anabolics
	Androgens
	Corticosteroids
	Corticotrophic hormones
	Norgestrels
	Oestrogens
	Progestogens
	Sex hormones
	Testosterones
Steroid-induced diabetes	Anabolics
	Androgens
	Corticosteroids
	Corticotrophic hormones
	Norgestrels
	Oestrogens
	Progestogens

Adverse drug reaction	Pharmacological group
Steroid-induced diabetes	Sex hormones
	Testosterones
Steroid-induced glaucoma	Anabolics
	Androgens
	Corticosteroids
	Corticotrophic hormones
	Norgestrels
	Oestrogens
	Progestogens
	Sex hormones
	Testosterones
Stevens–Johnson syndrome	4-methanolquinoline antimalarials
	4-quinolones
	Analgesics and anti-inflammatory drugs
	Anthelmintics
	Antibacterial agents
	Antiepileptics
	Antifungals
	Antivirals
	Carbazepine antiepileptics
	Chelating agents
	Class I antiarrhythmics
	Gastrointestinal agents
	Hydantoin antiepileptics
	Phenytoin
	Polyene antibiotics
	Sulphonamides
	Triazole antifungals
	Trimethoprim–sulphonamide combinations
	Xanthine oxidase inhibitors
Stomatitis	ACE inhibitors
	Analgesics and anti-inflammatory drugs
	Antibiotic antineoplastics
	Antifolate antineoplastics
	Antineoplastics
	Antiulcer agents
	Beta-2-selective stimulants
	Biguanide antimalarials
	Chelating agents
	Colony-stimulating factors
	Expectorants
	Fluorouracil
	Macrolides

Adverse drug reaction	Pharmacological group
Stomatitis	Medicinal enzymes Polyene antibiotics Pyrimidine antagonist antineoplastics
Striae atrophicae	Corticosteroids Corticotrophic hormones
Stricture of intestine	Medicinal enzymes
Stroke and cerebrovascular accident	ACE inhibitors Ergot alkaloids Ergot compounds Selective serotonin reuptake-inhibiting antidepressants
Subacute confusional state	Opioid analgesics
Subacute hepatitis – non-infectious	Retinoic acid dermatological agents
Subarachnoid haemorrhage	Oxytocic hormones
Subcutaneous sclerotic plaques	Antibiotic antineoplastics
Sudden death	Antiandrogens Antianginal vasodilators Lithium Mercurial diuretics
Suicidal	Retinoic acid dermatological agents
Suicidal ideation	Rauwolfia antihypertensives Selective serotonin reuptake-inhibiting antidepressants
Sulphuric acid – toxic effect	Mineral acids
Supraventricular ectopic beats	Anthracycline antibiotic antineoplastics
Sweating	Alpha-blocking vasodilators Antifolate antineoplastics Antiulcer agents Oestrogen antagonist antineoplastics Pilocarpine Pyrimidine antagonist antineoplastics Respiratory stimulants

Adverse drug reaction	Pharmacological group
Sweating	Selective noradrenaline reuptake-inhibiting antidepressants
Swelling at site of injection	Hyaluronic acid
	Organic iodinated contrast media
Syncope	Analgesics and anti-inflammatory drugs
	Antianginal vasodilators
	Antibiotic antituberculous agents
	Antidepressants
	Antiemetics
	Benzimidazole anthelmintics
	Catechol O-methyl transferase inhibitors
	Colony-stimulating factors
	Contrast media
	Corticotrophic hormones
	Cytoprotective agents
	Diamidine antiprotozoals
	Dopaminergic antiparkinsonian agents
	E series prostaglandins
	Ergolines
	H_1-antagonist antihistamines
	Lithium
	Neuroleptics
	Papaverine and analogues
	Salicylate analgesics
	Sedatives
	Skeletal muscle relaxants
	Tetracyclic antidepressants
	Tricyclic antidepressants
Synovitis and tenosynovitis	4-quinolones
Systemic lupus erythematosus	Aliphatic phenothiazine neuroleptics
	Centrally acting antihypertensives
	Class I antiarrhythmics
	Gastrointestinal agents
	Neuroleptics
	Sex hormones
	Tetracyclines
	Thiouracil antithyroid agents
	Vasodilator antihypertensives
Tachycardia	4-quinolones
	ACE inhibitors
	Aliphatic phenothiazine neuroleptics
	Alpha-adrenoceptor stimulants

Adverse drug reaction	Pharmacological group
Tachycardia	Alpha-blocking antihypertensives
	Alpha-blocking vasodilators
	Amphetamines
	Analgesics and anti-inflammatory drugs
	Anorectics
	Antianginal vasodilators
	Antidepressants
	Antiemetics
	Antimuscarinics
	Antineoplastics
	Aromatics
	Benzodiazepine antagonists
	Beta-adrenoceptor stimulants
	Beta-sympathomimetic vasodilators
	Beta-1-selective stimulants
	Beta-2-selective stimulants
	Butyrophenone neuroleptics
	Calcium antagonist vasodilators
	Central stimulants
	Chelating agents
	Cholinesterase reactivators
	Diagnostic agents
	Diphenylbutylpiperidine neuroleptics
	Dopaminergic antiparkinsonian agents
	E series prostaglandins
	Edetates
	Ergolines
	Ergot compounds
	Flupentixols
	Fluphenazine
	Ganglion-blocking antihypertensives
	Glycols
	H_1-antagonist antihistamines
	Haloperidols
	Immunosuppressants
	Inhalation anaesthetics
	Interleukins
	Isoprenaline
	Lipid-regulating agents
	Neuroleptics
	Parenteral anaesthetics
	Peripheral and cerebral vasodilators
	Phenothiazine neuroleptics
	Piperazine phenothiazine neuroleptics
	Piperidine phenothiazine neuroleptics
	Respiratory stimulants

Adverse drug reaction	Pharmacological group
Tachycardia	Sedatives
	Selective noradrenaline reuptake-inhibiting antidepressants
	Serotonin and analogues
	Skeletal muscle relaxants
	Smooth-muscle relaxants
	Sulphone antileprotics
	Sympathomimetics
	Tetracyclic antidepressants
	Theophylline xanthines
	Thioxanthene neuroleptics
	Thyroid agents
	Thyrotrophic hormones
	Tricyclic antidepressants
	Vasodilator antihypertensives
	Xanthine-containing beverages
	Xanthines
	Zuclopenthixols
Tachypnoea	Antivirals
Taste disturbance	4-quinolones
	ACE inhibitors
	Angiotensin-inhibiting antihypertensives
	Antifolate antineoplastics
	Antifungals
	Antineoplastics
	Antituberculous agents
	Antiulcer agents
	Antivirals
	Beta-2-selective stimulants
	Bisphosphonates
	Calcitonin
	Carbapenems
	Carbonic anhydrase inhibitors
	Centrally acting antihypertensives
	Cephalosporins
	Chelating agents
	Class I antiarrhythmics
	Class III antiarrhythmics
	Contrast media
	Diamidine antiprotozoals
	Disinfectants
	Gold salts
	H_1-antagonist antihistamines
	Macrolides
	Monobactams

Adverse drug reaction	Pharmacological group
Taste disturbance	Nitroimidazole antiprotozoals
	Organic iodinated contrast media
	Prophylactic antiasthmatics
	Sedatives
	Skeletal muscle relaxants
	Thyrotrophic hormones
	Vasodilator antihypertensives
	Xanthine oxidase inhibitors
Telangiectasia	Calcium antagonist vasodilators
Temporary blindness	Cinchona antimalarials
Temporary worsening of symptoms	Fluorouracil
	Oestrogen antagonist antineoplastics
	Pyrimidine antagonist antineoplastics
	Retinoic acid dermatological agents
	Sex hormones
Throat irritation	Corticosteroids
Throat pain	Chelating agents
	Serotonin and analogues
Thrombocythaemia	Carbapenems
	Erythropoietin
	Pyrimidine antagonist antineoplastics
	Retinoic acid dermatological agents
Thrombocytopenia	4-aminoquinoline antimalarials
	4-methanolquinoline antimalarials
	4-quinolones
	ACE inhibitors
	Alpha-blocking vasodilators
	Amidinopenicillins
	Aminopenicillanic derivatives
	Aminopenicillins
	Analgesics and anti-inflammatory drugs
	Antiandrogens
	Antibacterial agents
	Antibiotic antituberculous agents
	Antidepressants
	Antiepileptics
	Antifungals
	Antineoplastics
	Antipseudomonal penicillins
	Antiulcer agents
	Antivirals
	Benzylpenicillin and derivatives

Adverse drug reaction	Pharmacological group
Thrombocytopenia	Calcium antagonist vasodilators
	Carbacephems
	Carbapenems
	Carbazepine antiepileptics
	Carboxypenicillins
	Cardiac inotropic agents
	Central stimulants
	Cephalosporins
	Cephamycins
	Chelating agents
	Cinchona antimalarials
	Class I antiarrhythmics
	Class III antiarrhythmics
	Dermatological agents
	Diagnostic agents
	Diamidine antiprotozoals
	Direct-acting anticoagulants
	Gastrointestinal agents
	Heparinoids
	Histamine H_2 antagonists
	Hydantoin antiepileptics
	Imidazole antifungals
	Immunosuppressants
	Isoxazolyl penicillins
	Lincomycins
	Low-molecular-weight heparins
	Monobactams
	Natural penicillins
	Nitrofuran antimicrobials
	Oestrogen antagonist antineoplastics
	Opioid antagonists
	Oral hypoglycaemics
	Organic iodinated contrast media
	Oxacephalosporins
	Oxazolidinedione antiepileptics
	Penicillinase-resistant penicillins
	Phenoxymethylpenicillin and derivatives
	Phenoxypenicillins
	Phenytoin
	Platelet-activating factor antagonists
	Progestogens
	Pyrimidine antagonist antineoplastics
	Retinoic acid dermatological agents
	Salicylate analgesics
	Sedatives

Adverse drug reaction	Pharmacological group
Thrombocytopenia	Selective serotonin reuptake-inhibiting antidepressants
	Sex hormones
	Skeletal muscle relaxants
	Sulphonamides
	Sulphonylurea hypoglycaemics
	Tetracyclic antidepressants
	Thiazide diuretics
	Tricyclic antidepressants
	Trimethoprim–sulphonamide combinations
	Ureido penicillins
	Vasodilator antihypertensives
Thromboembolism	Carbazepine antiepileptics
	Direct-acting anticoagulants
Thrombosis of arteriovenous surgical shunt	Erythropoietin
Thyroid hormone tests high	Antineoplastics
	Antivirals
	Dermatological agents
	Interleukin 2
Thyroid hormone tests low	Antineoplastics
	Antivirals
	Dermatological agents
	Interleukin 2
Thyroid swelling	Thyrotrophic hormones
Thyrotoxicosis	Class III antiarrhythmics
	Iodides
	Iodine compounds
	Iodophors
Tics	Central stimulants
Tightening pain	Serotonin and analogues
Tingling sensation	Alpha-adrenoceptor stimulants
	Alpha-blocking vasodilators
	Antivirals
	Beta-blockers
	Calcitonin
	Carbonic anhydrase inhibitors
	Chelating agents
	Diagnostic agents

Adverse drug reaction	Pharmacological group
Tingling sensation	H₁-antagonist antihistamines
	HMG CoA reductase inhibitors
	Oestrogen antagonist antineoplastics
	Serotonin and analogues
	Sympathomimetics
Tinnitus symptoms	4-quinolones
	Analgesics and anti-inflammatory drugs
	Antibacterial agents
	Antibiotic antituberculous agents
	Antineoplastics
	Benzimidazole anthelmintics
	Calcium antagonist vasodilators
	Cinchona antimalarials
	Dermatological agents
	Ergot alkaloids
	Ergot compounds
	Haemostatics
	Mucolytics
	Salicylate analgesics
Tiredness	ACE inhibitors
	Alpha-blocking antihypertensives
	Alpha-blocking vasodilators
	Antiandrogens
	Antianginal vasodilators
	Antidepressants
	Antiepileptics
	Antifolate antineoplastics
	Antineoplastics
	Antivirals
	Beta-blockers
	Bisphosphonates
	Calcium antagonist vasodilators
	Colony-stimulating factors
	Ergolines
	GABA-related antiepileptics
	Gonadotrophic hormones
	Histamine H₂ antagonists
	Oestrogen antagonist antineoplastics
	Pilocarpine
	Sedatives
	Selective serotonin reuptake-inhibiting antidepressants
Tissue necrosis	Alkyl sulphonate antineoplastics
	Alkylating antineoplastics

Adverse drug reaction	Pharmacological group
Tissue necrosis	Anthracycline antibiotic antineoplastics
	Antibiotic antineoplastics
	Antifolate antineoplastics
	Antineoplastics
	Asparaginase antineoplastics
	Class II antiarrhythmics
	Diamidine antiprotozoals
	Ethyleneimine antineoplastics
	Fluorouracil
	Immunostimulants
	Immunosuppressants
	Interleukin 2
	Nitrogen mustards
	Nitrosoureas
	Organic iodinated contrast media
	Purine antagonist antineoplastics
	Pyrimidine antagonist antineoplastics
	Sulphur mustards
	Triazene antineoplastics
	Vinca alkaloid antineoplastics
Toxic encephalitis due to mercury	Mercurial dermatological agents
	Organic mercurial disinfectants
Toxic epidermal necrolysis	4-quinolones
	ACE inhibitors
	Analgesics and anti-inflammatory drugs
	Antibiotic antifungals
	Antiepileptics
	Antifungals
	Antivirals
	Carbacephems
	Carbapenems
	Carbazepine antiepileptics
	Cephalosporins
	Cephamycins
	HMG CoA reductase inhibitors
	Hydantoin antiepileptics
	Phenytoin
	Sulphonamides
	Thiazide diuretics
	Trimethoprim–sulphonamide combinations
	Xanthine oxidase inhibitors
Toxic optic neuropathy	Antituberculous agents

Adverse drug reaction	Pharmacological group
Tremor	4-quinolones
	Amphetamines
	Analgesics and anti-inflammatory drugs
	Anorectics
	Anthelmintics
	Antibiotic antituberculous agents
	Anticholinesterase parasympathomimetics
	Antidepressants
	Antiemetics
	Antiepileptics
	Antivirals
	Barbiturate anaesthetics
	Beta-adrenoceptor stimulants
	Beta-1-selective stimulants
	Beta-2-selective stimulants
	Central stimulants
	Class I antiarrhythmics
	Class III antiarrhythmics
	Corticosteroids
	Dopaminergic antiparkinsonian agents
	GABA-related antiepileptics
	Ganglion-blocking antihypertensives
	Gastrointestinal agents
	H_1-antagonist antihistamines
	Hydantoin antiepileptics
	Hydrazine monoamine oxidase-inhibiting antidepressants
	Immunosuppressants
	Isoprenaline
	Lithium
	Monoamine oxidase-inhibiting antidepressants
	Phenothiazine antihistamines
	Phenytoin
	Promethazines
	Respiratory stimulants
	Sedatives
	Selective serotonin reuptake-inhibiting antidepressants
	Skeletal muscle relaxants
	Sympathomimetics
	Tetracyclic antidepressants
	Tricyclic antidepressants
Ulcer of oesophagus	Analgesics and anti-inflammatory drugs
	Bisphosphonates
	Medicinal enzymes

Adverse drug reaction	Pharmacological group
Unspecified cell-type leukaemia	Alkyl sulphonate antineoplastics
Uraemia	Organic iodinated contrast media
Urinary retention	Analgesics and anti-inflammatory drugs Antimuscarinics Benzodiazepine sedatives Carbamate sedatives Cardiac inotropic agents Class I antiarrhythmics H_1-antagonist antihistamines Haemostatics Neuroleptics Phenothiazine antihistamines Promethazines Selective noradrenaline reuptake-inhibiting antidepressants Skeletal muscle relaxants
Urinary system symptoms	Skeletal muscle relaxants
Urinary tract infection	Anticholinesterase parasympathomimetics Antiulcer agents Lipid-regulating agents Smooth-muscle relaxants
Urine – abnormal coloration	4-quinolones Analgesics and anti-inflammatory drugs Anthraquinone glycosides Antibiotic antituberculous agents Antileprotics Antiprotozoals Carbapenems Dopaminergic antiparkinsonian agents Gastrointestinal agents Indanedione anticoagulants Nitroimidazole antiprotozoals
Urine albumin	Aromatics
Urine colour abnormal	Anthelmintics
Urine looks dark	Nitrofuran antiprotozoals
Urine protein abnormal	Anthelmintics
Urine urate raised	Antivirals Medicinal enzymes

Adverse drug reaction	Pharmacological group
Urticaria	4-methanolquinoline antimalarials
	ACE inhibitors
	Amidinopenicillins
	Aminopenicillanic derivatives
	Aminopenicillins
	Analgesics and anti-inflammatory drugs
	Anthelmintics
	Antibacterial agents
	Antibiotic antituberculous agents
	Antiemetics
	Antifungals
	Antineoplastics
	Antipseudomonal penicillins
	Antituberculous agents
	Antiulcer agents
	Antivirals
	Benzomorphan opioid analgesics
	Benzylpenicillin and derivatives
	Beta-2-selective stimulants
	Carbacephems
	Carbapenems
	Carboxypenicillins
	Central stimulants
	Cephalosporins
	Cephamycins
	Clofibrate and analogues
	Dichloroacetamide antiprotozoals
	Direct-acting anticoagulants
	Gastrointestinal agents
	Gold salts
	Gonad-regulating hormones
	Heparinoids
	Histamine H_2 antagonists
	Imidazole antifungals
	Immunosuppressants
	Isoxazolyl penicillins
	Laxatives
	Leukotriene inhibitors
	Low-molecular-weight heparins
	Macrolides
	Medicinal enzymes
	Methadone and analogues
	Monobactams
	Morphinan opioid analgesics
	Mucolytics
	Natural penicillins

Adverse drug reaction	Pharmacological group
Urticaria	Nitrofuran antimicrobials
	Nitroimidazole antiprotozoals
	Norgestrels
	Opioid analgesics
	Opioid peptides
	Opium alkaloid opioid analgesics
	Opium poppy substances
	Organic iodinated contrast media
	Penicillinase-resistant penicillins
	Pethidine and analogues
	Phenoxymethylpenicillin and derivatives
	Phenoxypenicillins
	Polyene antibiotics
	Progestogens
	Sedatives
	Sex hormones
	Skeletal muscle relaxants
	Thyrotrophic hormones
	Triazole antifungals
	Typhoid vaccines
	Ureido penicillins
Uterus rupture in/after labour	Oxytocic hormones
Uveitis	Antibiotic antituberculous agents
	Beta-blockers
	F series prostaglandins
Vaginal discharge	Gonad-regulating hormones
	Oestrogen antagonist antineoplastics
	Sex hormones
Vaginitis and vulvovaginitis	Cephalosporins
Vasculitis	Cardiac inotropic agents
Vasodilatation	Contrast media
	Organic iodinated contrast media
Venous embolus/ thrombus	Haemostatics
	Oestrogens
	Sex hormones
Ventricular ectopic beats	Antimalarials
	Beta-1-selective stimulants
	H_1-antagonist antihistamines

Adverse drug reaction	Pharmacological group
Ventricular fibrillation/flutter	Antianginal vasodilators Antimalarials Beta-blockers Calcium antagonist vasodilators H_1-antagonist antihistamines Inhalation anaesthetics Lipid-regulating agents
Vertigo	Alpha-blocking antihypertensives Analgesics and anti-inflammatory drugs Anthelmintics Antibiotic antituberculous agents Antiemetics Antifungals Antiulcer agents Benzodiazepine sedatives Benzomorphan opioid analgesics Carbamate sedatives Class III antiarrhythmics Clofibrate and analogues Dermatological agents Fat-soluble vitamins Gases Gonad-regulating hormones Methadone and analogues Morphinan opioid analgesics Opioid analgesics Opioid peptides Opium alkaloid opioid analgesics Opium poppy substances Pethidine and analogues Polymyxins Salicylate analgesics Sedatives Skeletal muscle relaxants Tetracyclines Vitamin D substances Vitamins Xanthine oxidase inhibitors
Vesicles	Antifungals
Vesicular eruption	Pyrimidine antagonist antineoplastics
Vestibular disorders	Aminoglycosides Antibacterial agents

Adverse drug reaction	Pharmacological group
Viral/chlamydial infection	Antivirals Corticosteroids Corticotrophic hormones Immunosuppressants Oestrogen antagonist antineoplastics
Virilism	Anabolics Androgens Medicinal enzymes Sex hormones Testosterones
Visual disturbances	Antiulcer agents Barbiturate antiepileptics
Visual symptoms	Antiandrogens Oxazolidinedione antiepileptics
Vitamin-B_{12}-deficiency anaemia	Biguanide hypoglycaemics Inhalation anaesthetics
Vitamin K deficiency	Bile acid-binding resins
Voice disturbance	Gases
Vomiting	4-aminoquinoline antimalarials 4-methanolquinoline antimalarials 4-quinolones 8-aminoquinoline antimalarials ACE inhibitors Alcoholic disinfectants Aldosterone inhibitors Alkyl sulphonate antineoplastics Alkylating antineoplastics Alpha-adrenoceptor stimulants Alpha-blocking antihypertensives Alpha-blocking vasodilators Amino acids Anabolics Analgesics and anti-inflammatory drugs Anthelmintics Anthracycline antibiotic antineoplastics Antiandrogens Antianginal vasodilators Antibacterial agents Antibiotic antifungals Antibiotic antineoplastics Antibiotic antituberculous agents Anticholinesterase parasympathomimetics

Adverse drug reaction	Pharmacological group
Vomiting	Antidepressants
	Antidiarrhoeals
	Antidiuretic hormones
	Antidotes
	Antiepileptics
	Antifolate antineoplastics
	Antifungals
	Antimalarials
	Antimony antiprotozoals
	Antimuscarinics
	Antineoplastics
	Antiprotozoals
	Antithyroid agents
	Antituberculous agents
	Antiulcer agents
	Antivirals
	Aromatics
	Asparaginase antineoplastics
	Aspartic acid
	Benzimidazole anthelmintics
	Benzodiazepine antagonists
	Benzomorphan opioid analgesics
	Beta-blockers
	Beta-sympathomimetic vasodilators
	Beta-1-selective stimulants
	Beta-2-selective stimulants
	Biguanide hypoglycaemics
	Bile acid-binding resins
	Bismuth salts
	Blood products
	Borates
	Calcitonin
	Carbacephems
	Carbapenems
	Carbazepine antiepileptics
	Cardiac glycosides
	Cardiac inotropic agents
	Catechol *O*-methyl transferase inhibitors
	Central stimulants
	Cephalosporins
	Cephamycins
	Chelating agents
	Chloramphenicols
	Class I antiarrhythmics
	Class II antiarrhythmics
	Class III antiarrhythmics

Adverse drug reaction	Pharmacological group
Vomiting	Class IV antiarrhythmics
	Colchicum alkaloids
	Colony-stimulating factors
	Contrast media
	Coumarin anticoagulants
	Cytoprotective agents
	Diagnostic agents
	Diamidine antiprotozoals
	Dichloroacetamide antiprotozoals
	Digitalis
	Dopaminergic antiparkinsonian agents
	E series prostaglandins
	Edetates
	Ergolines
	Ergot alkaloids
	Ergot compounds
	Essential amino acids
	Ethyleneimine antineoplastics
	Expectorants
	F series prostaglandins
	Fat-soluble vitamins
	Fluorouracil
	GABA-related antiepileptics
	Gastrointestinal agents
	Glucose tests
	Glycol and glycerol esters
	Glycols
	Gonad-regulating hormones
	Haemostatics
	Histamine H_2 antagonists
	HMG CoA reductase inhibitors
	Hydantoin antiepileptics
	Hydrazide antituberculous agents
	Hydroxynaphthoquinones
	Imidazole antifungals
	Immunosuppressants
	Indanedione anticoagulants
	Inhalation anaesthetics
	Iron compounds
	Laxatives
	Leukotriene inhibitors
	Lincomycins
	Lipid-regulating agents
	Lithium
	Macrolides
	Medicinal enzymes

Adverse drug reaction	Pharmacological group
Vomiting	Methadone and analogues
	Monobactams
	Morphinan opioid analgesics
	Neuroleptics
	Nitrofuran antimicrobials
	Nitrofuran antiprotozoals
	Nitrogen mustards
	Nitroimidazole antiprotozoals
	Nitrosoureas
	Oestrogen antagonist antineoplastics
	Oestrogens
	Opioid analgesics
	Opioid antagonists
	Opioid peptides
	Opium alkaloid opioid analgesics
	Opium poppy substances
	Oral hypoglycaemics
	Organic iodinated contrast media
	Oxazolidinedione antiepileptics
	Oxytetracyclines
	Parasympathomimetics
	Peripheral and cerebral vasodilators
	Pethidine and analogues
	Phenytoin
	Pilocarpine
	Platelet-activating factor antagonists
	Polyene antibiotics
	Posterior pituitary hormones
	Prophylactic antiasthmatics
	Purine antagonist antineoplastics
	Pyrimidine antagonist antineoplastics
	Respiratory stimulants
	Sedatives
	Selective serotonin reuptake-inhibiting antidepressants
	Serotonin and analogues
	Sex hormones
	Somatotrophic hormones
	Sulphonamides
	Sulphone antileprotics
	Sulphur mustards
	Sympathomimetics
	Tetracyclines
	Thyrotrophic hormones
	Triazene antineoplastics
	Trimethoprim and derivatives

Adverse drug reaction	Pharmacological group
Vomiting	Trimethoprim–sulphonamide combinations
	Typhoid vaccines
	Uricosuric agents
	Vasodilator antihypertensives
	Vinca alkaloid antineoplastics
	Vitamin B substances
	Vitamin D substances
	Vitamins
Water intoxication	Oxytocic hormones

CHAPTER 21

Insulins

TABLE 21.1 Insulin preparations currently marketed in the UK

Name of preparations	Species	pH	Physical state	Absorption and effect (hours)		
				Onset	Peak	Duration
Humalog	H	7.0–7.8	Solution	0.25	0.5–1.5	2–5
Humalog Mix25	H	7.0–7.8	Insulin lispro 25%, insulin lispro protamine suspension 75%	0.25	0.5–2	22
Human Actrapid	H	7.0	Solution	0.5	2.5–5.5	8
Human Insulatard	H	7.0	Isophane insulin	2	4–12	24
Human Mixtard 10	H	7.2–7.4	Soluble 10%, isophane 90%	0.5	2–12	24
Human Mixtard 20	H	7.2–7.4	Soluble 20%, isophane 80%	0.5	2–12	24
Human Mixtard 30	H	7.2–7.4	Soluble 30%, isophane 70%	0.5	2–12	24
Human Mixtard 40	H	7.2–7.4	Soluble 40%, isophane 60%	0.5	2–12	24
Human Mixtard 50	H	7.2–7.4	Soluble 50%, isophane 50%	0.5	2–12	24
Human Monotard	H	7.0	Insulin zinc suspension (amorphous 30%, crystalline 70%)	3	7–15	24
Human Ultratard	H	7.0	Crystalline insulin zinc suspension	4–8	8–24	24–28

Human Velosulin	H	7.0	Solution	0.5	1–3	8
Humulin I	H	6.9–7.5	Crystalline isophane insulin	0.5	2–8	22
Humulin Lente	H	7.0–7.8	Insulin zinc suspension (amorphous 30%, crystalline 70%)	1	3–9	23
Humulin M1	H	6.9–7.5	Soluble 10%, isophane 90%	0.5	1–12	22
Humulin M2	H	6.9–7.5	Soluble 20%, isophane 80%	0.5	1–12	22
Humulin M3	H	6.9–7.5	Soluble 30%, isophane 70%	0.5	1–12	22
Humulin M4	H	6.9–7.5	Soluble 40%, isophane 60%	0.5	1–12	23
Humulin M5	H	6.9–7.5	Soluble 50%, isophane 50%	0.5	1–12	22
Humulin S	H	7.0–7.8	Solution	0.5	1–6	12
Humulin Zn	H	7.0–7.8	Crystalline insulin zinc suspension	2	4–20	25
Hypurin Bovine Isophane	B	7.2	Isophane insulin	0.5–2	6–12	18–24
Hypurin Bovine Lente	B	7.3	Insulin zinc suspension (amorphous 30%, crystalline 70%)	2	8–12	30
Hypurin Bovine Neutral	B	7.0	Solution	0.5–1	2–5	6–8
Hypurin Bovine PZI	B	7.2	Protamine zinc sulphate suspension	4–6	10–20	24–36
Hypurin Porcine Biphasic Isophane	P	6.9–7.8	Soluble 30%, isophane 70%	0.5–1	4–12	18–24

TABLE 21.1 Insulin preparations currently marketed in the UK – cont'd

Name of preparations	Species	pH	Physical state	Absorption and effect (hours)		
				Onset	Peak	Duration
Hypurin Porcine Isophane	P	6.9–7.8	Isophane insulin	0.5–2	6–12	18–24
Hypurin Porcine Neutral	P	7.0	Solution	0.5–1	2–5	6–8
Lentard MC	P, B	7.0	Insulin zinc suspension (amorphous porcine MC insulin 30%, crystalline bovine MC insulin 70%)	3	7–16	24
Pork Actrapid	P	7.0	Solution	0.5	1–3	8
Pork Insulatard	P	7.3	Isophane insulin	2	4–12	24
Pork Mixtard 30	P	7.0	Soluble 30%, microcrystalline isophane insulin 70%	0.5	4–8	22

B = bovine, H = human, P = porcine.
Time for absorption and effect may be prolonged in patients with high titres of anti-insulin antibodies.

CHAPTER 22

Intravenous drug administration

B. Langfield, A. Mackeller

CALCULATION OF DOSE AND RATE OF ADMINISTRATION

CONCENTRATIONS

Concentrations of drug in solution may be expressed in four different ways:

Percentage weight in volume (% w/v)

Expressed as the number of grams (g) of solute (dissolved substance) in a total final volume of 100 millilitres (ml) of solution.

A 55% w/v solution means 55 g in 100 ml of solution.

Percentage volume in volume (% v/v)

Expressed as the number of millilitres (ml) of the diluted liquid when made up to a total final volume of 100 ml of a second liquid.

A 40% v/v solution means 40 ml in a total volume of 100 ml of liquid.

Ratios

These do not base the measurement on a fixed final volume of liquid or solvent.

1 in 1000 means 1 g in 1000 ml, i.e. 1 g/litre, which is equivalent to 1 mg/ml.

Molar solutions

The *mole* is a unit of mass that relates to the *molecular weight* or *relative molecular mass* (RMM) of a compound, or to the *relative atomic mass* (RAM) of an element.

Each molecule has a mass and its molecular weight or RMM is calculated by adding up the RAMs of all the atoms in the molecule.

A mole is the RMM expressed in grams.

A molar solution of a compound contains 1 mole of the compound (measured in grams) dissolved in 1 litre of solvent, usually water.

The RMM of sulphuric acid (H_2SO_4) is 98, so a molar solution of sulphuric acid consists of 98 g of pure sulphuric acid dissolved in 1 litre of water.

The *molarity* of a solution is the number of moles (measured in grams) of solute in 1 litre of solvent.

The abbreviation M is sometimes used for a molar solution. A 5 M (or 5 mol/l) sulphuric acid solution contains: $5 \times 98 = 490$ g of sulphuric acid in 1 litre of water.

DRIP RATE CALCULATIONS

A standard 'giving' set or 'solution' set will administer 20 drops per ml of clear fluid.

A blood giving set will administer 15 drops per ml of blood (or 20 drops per ml of clear fluid).

Some burettes will administer 60 drops per ml.

It is important to check the number of drops per ml delivered by the giving set on the outer packaging, as this may vary slightly between products.

The formula to calculate the drip rate required to deliver the correct volume to be administered is:

Number of drops per minute = Volume to be given (ml)
× Number of drops per ml delivered by the set/duration of the infusion (minutes).

Example

A drug is to be administered using a standard solution set at a rate of 50 mg/m^2 per min to a patient whose surface area is 1.6 m^2. The drug is a 4% w/v solution.

What drip rate should be used?

The patient requires $50 \times 1.6 = 80$ mg/min
A 4% w/v solution   = 4 g in 100 ml
                    = 4000 mg in 100 ml
                    = 40 mg in 1 ml

To obtain 80 mg divide the 1 ml by 40 mg and multiply by 80 mg:

$$= 80 \text{ mg in } 2 \text{ ml}$$

The patient needs 2 ml/min of the solution. Using the drip rate formula:

Number of drops/min $= 2 \text{ (ml)} \times 20/1 \text{ (minute)}$
         $= 40 \text{ drops/min.}$

DISPLACEMENT VALUES

When dry powder injections are reconstituted the powder displaces a certain volume of fluid, known as the *displacement value* or *displacement volume* of the drug. Errors will occur unless this displacement volume is considered when part-vials are used to administer doses, as frequently occurs in neonates and children when the doses are small. Displacement values can be found in the relevant data sheets or paediatric dosage books.

 The total final volume in the reconstituted vial is equal to the sum of the displacement value of the drug and the volume of diluent added. The volume of diluent added is generally reduced by a value equal to the displacement value.

Example

Dosage required: 50 mg/kg for a child weighing 8 kg. The 500 mg vial has a displacement value of 0.3 ml, and 5 ml water for injection is generally used to reconstitute the drug.

 What volume should be administered?

Displacement value of the 500 mg vial = 0.3 ml
Add 5−0.3 ml = 4.7 ml water to the vial to make a total volume = 5 ml,
giving a final dilution of 500 mg in 5 ml.
Dosage required = 50 × 8 = 400 mg
so 400 mg in 5/500 × 400 = 4 ml

The difference if the displacement value is not considered is:

Add 5 ml water to the 500 mg vial to make a total volume = 5.3 ml.

If 4 ml of this reconstituted drug is administered, the dose given to the patient will be:

500/5.3 × 4 = 377 mg,
23 mg less than prescribed.

RECONSTITUTION AND DILUTION

Awareness of possible interactions and knowledge of the basic steps to minimise or prevent these are essential. Interactions may occur between drugs, between the drug and the diluent or between the drug and the container.

DRUG STABILITY

Problems can arise from three main areas: chemical breakdown or the influence of light; the precipitation of the drug out of solution; or incompatibilities or interaction of the drug with the plastic tubing used in the administration set or solution bag.

When several drugs interact with one another, a multilumen central venous cannula can be used. Each drug enters the vein separately from the others through its own lumen and the rapid blood flow dilutes the drugs to prevent harmful interactions.

Chemical breakdown

Chemical breakdown of a single drug can happen in any of several ways, including:

- hydrolysis
- oxidation or reduction
- photolysis or light degradation.

Hydrolysis

Invariably, injectable drugs are made up in water or water-based solutions such as glucose or saline. In practice, degradation due to hydrolysis is not a significant problem. It may occur with drugs that are relatively unstable in aqueous solutions. These often need to be reconstituted immediately before use.

The pH of the solution is an important factor. Drugs that are not obviously acids or alkalis can have acidic or basic characteristics. For example, glucose 5% has a pH of approximately 4.0–4.2 (depending on the manufacturer).

Hydrolysis will often be accelerated by inappropriate pH changes, which can occur if a diluent (or a second drug) causes the solution to become more acidic or more alkaline. Even the small difference in pH between sodium chloride 0.9% and glucose 5% injections, for example, can dramatically affect the stability of some drugs such as amphotericin. pH changes can often be controlled by adding a 'buffer solution' to the infusion fluid.

Temperature can also affect the rate at which hydrolysis occurs; usually the higher the temperature, the faster the reaction. But as with pH effects, this is not a serious problem under normal clinical conditions.

Oxidation/reduction

Some drugs react with oxygen. Adrenaline (epinephrine), dopamine and ascorbic acid can react quite readily and, as with hydrolysis, the higher the temperature, the faster the reaction. Degradation can eventually occur over a period of time but, under normal clinical conditions, oxidation is not a problem.

Slight colour changes (usually pink) may occur with some drugs, e.g. dopamine and noradrenaline (norepinephrine). A minor discoloration usually represents minimal levels of oxidation. It is recommended that discoloured solutions are not used.

Reduction, or reaction with reducing agents, is similar. Thiamine is particularly prone to attack by reducing agents and the effect is greater at higher temperatures.

Photolysis or degradation by light

Natural daylight, specifically ultraviolet radiation, is the main cause of light-induced degradation. Examples of drugs prone to this are furosemide, nitroprusside, vitamin K, dacarbazine and amphotericin.

Fluorescent light is generally safe because it does not emit ultraviolet radiation. The exception is nitroprusside, which is very sensitive and is degraded rapidly by both fluorescent light and natural daylight. Therefore, light protection of the infusion bag and administration set is essential for nitroprusside.

Precipitation

A precipitate can block tubing, filters, cannulas or catheters and may lead to coronary or pulmonary emboli if administered to the patient. The rate at which a precipitate forms depends on time and temperature. Where precipitation is thought possible, the infusion must be inspected frequently and carefully.

pH effects

Insoluble drugs are rendered soluble by conversion to a salt. This makes them more sensitive to pH changes. Injections formulated using the compound itself rather than the salt of the compound are not affected by changes in pH. Insulin is one such example.

Acid drugs (which are made into salts of sodium, calcium or potassium) generally have an alkaline pH in solution. When alkaline injections are diluted with solutions of a lower pH, the pH of the overall solution will decrease. If the fall is too great and the solubility of the original drug in its acid form is low, a precipitate may form. Hence, if phenytoin, which has a pH greater than 9, is diluted, the minimum volume of diluent should be used.

Similarly, basic drugs (formulated as an acid salt such as hydrochloride, sulphate or nitrate) are soluble in acidic solutions. Dilution of these acidic salts with solutions of a higher pH will raise the pH and a precipitate may form. An example of a drug affected in this way is gentamicin.

 As a general rule, salts of acidic drugs in alkaline solutions are more likely to precipitate on dilution than the salts of basic drugs.

Other dilution effects

Some drugs are very poorly soluble in water and have to be dissolved or solubilised using co-solvents. These solubilisers include ethanol, polysorbates and propylene glycol. If the injection is diluted the co-solvent is also diluted and the drug may precipitate. An example of a drug affected in this way is diazepam.

Drug–drug co-precipitation

If two oppositely charged ions are mixed in solution, they may react to form an insoluble ion-pair. Examples of drugs at risk of such an interaction are gentamicin with heparin; furosemide with aminoglycosides.

Formation of an insoluble salt

Metals such as calcium, magnesium and iron will form an insoluble salt if allowed to mix with an acid drug.

Interaction with plastic component

Almost all containers, administration sets and components are made from plastics. A few drugs may bind to these plastics and this may affect the dose delivered. Often, these interactions can only be avoided by changing to polythene.

There are four types of process that can occur.

Adsorption

The drug binds to the surface of the plastic and does not penetrate any further.

The initial effect is a rapid and substantial drug loss from the solution. This occurs as the drug binds to the surface of the plastic. If this solution is run though a plastic/polyvinyl chloride (PVC) line, the dose of drug is initially reduced due to adsorption. Subsequently, the plastic surface becomes saturated and the delivery of the drug rapidly increases. Drugs affected in this way include insulin and interferons.

Insulin will adsorb on to any plastic, especially PVC and also on to glass. To minimise the effect, insulin should not be added to an infusion bag but should be given by syringe pump and the line flushed with the drug prior to use.

Absorption

The drug migrates into the plastic. This is a more common occurrence than adsorption. It is a slower process but eventually an equilibrium is established between the drug within the plastic and the drug in solution.

PVC is made pliable and flexible by incorporating a 'plasticiser' during its manufacture. This presents a particular problem with lipid-soluble drugs as they diffuse from the solution into the plasticiser within the plastic matrix. Examples of drugs affected are diazepam, chlorpromazine, nimodipine, carmustine.

Permeation

In this case, the drug migrates through the plastic to the outer surface, where it evaporates. Losses from permeation can be substantial and they continue throughout the period of administration because the plastic never becomes saturated. PVC presents the biggest problem. Examples of drugs affected are nitrates (glyceryl trinitrate, isosorbide dinitrate) and clomethiazole.

Many variables alter the magnitude of drug loss. These include drug concentration, flow rate, the surface area of the plastic, the type of plastic and the temperature.

Leaching

Leaching of the plasticiser into the solution can occur with PVC. The effect is not usually important except for ciclosporin infusions and storage of total parenteral nutrition regimens in PVC bags. Leaching from administration sets during infusion is relatively small but can occur from the rubber plungers of plastic syringes and may affect the stability of some drugs (e.g. asparaginase).

ADMINISTRATION

METHODS

There are three methods:

Bolus/intravenous push

Usually given undiluted over 3–5 minutes.

Intermittent infusion

Usually given over 10 minutes and up to over 6–8 hours.

Used as an alternative to bolus administration for regular dosing, where slower administration of a more dilute solution is required to avoid toxicity. For example, vancomycin must be given at a maximum rate of 10 mg/min to avoid red-man syndrome; erythromycin must be diluted to at least 5 mg in 1 ml to reduce the risk of thrombophlebitis.

Continuous infusion

The term is used when infusions are given continuously over 24 hours. The rate may be variable. Drugs delivered in this way include dopamine and heparin. Continuous infusions are used where a continuous or controlled therapeutic response is required for drugs with a short half-life or a narrow therapeutic window. If a drug has a short half-life, it will be eliminated from the body quickly. In most cases it can be assumed that no drug will remain in the body after a time interval of four half-lives. For example, it is essential to maintain adequate levels of heparin in the plasma over a 24-hour period to treat a thrombosis. The half-life of heparin is approximately 1 hour. Therefore, it must be infused continuously to maintain its therapeutic effect.

If a drug has a narrow therapeutic window, e.g. aminophylline, there is a narrow range of plasma concentrations between which the drug exerts a therapeutic effect without toxicity. It is vital to maintain the drug concentration in the plasma within this range.

THE ADMINISTRATION SET

The components that make up administration sets are shown in Figure 22.1. Manufacturers can provide any combination of components but, if requirements are special, then the cost may be higher for standard items. The components shown will vary from manufacturer to manufacturer and so this is not a comprehensive list.

A. Four-way lumen for central venous site, which can infuse four drugs separately, each with its own lumen

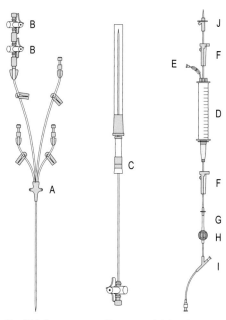

Fig. 22.1 Components making up an administration set.

B. Three-way stopcocks, also known as 'traffic lights', so that additional drugs can be infused into a lumen or a peripheral line
C. Cannula for peripheral site. The cannula has a steel inner needle that punctures the vein and is then withdrawn. The cannula has an extension line of its own and a three-way stopcock
D. 150 ml burette for neonatal infusions with a volumetric pump shown with an extra injection port
E. Air inlet port
F. Roller clamp for closing off any administration line
G. Silicone rubber insert in ordinary PVC tubing for use in neonatal infusions, because this rubber does not distort or 'creep' when compressed by the volumetric pump mechanism. Silicone rubber improves the accuracy of the administration rate
H. Pressure disc for measuring pressure in the administration set during an infusion. Used in sets for volumetric and syringe pumps
I. 'Y' connector (Y site) for entry of another drug into the line

J.   Spike for insertion into the fluid bag, shown with its own
     injection port.

INFUSION PUMPS

These can be grouped broadly into two types, which are summarised
in Table 22.1 (pp 420–421):

- Simple gravity drips
- Infusion pumps.

Simple gravity drips

These depend entirely on gravity to drive the infusion and generally
use the cheapest administration sets. They comprise a drip chamber
and use a roller clamp to control the flow rate, which is measured by
counting drops. They are suitable for infusing replacement fluids such
as simple electrolytes, which do not require any particular degree of
accuracy. The delivery pressure developed for infusion depends
entirely on the height above the infusion site of the liquid level in the
container; at about 1 m this pressure is 70 mmHg. The pressure in an
adult peripheral vein is about 25 mmHg so, provided there is not too
much resistance to flow through the cannula, the infusion will run
satisfactorily. The risk of extravasation is minimised by the use of low
delivery pressures.

    Limitations include the following:

- The tubing can distort and flatten within the roller clamp over
  time
- The clamp position can be disturbed
- High fluctuations in venous pressure can reduce the flow rate
- The size of drops can vary with the fluid being infused
- The delivery pressures may be insufficient to provide arterial
  infusions and to deliver viscous fluids into a peripheral vein
- An open roller clamp may free-flow without warning.

Infusion pumps

Infusion pumps are powered devices that provide the desired flow by
a positive pumping action. They include:

Volumetric pumps

The desired flow rate is set in millilitres per hour. A drop sensor may
be present for the purpose of indicating an empty infusion bag or for
detecting inaccuracies in the flow rate.

    Volumetric pumps achieve good delivery accuracy over a wide
range of flow rates. They have safety features with alarms, e.g. to

detect vascular occlusions and the presence of air bubbles in the infusion fluid. They can be used for both venous and arterial infusions and when the fluid reservoir is nearly empty they will automatically revert to a low delivery rate to keep the vein open. However, they are more expensive than other pumps and may require dedicated administration sets recommended by the manufacturers. It can sometimes be possible to insert the wrong set and the pump may still appear to work correctly.

Syringe pumps ('syringe drivers')

These are devices in which a syringe or cartridge containing the solution to be infused is secured in the pump and a plunger is driven forward at a predetermined rate to achieve the desired infusion rate. The flow rate may be set in millilitres per hour, millimetres (mm) per hour or millimetres per 24 hours.

Syringe pumps are used to administer drugs in concentrated solutions where fluid balance is important and/or when the rate of administration needs to be carefully controlled.

Modern syringe pumps have the same safety features as their volumetric counterparts and their administration sets are simple and relatively inexpensive. However, older models have insufficient safety features to minimise the possibility of free flow.

Mechanical backlash – the delay between starting the pump and achieving the constant infusion rate – is inherent in the pump mechanism. This delay can be therapeutically significant at very low infusion rates during the backlash period, hence the need for the use of two pumps used concurrently for infusion of inotropes. The most modern designs incorporate mechanisms to compensate for backlash.

Most syringe drivers require a specific brand or brands of syringe, due to the variation in the bore size of the syringes.

Patient-controlled analgesia (PCA) pumps

These are devices in which the patient is able to initiate a bolus dose of the infusion solution for the relief of pain. Patients are prevented from altering the setting of the pump and preprogrammed restraints are placed on the parameters of the boluses. In addition, a basal rate delivery of solution outside the control of the patient may be provided.

Pumps for ambulatory use

These are small and light enough to be carried around by the patient without unduly interfering with everyday activities.

Anaesthesia pumps

These are syringe pumps suitable for the administration of anaesthetic agents. They are unsuitable for any other use.

Multipurpose pumps

These pumps can be made to perform as one of the above pumps.

Other devices

These include non-electrically powered devices that do not have electrically generated alarm signals. Some of them are charged with a syringe and then deliver their output more or less continuously, with flow being controlled by a flow-regulating means such as a capillary tube. This type of pumping device may use an elastomeric membrane that, once expanded, provides sufficient force to drive the infusion. Applications include PCA and emergency situations.

The performance of non-electrically powered devices is generally inferior to the devices mentioned above but they may have other advantages, such as simplicity and the ability to operate in difficult environments.

Spring-driven, clockwork and gas-powered infusion devices are available but will not be discussed here.

Flow regulators are manually set, non-powered devices that appear in a variety of forms and clamp on to or are inserted in the line. They usually have a rotary dial to give an indication of expected flow rate. Some of these devices claim to compensate for venous back pressure and maintain consistent flow.

TABLE 22.1 Advantages and disadvantages of different pump types

Pump type	Advantages	Disadvantages
Simple gravity drip	Lowest cost Familiar to all staff Simple to set up Infusion of air less likely Minimises risk of extravascular infusion	Cannot be used for arterial infusions Requires frequent observation and adjustment Variability of drop size Infusion rates limited, especially with viscous fluids and small catheters

TABLE 22.1 Advantages and disadvantages of different pump types – cont'd

Pump type	Advantages	Disadvantages
		Risk of free flow (open roller clamps)
		User may need to calculate drop rate
Volumetric pumps	Calibrated in ml/h	More expensive than most other pumps
	Good volumetric accuracy	Some require dedicated sets*
	Wide flow rate range	Some can be complicated to set up
	Many features and facilities designed to ensure very safe operation	Incorrect set* can be loaded and pump appears to work
	Comprehensive alarm systems	
	Air-in-line detection	
	Many have low occlusion alarm pressure settings	
	Some have delivery pressure sensors	
	Secondary infusion facility often available	
	Can be used for both venous and arterial infusions	
	Neonatal versions available	
Syringe pumps	Usually calibrated in mm/h or mm/24h	Free flow possible on older models without plunger clamps
	Smooth and precise delivery at low flow rates	There can be problems with mechanical backlash
	Easy to operate	Occlusion alarm pressure settings on earlier models are sometimes rather high, which would result in a poor occlusion response
		Earlier models prone to incorrect fitting of syringe
		Danger of setting wrong rate. User must ensure whether pump is calibrated per hour or or per 24h

*A number of volumetric pumps use low-cost standard solution sets, but it is important to note that the pump must be configured correctly for the specific set.

RISK CLASSIFICATION OF INFUSION PUMPS

The Department of Health has specified the performance and functions that an infusion pump must meet in order to be classified under one or more of the following risk categories (Medicines Device Agency 1995):

a. neonatal risk
b. high-risk
c. lower-risk
d. ambulatory risk.

- *a. Neonatal risk infusion pumps,* for infusions to neonates, require equipment of high accuracy and consistency of flow with 0.1 ml/h increments, low occlusion alarm times and very low bolus on release of occlusion. Comprehensive alarm displays that identify the precise problem and safety interlocks to prevent tampering while running are important
- *b. High-risk infusion pumps* are used for high-risk infusions to adults, for drugs such as dopamine, dobutamine and cytotoxics. This category requires high accuracy and consistency of flow, good occlusion alarm response, comprehensive alarm displays that identify the precise problem, and safety interlocks.

Both neonatal and high-risk pumps should have internal rechargeable battery back-up with a memory of parameters displayed so that vital data are not lost due to inadvertent switch off.

Neonatal and high-risk infusion pumps must be accurate to within 5% of the set rate when measured over a 60-minute period. They must also satisfy short-term minute-to-minute requirements that determine smoothness and consistency of flow rate. These pumps must not suck back during infusion, there should not be significant periods of zero flow and the flow rate should not have large fluctuations.

- *c. Lower-risk infusion pumps,* for lower-risk infusion to adults but not to neonates, cover the infusion of simple electrolytes and antibiotics. The equipment does not need to be so accurate and consistent in output and need have only rudimentary alarm and safety systems. Battery back-up is not essential
- *d. Ambulatory infusion pumps.* The Department of Health has not yet assessed the risk associated with these. These pumps include all infusion equipment, which may be worn on the person so that normal activities can be continued while the infusion is being given. The equipment will often be battery-powered but clockwork mechanisms, elastomeric membranes or gas-powered devices can also be used.

DRUGS

To ensure safe administration of infusions, drugs can be classified into matching risk categories (Pickstone et al 1995). This classification is based on the perceived level of risk in the administration of that drug. This risk level may also be influenced by factors such as the environment in which the drug is being used. Once the risk level of a drug has been defined, this can be matched to the performance and functions of the different categories of infusion pump. Safe administration can then be ensured if the drug is administered using a pump of the same or higher risk level.

FILTERS

For a small selection of drugs, e.g. flucytosine, mannitol, phenytoin and tetracycline, manufacturers recommend that in-line filters are used when administering the drug. This is because there may be particulate deposits in the vial (e.g. tetracycline) or because the solution is prone to precipitation (e.g. phenytoin).

The pore size of the filter required varies between products. Most standard solution administration sets contain a 15 micron (μm) filter. However, if a smaller pore size is required, a separate filter must be connected into the administration set. For example, phenytoin requires a 0.22–0.55 μm filter.

 In-line filters should only be used once.

REFERENCES

Medicines Devices Agency 1995 Device bulletin infusion systems. MDA DB 9503, May 1995. Medicines Devices Agency, London

Pickstone M, Auty B, Jacklin A et al 1995 Intravenous infusion of drugs: part 2. A new safety protocol for intravenously infused drugs. British Journal of Intensive Care 5: 17–24

CHAPTER 23

Sodium content of injectable drugs

B. Langfield

Table 23.1 lists the sodium content (in millimoles) of injectable drugs. Where there is more than one strength of ampoule/vial, the differing sodium contents have been given whenever differences exist.

TABLE 23.1 Sodium content of injectable drugs

Drug	Sodium content
Abciximab	0.15 mmol/2 mg
Acetazolamide	2.36 mmol/500 mg
Acetylcysteine	12.78 mmol/2 g
Aciclovir	1.16 mmol/250 mg
Adenosine	0.154 mmol/3 mg
Adrenaline (epinephrine) (Martindale)	0.118–0.148 mmol/ml
L-alanyl-L-glutamine	Nil
Albumin 5%	130–160 mmol/l
Albumin 20%	
Alemtuzumab	0.05–0.5 mmol/30 mg
Alfentanil	0.39 mmol/500 µg 0.36 mmol/5 mg
Alteplase (Actilyse)	Nil
Alprostadil	Nil
Amikacin	0.14 mmol/100 mg 0.72 mmol/500 mg
Amifostine	Nil
Aminophylline	Nil
Amiodarone	Nil
Amoxicillin	3.3 mmol/1 g vial
Ampicillin	1.47 mmol/500 mg
Amphotericin (Fungizone)	<0.5 mmol/50 mg

TABLE 23.1 Sodium content of injectable drugs – cont'd

Drug	Sodium content
Amphotericin lipid (Abelcet)	Nil
Amphotericin liposomal (AmBisome)	0.4 mmol/50 mg
Aprotinin	0.154 mmol/ml
Atenolol	1.26–1.76 mmol/ml
Atosiban	Nil
Atracurium	Nil
Ascorbic acid	2.9 mmol/100 mg
Atropine sulphate (Min-I-Jet)	4.5 mmol/100 µg
Azathioprine	0.2 mmol/50 mg
Aztreonam	Nil
Basiliximab	0.021 mmol/10 mg vial 0.042 mmol/20 mg vial
Benzatropine	0.15 mmol/1 mg
Benzylpenicillin	1.68 mmol/600 mg 3.36 mmol/1.2 g
Bumetanide	0.01 mmol/500 µg
Buprenorphine	Nil
C1 esterase inhibitor	0.146–0.207 mmol/50 mg
Caffeine citrate	136 mmol/l
Calcitonin (salmon)/salcatonin	0.13 mmol/ml
Calcium chloride	Negligible
Calcium folinate (Mayne Pharma)	*15 mg/2 ml:* 0.2 mmol/ml
Calcium levofolinate	0.13 mmol/10 mg
Calcitriol	Negligible
Caspofungin	0.028 mmol/50 mg 0.04 mmol/70 mg
Cefotaxime	2.09 mmol/g
Cefradine	Nil
Ceftazidime	2.3 mmol/g
Cefuroxime	1.8 mmol/750 mg
Chloramphenicol sodium succinate	3.14 mmol/g
Chloroquine	No information available
Chlorphenamine	No information available

TABLE 23.1 Sodium content of injectable drugs – cont'd

Drug	Sodium content
Chlorpromazine	Negligible
Ciclosporin	Nil
Cimetidine	Nil
Ciprofloxacin	15.4 mmol/200 mg
Clarithromycin	<0.5 mmol/500 mg
Clindamycin	Negligible
Clonazepam	Nil
Clonidine	0.15 mmol/150 µg
Co-amoxiclav (Augmentin)	1.35 mmol/600 mg 2.7 mmol/1.2 g
Colistimethate sodium (Colomycin)	<0.5 mmol/500 000 unit and 1 000 000 unit vials
Co-trimoxazole	1.64 mmol/480 mg
Cyclizine	Nil
Dantrolene	0.08 mmol/20 mg
Desferrioxamine	Nil
Desmopressin	0.15 mmol/ml
Dexamethasone sodium phosphate	0.021 mmol/ml
Diamorphine hydrochloride	Nil
Diazepam emulsion (Diazemuls)	0.004 mmol/2 ml
Diclofenac	0.273 mmol/75 mg
Digoxin (Glaxo SmithKline)	0.0252 mmol/ml
Dicobalt edetate	Nil
Digoxin-specific antibody fragments (Digibind)	≈0.48 mmol/38 mg vial
Disodium folinate	<0.325 mmol/54.65 mg
Dipyridamole	Nil
Dobutamine	Nil
Dopamine	<2.1 mmol/200 mg
Dopexamine	0.09 mmol/50 mg
Doxapram	Nil
Edrophonium	0.165 mmol/ml
Esomeprazole	0.1 mmol/40 mg vial
Epoetin-beta (NeoRecormon)	Negligible

TABLE 23.1 Sodium content of injectable drugs – cont'd

Drug	Sodium content
Epoprostenol	No information
Erythromycin	Nil
Esmolol	2.87 mmol/2.5 g, 0.473 mmol/100 mg
Fentanyl	0.3 mmol/l
Filgrastim	Negligible
Flucloxacillin	0.55 mmol/250 mg 1.1 mmol/500 mg 2.2 mmol/g
Fluconazole	0.154 mmol/ml
Foscarnet sodium	15.6 mmol/g
Furosemide	≈0.16 mmol/10 mg
Gelofusine	154 mmol/l
Gentamicin	0.034 mmol/40 mg
Glucagon	Nil
Glyceryl trinitrate (Mayne Pharma)	Nil
Glycopyrronium	0.15 mmol/ml
Gonadorelin	Nil
Granisetron	0.15 mmol/1 mg 1.17 mmol/3 mg
Heparin (Monoparin/Multiparin, CP)	*1000 units/ml:* 0.025–0.032 mmol/ml *5000 units/ml:* 0.125–0.16 mmol/ml *25 000 units/ml:* 0.625–0.8 mmol/ml
Heparin (Leo)	*1000 units/ml:* 0.21 mmol/ml *5000 units/ml:* 0.13 mmol/ml *25 000 units/ml:* 0.65 mmol/ml
Hydralazine	Nil
Hydrocortisone sodium succinate	0.5 mmol/100 mg
Hydrocortisone sodium phosphate	0.66 mmol/ml
Iloprost	0.08 mmol/0.5 ml
Imipenem with cilastatin	1.7 mmol/500 mg
Indometacin	0.003 mmol/1 mg

TABLE 23.1 Sodium content of injectable drugs – cont'd

Drug	Sodium content
Iron dextran (CosmoFer)	Nil
Iron sucrose (Venofer)	Nil
Isoniazid	Nil
Itraconazole	Nil
Ketorolac trometamol	0.07 mmol/10 mg ampoule 0.13 mmol/30 mg ampoule
Labetalol	Negligible
Lenograstim	Negligible
Levomepromazine (methotrimeprazine)	0.119 mmol/ml
Linezolid	5 mmol/300 ml
Meropenem	3.9 mmol/g
Methylprednisolone sodium succinate	2.01 mmol/g
Metoclopramide	0.1 mmol/10 mg
Metoprolol	0.8 mmol/5 mg
Metronidazole (Flagyl)	13.6 mmol/100 ml
Midazolam	0.14 mmol/ml
Milrinone	Nil
Morphine sulphate	Negligible
Muromonab CD3	≈0.88 mmol/5 mg
Netilmicin	0.223 mmol/15 mg 0.106 mmol/50 mg 0.038 mmol/100 mg 0.058 mmol/150 mg 0.077 mmol/200 mg
Neostigmine	0.115 mmol/2.5 mg
Octreotide	0.029 mmol/ml
Ofloxacin	15.4 mmol/200 mg
Omeprazole	0.13–0.15 mmol/40 mg
Ondansetron	0.16 mmol/2 mg
Pabrinex I/V High potency	2.95 mmol per combined pair ampoule
Pancuronium	0.15 mmol/ml
Papaveretum BP	≈0.016 mmol/ml
Pentamidine (pentamidine isetionate)	Nil

TABLE 23.1 Sodium content of injectable drugs – cont'd

Drug	Sodium content
Phenoxybenzamine	Nil
Phentolamine mesylate	Negligible
Phenytoin sodium	0.18 mmol/50 mg
Phytomenadione (vitamin K) (Konakion MM)	0.115 mmol/10 mg
Potassium chloride	Nil
Potassium phosphate (Martindale)	0.011 mmol/ml
Potassium phosphate (Torbay)	Nil
Propranolol	Nil
Remifentanil	Nil
Rifampicin	<0.5 mmol/vial
Rituximab	0.03 mmol/ml (7.35 mg/ml) 0.15 mmol/ml (9 mg/ml)
Salbutamol	0.15 mmol/ml
Sodium bicarbonate 1.26%	150 mmol/1 litre
Sodium clodronate concentrate	0.45 mmol/60 mg
Sodium chloride 0.9%	150 mmol/1 litre
Sodium fusidate	3.1 mmol/500 mg
Sodium nitroprusside	0.34 mmol/50 mg
Sodium valproate	2.40 mmol/400 mg
Sotalol	0.4 mmol/40 mg
Streptokinase	No information
Sulfadiazine	4 mmol/g
Suxamethonium	Nil
Synercid	16 mmol/500 mg vial
Tazocin (piperacillin with tazobactam)	4.69 mmol/2.25 g vial 9.37 mmol/4.5 g vial
Teicoplanin	<0.5 mmol/200 mg and 400 mg vial
Terlipressin	Nil
Tetracosactide	0.14 mmol/3.32 mg
Thiopental sodium	1.89 mmol/550 mg vial
Timentin (ticarcillin with clavulanic acid)	5.3 mmol/g
Tirofiban	164 mmol/12.5 mg

TABLE 23.1 Sodium content of injectable drugs – cont'd

Drug	Sodium content
Tobramycin (Medimpex UK)	0.0155 mmol/40 mg
Tranexamic acid	Nil
Trastuzumab	Nil
Tropisetron	0.15 mmol/ml
Vancomycin	Nil
Vasopressin (synthetic)	No information available
Verapamil	No information available
Vitamins B and C (Pabrinex I/V High potency)	2.95 mmol per combined pair ampoule
Voriconazole	9.62 mmol/200 mg vial
Zoledronic acid	0.279 mmol/4 mg

Laboratory tests

A. Willson, A. Kostrzewski

In the tables that follow, we have quoted reference ranges for commonly performed tests. Many of these, for example serum potassium and sodium or red and white blood cell counts, vary little from hospital to hospital. Others may be affected by the characteristics of the indigenous population or by the test method used. The latter is particularly true of enzyme assays and so it is worth checking these tables against those used locally.

Typically, a reference range represents the mean result observed ± 2 standard deviations, so a small percentage of the population will normally be outside this range even when healthy. The role of laboratory tests is therefore to screen for possible disease, to confirm a clinical diagnosis or to follow the course of a disease process. They can never be regarded as a diagnosis in themselves.

CLINICAL CHEMISTRY

FLUID BALANCE (Table 24.1)

Water accounts for approximately 60% (approx. 42 litres) of body weight. There is less water in women, 55% of body weight, owing to a higher body fat content – adipose tissue contains very little water. The metabolisms of sodium and water are closely linked both physiologically and clinically.

The osmolalities of the intracellular fluid (approx. 28 litres) and extracellular fluid (approx. 14 litres) determine the distribution of water between compartments. In health the osmolality of plasma is approximately 285 mmol/kg.

UREA AND ELECTROLYTES

The interpretation of the tests of urea and electrolytes is described in Table 24.2.

TABLE 24.1 Fluid balance over 24 hours in a healthy adult

	Intake (ml)	Output (ml)
Oral fluids	1500	
Water in food	600	
Endogenous water production	400	
Losses		
Skin		500
Lungs		400
Faeces		100
Kidney		1500
Total	**2500**	**2500**

ACID–BASE BALANCE

The pH of blood is normally maintained between 7.35 and 7.45. It represents a balance between alkali (mainly bicarbonate, HCO_3^-) and acid (mainly carbonic acid, H_2CO_3), where the alkali is kept in excess. Hydrogen ions are generated by many of the metabolic reactions in the body and, in the presence of oxygen, are removed from metabolic coenzymes to produce water. The dehydrogenated coenzymes are then able to participate in further reactions. When the blood pH is disturbed, metabolic reactions are impaired and death is likely to result when blood pH is outside the range 6.9–7.9. Tests of acid–base balance are listed in Table 24.3.

Other ion pairs are sometimes important. If tissue oxygenation is poor, for example after an infarct or in vascular insufficiency, hydrogen ions are not cleared in the usual way and pyruvate is reduced to lactate. Lactic acid builds up and is only cleared when oxygen is once again available.

Homeostasis

Balance is preserved by the interplay of several systems, most of which are capable of some adjustment in a disturbed environment. The lungs supply oxygen to tissues and expel carbon dioxide, so converting carbonic acid to water. In acidosis, or if there is an increase in carbon dioxide in the blood, respiratory rate increases. Erythrocytes mop up small amounts of carbon dioxide in exchange for bicarbonate and will rectify small acidotic disturbances, but their capacity is limited. They rely on regular 'rejuvenation' by healthy lungs and even then will make little contribution to correcting a severe imbalance.

TABLE 24.2 Urea and electrolytes

Test	Reference range	Interpretation
Bicarbonate	22–29 mmol/l	See Table 24.3. Danger levels are <10 mmol/l or >40 mmol/l
Calcium	2.25–2.6 mmol/l	Adjust result for hypoproteinaemia: add 0.02 mmol/l for every g/l of serum albumin below 40 g/l
		⚠ **Above 3.50 mmol/l = medical emergency, danger of cardiac arrest.**
		2.6–3.5 mmol/l, treat once diagnosis is made to avoid renal damage. Hydration plus other measures if needed. Below 2.25 usually symptom-free. Give oral vitamin D ± calcium if needed. Tetany usually only below 1.6 mmol/l. Low calcium levels are found in patients with hypomagnesaemia
Chloride	95–105 mmol/l	Don't bother, it tells you very little
Glucose	3.3–7.8 mmol/l (fasting)	Random venous plasma glucose ≥11.1 mmol/l or a venous plasma level above 7.8 mmol/l after overnight fast suggests diabetes mellitus. Equivocal results are clarified with glucose tolerance test. Level should return below 6.7 mmol/l 2 hours after 75 g challenge for venous or capillary whole blood
Magnesium	0.7–1.2 mmol/l	Hypomagnesaemia has similar symptoms to hypocalcaemia. Especially likely with severe diarrhoea. Measurement indicated in normocalcaemic tetany. Hypermagnesaemia results in loss of muscle tone: occurs in renal failure, especially if magnesium salts have been given. Symptoms above 2.5 mmol/l may cause cardiac arrhythmias

TABLE 24.2 Urea and electrolytes – cont'd

Test	Reference range	Interpretation
Phosphate	0.8–1.4 mmol/l	Disturbed phosphate levels are rarely symptomatic in themselves but may affect calcium metabolism
Potassium	3.5–5.3 mmol/l	⚠ **Levels above 6.5 mmol/l may be dangerous and should be treated as an emergency, first with calcium and then with, for example, dextrose and insulin. This condition is often precipitated by acidosis, which must be treated.**

Levels below 2.5 mmol/l usually result in muscle weakness and supplements are required. Alkalosis may also result. Mild hypokalaemia is rarely symptomatic |
Protein	50–70 g/l (total)	Albumin exerts substantial osmotic pressure and levels below 20 g/l usually result in oedema
	35–55 g/l (albumin)	Hypoalbuminaemia may reflect haemodilution, nephropathy, cirrhosis or catabolism. Total protein is composed of albumin plus globulins. In cirrhosis, globulin levels may rise because of reticuloendothelial hyperplasia. Hyperalbuminaemia may occur with haemoconcentration but is not usually of clinical interest
Sodium	133–149 mmol/l	Abnormal sodium levels should almost always be interpreted as water imbalance. Hence hypernatraemia usually reflects

TABLE 24.2 Urea and electrolytes – cont'd

Test	Reference range	Interpretation
		excess fluid loss or inadequate intake. Absolute sodium excess occurs with steroid therapy and in renal failure. Symptoms of confusion, then coma, above 155–160 mmol/l. Give dextrose infusion (dialysis for absolute sodium excess). Hyponatraemia usually reflects haemodilution due to cardiac or renal failure and hypoalbuminaemia. Symptoms of weakness below 120 mmol/l; confusion likely below 100 mmol/l. Mild hyponatraemia usually symptom-free. Treat with water deprivation, mannitol or, for excess antidiuretic hormone, demeclocycline
Urea	2.5–6.5 mmol/l	Levels above 10 mmol/l may reflect renal failure, catabolic states, haemorrhage or high dietary protein. For pharmacists, indicates need to check other indicators of renal function (see appropriate table)
Zinc	10–23 μmol/l	May be low in hypoalbuminaemic state. Used to evaluate nutrition inadequacy in enteral or parenteral nutrition, diabetes and wound healing

The most potent mechanism for adjusting pH is in the kidney. Normally, bicarbonate is filtered in the glomerulus and an equal amount is put back into the blood from the tubular cells. In acidosis, bicarbonate continues to be secreted into the blood while hydrogen ions are lost in the urine. Hence there is a net gain in extracellular bicarbonate and loss of hydrogen ions. This mechanism is stimulated by a rise in blood carbon dioxide or carbonic acid.

Potassium

Sodium conservation by the kidney and the sodium pump at cell walls exchanges sodium ions for potassium or hydrogen ions. There is free competition between these two species and balance may be disturbed if there is a lack or preponderance of one or the other. For example,

TABLE 24.3 Tests of acid–base balance

Test	Reference range	Interpretation
Blood pH	7.35–7.45	This is the main indicator of immediate danger to life. Outside this range, metabolic function throughout the body is impaired. Blood pH reflects the ratio of acid to base and not absolute concentration. It may therefore mask a defect for which the body has compensated
Base excess	–3 to +3 mmol/l	Reflects the amount of acid required to titrate blood back to pH 7.4. It therefore adds little more than knowledge of pH
Bicarbonate	22–29 mmol/l	This is the absolute amount of bicarbonate present in the blood and reflects renal and metabolic function
Pco_2	4.5–6.0 kPa (34–45 mmHg)	This is the partial pressure of carbon dioxide in blood and, since it is in equilibrium with carbonic acid, reflects the absolute amount of acid in the blood (except where there is a significant amount of lactic acid). It is the indicator of respiratory function (carbonic acid is not measured directly as it is volatile and present only in small concentrations)
Standard bicarbonate	22–27 mmol/l	This is a measurement of bicarbonate plus related alkalis conducted at Pco_2 of 40 mmHg. Comparison with the actual bicarbonate level permits assessment of the relative contributions of the erythrocytes and kidneys

metabolic acidosis will increase the concentration of hydrogen ions and hence the amount cleared from the blood at these two sites. Since the amount of sodium exchanged is unaltered, clearance of potassium will be diminished and hyperkalaemia results. Conversely, alkalosis can produce a relative hypokalaemia.

This may lead to a problem of interpretation. If hydrogen and potassium ion concentrations are both abnormal, which was the primary disturbance? In the absence of a known cause, it is reasonable to assume that an acidosis with hyperkalaemia has been set up by a primary acidosis, since primary hyperkalaemia is relatively uncommon. On the other hand, hypokalaemia is more likely than primary alkalosis.

Acidosis

Respiratory acidosis is a result of accumulation of carbon dioxide: a raised carbonic acid concentration is caused by depressed respiration. The disturbed acid:alkali ratio is a result of increased acid. Metabolic acidosis, on the other hand, occurs due to a net fall in bicarbonate ions. These may be lost by poorly functioning kidneys or be used up in buffering excessive hydrogen ions from the tissues. The imbalance here is due to a decrease in alkali.

When pH is disturbed by a malfunction of one system, other mechanisms attempt to compensate. A respiratory alkalosis will cause the kidneys to excrete hydrogen ions and so a rise in pH is achieved by a net increase in bicarbonate ions. Conversely, when plasma bicarbonate is diminished by a metabolic acidosis, the lungs will attempt to restore normal pH by exhaling more carbon dioxide. In general, the kidneys are more effective in compensating for acid–base defects than are the lungs.

Ketoacidosis

This is distinguished from other types of metabolic acidosis by its cause and several concurrent electrolyte disturbances. Insulin lack leads to hyperglycaemia and thus osmotic diuresis and profound dehydration. Also, intracellular metabolism switches to fat with ketones and acid byproducts. Acidosis produces secondary hyperkalaemia. Treatment is with insulin and rehydration, plus careful attention to potassium levels.

Alkalosis

Overbreathing may precipitate alkalosis by reducing the carbon dioxide level of the blood and hence the carbonic acid concentration. Production of bicarbonate by the kidneys will be slowed and the pH corrected.

Rarely, metabolic alkalosis can occur, for example in severe potassium depletion or pyloric stenosis. The lungs do not compensate for this state.

The interrelation of acid–base disturbances and the ability of the body to compensate for primary imbalances make the interpretation of results exceedingly difficult. Nonetheless, it is important to identify the primary disturbance so that the correct diagnosis and therapy can be found.

Acid–base disturbances

The common disturbances of acid–base balance, both acutely and after compensation, are described in Table 24.4.

LIVER FUNCTION TESTS (Table 24.5)

On a simplified level, abnormal liver function can be divided into three types.

Acute cellular damage

This occurs with acute hepatitis or toxicity to the liver. The main effect is that enzymes normally present in large amounts in liver cells and in relatively small amounts in serum leach out of the now permeable liver cell walls. These are mainly alanine and aspartate transaminase (ALT and AST), and they appear in massively increased quantities in the blood. A second effect is that the liver fails to clear bilirubin from the blood and so it builds up in its unconjugated form.

Chronic cellular damage

After long-term insults to the liver, as with alcohol-induced cirrhosis, cells pass through the stage described above and eventually die. They are replaced by fibrous tissue. Hence, transaminase levels are often normal but the elements of the blood which the liver is responsible for producing occur in small concentrations. Cirrhosis is thus characterised by hypoalbuminaemia and an increased prothrombin time, resulting from a reduction of clotting factors.

Cholestasis

Blockage of the bile duct may be mechanical or due to chemical action. Many drugs produce this effect. The result is that many substances normally excreted in the bile build up in the liver and appear in the blood. Conjugated bilirubin and alkaline phosphatase (ALP) are the most useful to measure. Another enzyme, gamma-glutamyl transferase (GGT), behaves similarly but is a less reliable indicator of disease since it is subject to induction. It will, for example, show increased serum levels after exposure to several drugs or a significant alcohol load.

The differential diagnosis of liver disease relies on the relative disturbance of each of these indicators, as well as on other tests.

TABLE 24.4 Acid–base disturbances

Disturbance		Acute change	After compensation
Respiratory acidosis			
CO$_2$ not cleared by the lungs. Chronic obstructive airways or barbiturate or opiate poisoning	pH	↓	
	Pco$_2$	↑	↑
	HCO$_3^-$		↑
	Standard HCO$_3^-$	↓	↑
	K$^+$		↑
Respiratory alkalosis			
Excessive CO$_2$ clearance by lungs. Hysterical overbreathing, CNS lesion or salicylate poisoning	pH	↑	
	Pco$_2$	↓	↓
	HCO$_3^-$		↓
	Standard HCO$_3^-$	↑	↓
	K$^+$		↓
Metabolic acidosis			
	pH	↓	– or ↓
Excessive lactic acid production or base loss.	Pco$_2$	↓	↓
Anaerobic metabolism, e.g. circulatory failure, renal disease, ketoacidosis	HCO$_3^-$	↓	↓
	Standard HCO$_3^-$	↓	↓
	K$^+$	↑	↑
Metabolic alkalosis			
	pH	↑	↑
Secondary to potassium depletion or loss of gastric acid. Chronic diuretic therapy or pyloric stenosis	Pco$_2$	–	–
	HCO$_3^-$	↑	↑
	Standard HCO$_3^-$	↑	↑
	K$^+$	↓	↓

TABLE 24.5 Liver function tests

Test	Reference range*	Interpretation
Alanine transaminase (ALT or SGPT)	5–30 IU/l	Markedly raised in hepatocellular damage. Mildly raised in cholestasis and sometimes in cirrhosis. Also raised after circulatory failure with hypoxia
Albumin	35–55 g/l	Levels below 20 g/l usually result in oedema. Also decreased in haemodilution, nephropathy and catabolism. Hypoalbuminaemia of hepatic origin indicates chronic damage, e.g. cirrhosis
Alkaline phosphatase (ALP)	20–100 IU/l	Markedly raised in cholestasis. Mildly raised in hepatocellular damage. Also raised in diseases of bone, e.g. osteomalacia, Paget's disease and carcinoma. Also present in placenta and so raised in third trimester of pregnancy
Aspartate transaminase (AST or SGOT)	5–40 IU/l	Markedly raised in hepatocellular damage. Mildly raised in cholestasis and sometimes in cirrhosis. Also raised after circulatory failure with hypoxia. Present in cardiac and skeletal muscle and so raised after infarction and muscle trauma
Bilirubin (total bilirubin)	2–20 mmol/l	Raised in cellular damage of the liver and cholestasis. Also raised in haemolytic states
Bilirubin (direct)	<3 μmol/l	Measures conjugated bilirubin. Raised level can indicate source of hepatic failure
Gamma-glutamyl transferase (GGT)	5–45 IU/l	Markedly raised in cholestasis. Raised in cellular damage, during therapy with enzyme-inducers such as phenobarbital and phenytoin, and after substantial alcohol intake

TABLE 24.5 Liver function tests – cont'd

Test	Reference range*	Interpretation
Prothrombin ratio	1–1.2	Coagulation factors normally made in hepatic parenchyma. Prothrombin ratio will be raised in severe, usually chronic, liver damage. This change is resistant to vitamin K supplements. Also raised in cholestasis when absorption of vitamin K is impaired. In this case, prothrombin time can be shortened with intravenous vitamin K or an oral, water-soluble analogue

*Reference ranges are particularly variable for most of these tests depending on the method and conditions of assay.
SGPT = serum glutamic pyruvic transaminase;
SGOT = serum glutamic oxaloacetic transaminase.

Bilirubin is usually measured as total (free plus conjugated) and is only differentiated if other tests are equivocal.

KIDNEY FUNCTION TESTS (Table 24.6)

Tests of renal function attempt to estimate the glomerular filtration rate (GFR), which is normally in the range of 100–140 ml/min. A reduction implies that a proportion of nephrons have closed down and so clearance of nitrogenous waste, drug metabolites and other mainly polar substances is similarly diminished.

A reliable estimate of GFR is extremely useful for the adjustment of drug therapy if this relies on renal excretion. Methods usually rely on observing a substance that is totally cleared by the glomerulus and not subject to reabsorption. An intravenous dose of insulin can be administered and serum and urinary concentrations measured to calculate clearance. Although the answer is likely to be very accurate, this method is too inconvenient for routine use.

An endogenous substance that is produced by the body at a constant rate should exhibit a constant plasma concentration unless its elimination is altered. Therefore, urea and creatinine levels are often monitored. They are cleared by the glomerulus, and an elevated concentration implies diminished excretion.

TABLE 24.6 Kidney function tests

Test	Reference range	Interpretation
Creatinine clearance	97–140 ml/min (males) 85–125 ml/min (females)	This is the best quantitative estimate of GFR using an endogenous indicator. It is not susceptible to theoretical errors, but accuracy of 24-hour urine collection and urinary creatinine assay are limiting factors
Creatinine concentration	50–120 μmol/l (males) 40–100 μmol/l (females)	Levels elevated in catabolism and pregnancy. Otherwise, should be adjusted according to age, sex and weight (see text). For example, a level of 100 μmol/l would reflect healthy kidneys in a young male adult but severe renal impairment in the elderly
Urea (blood urea nitrogen, BUN)	1–5 mmol/l	Levels above 10 mmol/l probably reflect renal impairment, although trends within an individual are more instructive than isolated measurements. For the clinician, urea remains an invaluable index of disease state

Urea

This is a breakdown product of protein metabolism and raised levels (*uraemia*) are an important sign of renal failure. However, a constant production rate cannot be assumed and levels may also be elevated by high protein meals, tissue damage and catabolism. Although urea levels are of utmost interest to the clinician, they are poor quantitative indicators for pharmacokinetic estimations.

Creatinine

This is a product of muscle breakdown and in normal anabolic states is produced at a constant and reliable rate. It is, therefore, more useful than urea. Several investigators have noted that muscle turnover is variable according to age, sex and body weight and many nomograms and formulae have been produced to improve estimates of GFR based on serum creatinine concentrations. The following formula is often used:

Creatinine clearance (ml/min) = 1.23 (males) or 1.04 (females)
× (140 – age in years) × (weight in kg*)/[Serum creatinine in
μmol/l] = approx. GFR.

The creatinine clearance formula does not apply to
children, in pregnancy, when there is marked catabolism
or when renal function is rapidly changing.

Where a more accurate determination is required, creatinine
clearance can be measured directly by taking a serum creatinine level
in conjunction with measurement of creatinine in a 24-hour urine
sample.

HEART (Table 24.7)

Diagnosis of myocardial infarction depends upon three main elements: an appropriate history, ECG changes and elevation of certain serum enzyme levels. The absence of one sign does not exclude infarction since, for example, a history is not always available and ECG and enzyme changes do not always take place. Most clinicians would therefore accept two out of three signs.

Creatinine kinase (CK) and aspartate transaminase are both present in cardiac muscle and, following damage, appear in the blood in greatly elevated concentrations. The degree of elevation is a rough

TABLE 24.7 Enzyme elevation after myocardial infarction

	CK	AST	HBD
Onset of rise (hours)	4–12	6–12	8–24
Peak (hours)	20–40	20–40	30–70
Duration of rise (days)	2–5	2–6	5–12
Extent of rise	up to 10x	up to 8x	up to 6x

CK has two subunits, M and B; this gives three isoenzymes:
BB – from brain, MM – from skeletal muscle, and MB – from the
heart (CK-MB). CK-MB starts to rise 4–6 hours postinfarct and peaks
at 24 hours. CK–MB = <25u/l and <6% of total CK.

*If obese, use ideal body weight (IBW). Obese patients are more than 20% of
IBW. To calculate IBW in kg: Males = 50 + (2.3h), Females = 45.5 + (2.3h),
where h is the number of inches the patient is over 5 foot high (in metric units:
1 inch = 2.5 cm; 5 foot = 1.50 meter).

index of the extent of damage. Because neither enzyme is tissue-specific (CK also occurs in skeletal muscle and AST in the liver, erythrocytes, skeletal muscle and kidney), most laboratories monitor a further enzyme known as hydroxybutyrate dehydrogenase (HBD or LD_1). This is a coenzyme of lactate dehydrogenase and is a specific monitor of cardiac damage. Measurement of lactate dehydrogenase itself contributes little, as it is distributed around the body in a similar pattern to AST.

A sustained elevation of AST plus a rise in ALT following infarction usually indicates a secondary involvement of the liver.

Cardiac enzymes are usually measured as soon as possible after the suspected infarct and their course is followed during the recovery phase. In the absence of re-infarction, levels should subside in the times indicated in Table 24.7.

MISCELLANEOUS LABORATORY TESTS

Some notes on the interpretation of selected laboratory tests are given in Table 24.8.

DRUGS THAT INTERFERE WITH LABORATORY TESTS

Certain drugs may interfere with the results of laboratory tests. These are listed in Table 24.9.

DRUGS THAT CAUSE ELECTROLYTE DISTURBANCES

These are listed in Table 24.10.

HAEMATOLOGY

Automated blood counts are virtually routine for patients coming into hospital. These results, and the results of more specialised tests, may be useful for pharmacists. They may form the basis for drug therapy, e.g. iron and vitamin supplements, or they may be an index of disease progress, e.g. leukaemia. Alternatively, they may demonstrate drug toxicity.

TABLE 24.8 Miscellaneous laboratory tests

Test	Reference range	Interpretation
Alpha-1-antitrypsin	2–4 g/l	Phenotyping done on those with low levels. Can be useful in some cases of cirrhosis and emphysema
Amylase (serum)	60–300 U/l*	Derived from the pancreas and usually raised in acute pancreatitis or in abdominal trauma. Sometimes raised in renal failure when clearance is impaired
Cortisol suppression test	200 nmol/l	Measured on the morning following a 2 mg dexamethasone dose. Failure to suppress cortisol usually indicates adrenal hyperplasia or tumour. Assay cross-reacts with prednisolone
CSF (glucose)	2.8–4 mmol/l	Infections of CSF are often characterised by raised protein and reduced glucose. Both may be raised after haemorrhage. Visual and microbiological examination are essential
CSF (protein)	0.2–0.5 g/l	
Folate (serum)	5–15 µg/l	Depressed serum folate should not be used as an absolute diagnosis of folate deficiency, since it is determined by recent dietary history. Body stores of folate are sufficient for 3–4 months and RBC levels are the best guide to these store levels.
Folate (RBC)	150–600 µg/l	
Iron (serum)	10–30 µmol/l (men) 7–25 µmol/l (women)	True iron deficiency produces a low serum iron and raised binding capacity (IBC or TIBC). Both indices are lowered in, for example, rheumatoid arthritis
Iron-binding capacity (serum)	45–72 µmol/l	
Lipids: cholesterol (total)	<5.2 mmol/l	Triglyceride levels must be taken after a fast of at least 12 hours since the level is dependent on diet. Apart from the primary hyperlipidaemias and their

TABLE 24.8 Miscellaneous laboratory tests – cont'd

Test	Reference range	Interpretation
		cardiovascular sequelae, hypercholesterolaemia can be caused by diabetes, nephrotic syndrome and biliary obstruction; hypertriglyceridaemia can accompany diabetes, nephritic syndrome pancreatitis, alcohol and oral contraceptives
cholesterol (HDL)	Male 0.9–2.0 mmol/l Female 1.0–2.3 mmol/l	Low levels of HDL are associated with a high risk of myocardial infarction
triglycerides (fasting)	<2.0 mmol/l	Triglyceride values increase with ageing
Osmolality serum	285–295 mOsm/kg	↑ Fluid depletion ↑ Fluid excess
Thyroxine (total)	60–140 mmol/l	↑ Hyperthyroidism (Graves' disease) can be confirmed with TRH challenge ↓ Hypothyroidism should be confirmed with TSH measurement and possibly a TRH challenge. Thyroxine levels may be decreased by salicylates and phenytoin through binding displacement
Free T_4	10–25 pmol/l	
Free T_3	5–10.2 pmol/l	
Urate (serum)	Male 0.24–0.48 mmol/l Female 0.16–0.36 mmol/l	↑ May lead to gout. May be due to increased production, e.g. from hereditary purine metabolic defect and carcinoma, or from diminished excretion, e.g. in glomerular failure, acidosis and with diuretics
Vitamin B_{12} (serum)	160–900 ng/l	↑ Leads to macrocytic anaemia and peripheral neuropathy. May be due to diet deficiency, pernicious anaemia, ileitis or short-bowel syndrome. Stores normally last for 2–4 years. Cause can be verified by the Schilling test

*Large variation between labs.
CSF = cerebrospinal fluid; HDL = high-density lipoprotein; IBC = iron-binding capacity; RBC = red blood cells; T_3 = triiodothyronine; T_4 = thyroxine; TIBC = total iron-binding capacity; TRH = thyrotrophin-releasing hormone; TSH = thyroid-stimulating hormone.

TABLE 24.9 Drugs that interfere with laboratory tests

Test	Effect	Drug	In vivo (V) or in vitro (T)
Alanine transaminase	+	Amitriptyline	V
	+	Amphotericin B	V
	+	Erythromycin	V
	+	Halothane	V
	+	Isoniazid	V
	+	Levodopa	V
	+	Nalidixic acid	V
	+	Nitrofurantoin	V
	+	Phenytoin	V
	+	Rifampicin	V
	+	Salicylate	V
	+	Streptokinase	V
	+	Sulphonamides	V
	+	Valproate	V
Alkaline phosphatase	−	Acetylcysteine	T
	+	Carbamazepine	V
	−	Clofibrate	V
	+	Disulfiram	V
	−	EDTA	V
	+	Erythromycin	V
	+	Methyldopa	V
	+	Nitrofurantoin	V
	−	Nitrofurantoin	T
	+	Phenytoin	V
	+	Rifampicin	V
	+	Sulphonamides	V
	−	Zinc salts	T
Amylase	+	Asparaginase	V
	+	Corticosteroids	V
	+	Fat emulsions	T
	+	Furosemide	V
	+	Metformin	V
	+	Morphine	V
	+	Pancreatic enzymes	T
	+	Valproate	V
Aspartate transaminase	+	Cimetidine	V
	+	Erythromycin	V
	+	Halothane	V
	+	Isoniazid	V
	+	Levodopa	V
	+	Mercaptopurine	V
	+	Methyldopa	V
	−	Metronidazole	V
	+	Nitrofurantoin	V
	+	Paracetamol	T
	+	Paracetamol	V
	+	Phenytoin	V

TABLE 24.9 Drugs that interfere with laboratory tests – cont'd

Test	Effect	Drug	In vivo (V) or in vitro (T)
	+	Rifampicin	V
	+	Salicylate	V
	+	Streptokinase	V
	+	Sulphonamides	V
	+	Valproate	V
Bilirubin	+	Carbamazepine	V
	+	Chlordiazepoxide	V
	+	Cimetidine	V
	+	Disulfiram	V
	+	Erythromycin	V
	+	Fluphenazine	V
	+	Fusidic acid	V
	+	Halothane	V
	+	Ibuprofen	V
	+	Imipramine	V
	+	Mercaptopurine	V
	+	Methyldopa	T
	+	Methyldopa	V
	+	Nitrofurantoin	V
	+	Oral contraceptives	V
	+	Phenothiazines	V
	+	Phenytoin	V
	−	Pindolol	T
	+	Quinidine	V
	+	Rifampicin	T
	+	Rifampicin	V
	+	Sulfamethoxazole	V
	+	Sulfasalazine	V
	+	Theophylline	T
Calcium (see also Table 24.10)	+	Hydralazine	T
Cholesterol	+	Chenodeoxycholic acid	V
	+	Chlorpromazine	T
	+	Chlorthalidone	V
	−	Cholestyramine	V
	+	Corticosteroids	T
	+	Corticosteroids	V
	+	Hydrochlorothiazide	V
	+	Iodides	T
	+	Levodopa	V
	−	Neomycin	V
	−	Nitrates	T
	+	Oral contraceptives	V
	+	Phenytoin	V
	−	Prazosin	V
	+	Vitamin C	T

TABLE 24.9 Drugs that interfere with laboratory tests – cont'd

Test	Effect	Drug	In vivo (V) or in vitro (T)
Glucose (blood) (See also Table 24.10)	–	Aspirin	V
	+	Chlorpromazine	V
	+	Chlorthalidone	V
	–	Clofibrate	V
	+	Corticosteroids	V
	–	Cyproheptadine	V
	+	Fructose	T
	–	Guanethidine	V
	+	Isoprenaline	V
	+/–	Levodopa	T
	+	Levodopa	V
	+	Lithium	V
	+	Metoprolol	V
	+	Oral contraceptives	V
	+	Phenytoin	V
	+/–	Propranolol	V
	–	Tetracycline	T
	+	Thiazides	V
Glucose (urine)	+	Acetazolamide	V
	+	Aspirin	T
	+	Cephalosporins	T
	+	Chloral	T
	+	Corticosteroids	V
	+	Fructose	T
	+	Glucagon	V
	+	Hydralazine	T
	+	Isoniazid	T
	+/–	Levodopa	T
	+	Methyldopa	T
	+	Nalidixic acid	T
	+	Oxazepam	T
	+	Penicillin (large dose)	T
	+	Probenecid	T
	+	Streptomycin	T
	+/–	Tetracycline	T
	+	Thiazide	V
	+/–	Vitamin C	T
Urea (see also Table 24.10)	+	Acetohexamide	T
	+	Methoxyflurane	V
	–	Streptomycin	T
	+	Sulphonylureas	T
	+	Tetracycline	V
	+	Thiazides	V
	+	Trimethoprim	V

TABLE 24.9 Drugs that interfere with laboratory tests – cont'd

Test	Effect	Drug	In vivo (V) or in vitro (T)
Uric acid	+	Acetazolamide	V
	+	Acetylcysteine	T
	+	Aspirin	V
	+/–	Clofibrate	V
	+	Ethambutol	V
	+	Furosemide	V
	+	Hydralazine	T
	+	Levodopa	T
	+	Levodopa	V
	+	Methyldopa	T
	+	Propranolol	V
	+	Thiazides	V
	+	Vitamin C	T

BLOOD SCREENING

Erythrocytes

Routine screening of erythrocytes is often performed using a Coulter Counter technique combined with microscopy. These tests demonstrate the size, number and colour of red blood cells, whether they are of normal shape and the percentage of young cells (reticulocytes).

Iron deficiency results in pale or hypochromic cells and these are normally smaller than usual. Deficiency of vitamin B_{12} or folate does not affect the nature of cytoplasm but reduces the frequency of cell division in the marrow. The red cells are therefore larger (macrocytic), but have a normal colour. A marrow biopsy demonstrates that red cell precursors are also larger than normal (megaloblasts). When folate and iron deficiencies combine, red cells are both macrocytic and hypochromic.

Conditions such as the thalassaemias, where abnormal haemoglobin chains are incorporated into erythrocytes, result in an abnormal shape of the cell as well as deficiencies in oxygen transport.

Erythrocytes normally have a life of 100–120 days and are eventually destroyed by the macrophages. For the first day or so they contain the remnants of a cell nucleus and after staining can be recognised as reticulocytes. Hence, normal production and destruction of erythrocytes are characterised by a reticulocyte count around 1%. If there is marrow aplasia and production is suppressed, the count will often be low. Alternatively, if erythrocytes are prematurely destroyed by macrophages, e.g. in macrocytosis or a haemoglobinopathy, the proportion of reticulocytes in the circulation will increase. There may be an accompanying increase in serum bilirubin as a result of increased

TABLE 24.10 Drugs that cause electrolyte disturbances

Electrolyte	Drug	Effect	Mechanism
Calcium	Acetazolamide	↓	↓ Renal reabsorption
	Aminoglycosides	↓	↓ Renal reabsorption (rare)
	Calcitonin	↓	↓ Resorption of bone
	Calcium salts	↑	
	Corticosteroids	↓	↓ Gastrointestinal absorption, resorption of bone and renal absorption
	Lithium	↑	↑ Parathyroid hormone (rare)
	Magnesium salts	↓	↓ Gastrointestinal absorption
	Mithramycin	↓	Parathyroid hormone antagonism
	Oestrogens	↓	?
	Oral contraceptives	↓	↓ Albumin synthesis
	Parathyroid hormone	↑	↑ Gastrointestinal absorption, resorption of bone and renal reabsorption
	Phenobarbital/phenytoin	↓	↑ Vitamin D metabolism
	Phosphates	↓	↓ Gastrointestinal absorption
	Tamoxifen	↑	? (rare)
	Thyroid hormones	↑	↑ Resorption of bone
	Vitamin D	↑	↑ Gastrointestinal absorption, resorption of bone and renal reabsorption
Glucose	Alcohol	↓ ↑ (less often)	↓ Gluconeogenesis ↑ Glycogenolysis
	Clonidine	↓	↓ Insulin secretion
	Corticosteroids	↑	↑ Gluconeogenesis + antagonise insulin
	Diuretics (not spironolactone)	↑	↓ Glucose tolerance

TABLE 24.10 Drugs that cause electrolyte disturbances – cont'd

Electrolyte	Drug	Effect	Mechanism
	Isoniazid	↑	↑ Gluconeogenesis
	Levodopa	↓	↑ Glucagon secretion
	Oral contraceptives	↑	↓ Glucose tolerance
	Phenytoin	↑	↓ Insulin secretion (rare)
	Propranolol	↑	↑ Glycogenolysis
		↑ (less often)	↓ Insulin secretion
	Salicylates	↓	↑ Glucose uptake (high doses)
	Theophylline	↑	↑ Glycogenolysis and gluconeogenesis
		↓	↑ Insulin secretion
Magnesium	Aminoglycosides	↓	Toxic tubular damage
	Amphotericin B	↓	Toxic tubular damage
	Cisplatin	↓	Toxic tubular damage
	Digoxin	↓	↑ Renal loss
	Furosemide	↓	↑ Renal loss
	Lithium	↑	? (rare)
	Magnesium salts	↑	
	Thiazides	↓	↑ Renal loss (less than with furosemide)

Phosphate	Aluminium salts	↓	↓ Absorption
	Corticosteroids	↓	↓ Resorption of bone
	Nutrition in malnourished subjects	↓	↑ Cellular uptake
	Thiazides	↓	?
Potassium	Aminoglycosides	↓	Toxic tubular damage
	Amphotericin B	↓	Toxic tubular damage
	Bicarbonates	↓	↑ Cell uptake + renal loss
	Captopril	↑	↓ Renal loss (aldosterone production)
	Carbenoxolone	↓	↑ Renal loss (aldosterone-like)
	Corticosteroids	↓	↑ Renal loss (aldosterone-like)
	Cytotoxics	↑	Rapid cell lysis
	Dinoprost	↓	↑ Renal loss (prostaglandin agonist)
	Fludrocortisone	↓	↑ Renal loss (aldosterone-like)
	Furosemide	↓	↑ Renal loss
	Indometacin	↑	↓ Renal loss (prostaglandin antagonist)
	Insulin + glucose	↓	↑ Cell uptake
	Laxatives	↓	↓ Reabsorption from gastrointestinal tract
	Levodopa	↓	↑ Renal loss (reduced by carbidopa and benserazide)
	Penicillins (large dose)	↓	Secondary to renal excretion of large amounts of anionic penicillin
	Salbutamol (IV)	↓	↑ Cell uptake + ↑ renin secretion
	Spironolactone	↑	↑ Renal uptake (aldosterone antagonist)
	Succinylcholine	↑	Transient loss of intracellular potassium
	Thiazides	↓	↑ Renal loss

TABLE 24.10 Drugs that cause electrolyte disturbances – cont'd

Electrolyte	Drug	Effect	Mechanism
Sodium	Carbamazepine	↓	May ↑ antidiuretic hormone (ADH) production
	Chlorpropamide	↓	Augmentation of ADH
	Corticosteroids	↑	↑ Renal reabsorption
	Cyclophosphamide	↓	↓ Water excretion
	Demeclocycline	↑	Inhibition of ADH
	Indometacin	↓	↓ Renal loss (prostaglandin antagonist)
	Laxatives	↓	↑ gastrointestinal water loss in excess of sodium
	Lithium	↓	↑ Renal water loss in excess of sodium
		↑	↑ Renal sodium loss
	Oxytocin	↓	ADH-like action
	Phenytoin	↑	Inhibition of ADH
	Thiazides	↓	↑ Renal loss in excess of water
	Tolbutamide	↓	Augmentation of ADH (less than with chlorpropamide)
	Vincristine	↓	↑ ADH production
Urea	Allopurinol		These drugs have all been reported to be nephrotoxic and are therefore capable of producing uraemia. Cytotoxic agents may also produce uraemia through rapid tissue breakdown
	Aminoglycosides		
	Amphotericin B		
	Busulphan		
	Carbamazepine		
	Cephalosporins		

Colistin
Furosemide
Gold
Methotrexate
Methyldopa
Mithramycin
Mitomycin C
Penicillamine
Phenindione
Phenylbutazone
Phenytoin
Probenecid
Radio-contrast media
Salicylates
Stibophen
Sulphonamides
Tetracyclines
Vancomycin

TABLE 24.11 Function of blood cells

Test or cell name	Reference range	Description or function	Interpretation
Basophils	$0.01-0.1 \times 10^9/l$ (0.1% of WBC)	Identical to mast cells, which they eventually become	↑ (Basophil leukocytosis) in granulocytic leukaemia or sometimes in ulcerative colitis
Eosinophils	$0.04-0.4 \times 10^9/l$ (1-4% of WBC)	Appear similar to neutrophils but feature in allergic response and defence against parasites	↑ (Eosinophilia) in atopic asthma, hay fever etc., amoebiasis and worm infestation, some lymphomas and skin disease
ESR	0-9mm/h (men) 0-20mm/h (women)	Erythrocyte sedimentation rate (rate of all of red cells in anticoagulated specimen)	It should be slow. ↑ in infections and some inflammatory diseases. Like pyrexia, it is a non-specific indicator but can be used to discover or follow a disease process
Ferritin	Male 15-300µg/l Female 15-200µg/l		May be normal in presence of iron deficiency due to acute-phase reaction. Useful in differential diagnosis of hypochromic, microcytic anaemias. Decreased in iron-deficiency anaemia and increased in iron overload
Hb	14-18g/dl (men) 12-16g/dl (women)	Haemoglobin concentration	Symptomatic below 9-10g/dl. If chronic, may lead to cardiomegaly; decreased by haemorrhage, iron deficiency, marrow depression or increased haemolysis (e.g. macrocytic or haemolytic anaemia, haemoglobinopathies)
HbA1c	<6%		Indicator of glycaemic control over the preceding 2 months

Carboxy-Hb	<1.5%		Can be up to 10% in smokers. Toxic levels >20%, can be lethal if >50%
Hct (haematocrit)	39–54% (men) 36–47% (women)	Packed cell volume of anticoagulated blood	Crude indicator of red cell volume. More specific information is derived from RBC and MCV
Lymphocytes	1.3–3.55 × 10⁹/l (20–35% of WBC)	B cells responsible for immunity against foreign (mainly bacterial) cells through production of immunoglobulins. T cells act as helpers to B cells and provide cell-mediated immunity against intracellular organisms (e.g. viruses, fungi and protozoa) and foreign cells (e.g. grafts)	↑ (Lymphocytosis) mononucleosis, viral infections, tuberculosis, toxoplasmosis, some leukaemias and autoimmune diseases ↓ (Lymphopenia) in marrow failure or with, for example, corticosteroids and azathioprine
MCH	27–32 pg	Mean cell haemoglobin: indicates weight in each cell	Determined by MCV and MCHC, which give more useful information
MCHC	32–36 g/dl	Mean cell haemoglobin concentration: indicates quality of the cytoplasm regardless of cell size	↓ (Hypochromic) especially in iron deficiency but also in inflammatory disease (e.g. rheumatoid arthritis, thalassaemia, sideroblastic anaemia)
MCV	82–95 fl	Mean cell volume	↓ (Microcytic) in iron deficiency ↑ (Macrocytic) in folate or vitamin B₁₂ deficiency, liver disease, after alcohol and some cytotoxics
Monocytes (macrophages)	0.1–0.8 × 10⁹/l (1.8% of WBC)	Large phagocytes	↑ (Monocytosis) in tuberculosis, endocarditis and typhoid fever. Also in lymphoma and leukaemia

TABLE 24.11 Function of blood cells – cont'd

Test or cell name	Reference range	Description or function	Interpretation
Neutrophils	$2.2–7 \times 10^9/l$ (45–75% of WBC)	Attracted to sites of inflammation and infection; phagocytosis of foreign cells or defective host cells and killing of bacterial cells	↑ (Neutrophil leukocytosis) especially in bacterial infections and inflammation but also in carcinoma, leukaemia and metabolic disorders such as gout and acidosis ↓ (Neutropenia) in viral infections, autoimmune disease or marrow failure, or after many drugs (e.g. phenylbutazone, chlorpromazine, chloramphenicol, phenytoin)
Platelets (thrombocytes)	$100–400 \times 10^9/l$	Mechanical plugging of haemorrhage and initiation of coagulation	↓ (Thrombocytopenia) in marrow failure or toxicity, leukaemia, splenomegaly or if destruction is increased in immune thrombocytopenic purpura
RBC	$4.5–6 \times 10^{12}/l$ (men) $4.3–5.5 \times 10^{12}/l$ (women)	Red blood cell (count)	↑ In fluid depletion, polycythaemia ↓ In fluid overload, macrocytic anaemia, marrow aplasia, haemolytic anaemia
Retics	$0.5–1.5\%$	Proportion of young red cells (reticulocytes)	Should be raised as a response to blood loss or anaemia. May remain low in iron, folate or vitamin B_{12} deficiency, carcinoma, marrow hypoplasia or malnutrition
WBC	$4–11 \times 10^9/l$	White blood cell (count)	↑ (Leukocytosis) usually indicates infection. Marked increase may indicate malignancy ↓ (Leukopenia) may be due to drugs, some infections and hypersensitivity reactions. Differential counts essential

haemoglobin breakdown. Similar changes, but to a more dramatic extent, are seen in haemolytic anaemias.

Anaemia

Anaemias are conditions of the blood where there are quantitative or qualitative changes of the erythrocytes.

Leukocytes

White blood cells (leukocytes) may be classified microscopically into two groups according to whether they contain granules in the cytoplasm. The granulocytes are further subdivided according to the staining characteristics of the granules (hence neutrophils, basophils and eosinophils). Two distinct types of cell comprise the agranulocytes, these being the monocytes (macrophages) and lymphocytes. The latter is the only class of leukocyte that does not exhibit phagocytic activity. The functions of the various types of cell are summarised in Table 24.11.

Coagulation tests

The most common test performed is the prothrombin time (PTT), which tests the extrinsic and common coagulation pathways. A normal result is 10–14 seconds. It may be expressed with reference to a standard preparation and a normal prothrombin ratio is in the range 1–1.2. When a patient is anticoagulated, the aim is to achieve a ratio of around 2. Most laboratories will accept a value between 1.5 and 4.

An alternative – the Thrombotest – has a normal range of 60–100% while the target range for anticoagulation is 5–17%. The activated partial thromboplastin time or kaolin–cephalin time (APTT, PTTK or KCT) is a test of intrinsic clotting pathways with a normal range of 30–40 seconds. Prolongation of this time is usually due to clotting factor deficiency. The test is used to monitor heparin therapy when it should achieve between 1.5 and 2.5 times the normal value.

CHAPTER 25

SI units for clinical chemistry

TABLE 25.1 Conversion from traditional to SI units

Test	Unit	To SI unit
Acid phosphatase (King–Armstrong)	0.56 KA	= 1 IU/l
Amylase		1 IU/l
Aspartate transminase (AST or SGOT)		IU/l
Blood gases: P_{CO_2} P_{O_2}	mmHg × 0.133 mmHg × 0.133	= 1 kPa = 1 kPa
Blood hydrogen ion concentration	pH is a log unit so no easy conversion	nmol/l
Serum albumin	g/100 ml × 10	= g/l
Serum bicarbonate	1 mEq/l	= 1 mmol/l
Serum bilirubin	mg/100 ml × 17.1	= 1 mmol/l
Serum calcium	mg/100 ml × 0.25	= 1 mmol/l
Serum chloride	1 mEq/l	= 1 mmol/l
Serum creatinine	mg/100 ml × 88.4	= 1 μmol/l
Serum globulin	g/100 ml × 10	= g/l
Serum glucose	mg/100 ml × 0.055	= mmol/l
Serum iron	mg/100 ml × 0.18	= μmol/l
Serum magnesium	mEq/l × 0.5	= mmol/l
Serum phosphate (inorganic)	mg/100 ml × 0.32	= mmol/l
Serum potassium	mEq/l	= mmol/l
Serum sodium	mEq/l	= mmol/l
Serum triglycerides	mg/100 ml × 0.011	= mmol/l
Serum urate	mg/100 ml × 0.17	= mmol/l
Serum urea	mg/100 ml × 0.17	= mmol/l

TABLE 25.1 Conversion from traditional to SI units – cont'd

Test	Unit	To SI unit
Total iron-binding capacity	mg/100 ml × 0.18	= μmol/l
Urinary calcium	mg/24 h × 0.025	= mmol/24 h
Urinary creatinine	mg/24 h × 0.0088	= mmol/24 h
Urinary phosphate	mg/24 h × 0.032	= mmol/24 h
Urinary urea	g/24 h × 16.6	= mmol/24 h

SGOT = serum glutamic oxaloacetic transaminase.

CHAPTER 26

Pharmacokinetics in clinical practice

S. Dhillon

Basic skills and knowledge of applied pharmacokinetics are required by clinical pharmacists in routine practice. The principles of pharmacokinetics are fundamental to the pharmacist's ability to design an appropriate dosage regimen for a patient that ensures maximal efficacy and minimal toxicity. Pharmacists should be able to:

- apply one-compartment pharmacokinetics to single and multiple dosing following the intravenous and oral administration of drugs
- state the rationale for using therapeutic drug monitoring (TDM) and applied clinical pharmacokinetics to optimise drug therapy in routine clinical practice
- identify drugs that should routinely be monitored
- apply the basic principles of interpretation of serum drug concentrations in practice
- apply one-compartment pharmacokinetics to describe steady-state serum drug concentrations following oral dosing.

Pharmacokinetics provides a mathematical basis for assessing the time course of drugs and their effects in the body. It enables the following processes to be quantified:

Absorption
Distribution
Metabolism
Excretion

It is these pharmacokinetic processes, often referred to as **ADME**, that determine the drug concentration in the body. It is the application of pharmacokinetics to these basic parameters of drug handling that enables the design of an appropriate dosage regimen.

Ideally the drug concentration of a drug should be measured at the site of drug action, i.e. at the receptor. However, because the receptor is inaccessible, drug concentrations are normally measured in whole blood from which serum or plasma is generated. Other body fluids such as saliva, urine and cerebrospinal fluid are sometimes used. It is assumed that drug concentrations in these fluids are in equilibrium with the drug concentration at the receptor. Drug concentrations refer to total drug concentration, i.e. a combination of bound and free drug concentrations that are in equilibrium with each other. In clinical practice the drug concentration is measured in serum or plasma.

For most drugs routinely monitored in practice one assumes a first-order rate for the processes of ADME, i.e. the amount of a drug A is decreasing at a rate that is proportional to the amount of drug A remaining in the body. Therefore, the rate of elimination of drug A can be described as:

$$dA/dt = -kA$$

where k is the first-order rate constant.

The reaction proceeds at a rate that is dependent on the concentration of drug A present in the body. Most drugs used in clinical practice at therapeutic doses follow first-order elimination processes. However, in overdose situations they may show saturation and follow zero-order elimination. Some drugs in therapeutic doses show zero-order elimination processes and it requires the application of Michaelis–Menten kinetics to interpret these drugs in clinical practice. Examples are phenytoin, high-dose salicylates and high-dose theophyllines (mainly reported in paediatrics).

PHARMACOKINETIC MODELS

Pharmacokinetic models are hypothetical structures that are used to describe the fate of a drug in a biological system following its administration.

ONE-COMPARTMENT MODEL

Following drug administration, the body is depicted as a kinetically homogeneous unit. This assumes that the drug achieves instantaneous distribution throughout the body and that the drug equilibrates instantaneously between tissues. Thus the drug concentration–time profile shows a monoexponential decline and can be described using the equation below. It is important to note that this does not imply that the drug concentration in plasma is equal to the drug concentration in the tissues. However, changes in the plasma concentration quantitatively reflect changes in the tissues.

The equation to describe the change in Cp_t (drug concentration at any time t) describes monoexponential decay.

$$Cp_t = Cp°e^{-kt}$$

where $Cp°$ is the initial concentration at time 0 h and k is the first-order elimination rate constant.

TWO-COMPARTMENT MODEL

This model resolves the body into central and peripheral compartments. These compartments have no physiological or anatomical meaning; however, it is assumed that the central compartment comprises tissues that are highly perfused, such as heart, lungs, kidneys, liver and brain. The peripheral compartment comprises less well-perfused tissues such as muscle, fat and skin. Drugs such as gentamicin, theophylline and digoxin show a two-compartment model. However, in practice one-compartment kinetics can be used to describe the serum concentration–time profile, providing the samples are taken after the distribution phase is complete.

PHARMACOKINETIC PARAMETERS

The following section will describe the basic pharmacokinetic parameters for a one-compartment model and their application in clinical practice.

ELIMINATION RATE CONSTANT

The elimination rate constant can be used to calculate the fraction of a dose eliminated per unit of time. For a one-compartment model the elimination of the drug is described by a first-order process.

VOLUME OF DISTRIBUTION

The volume of distribution is defined as the volume of plasma in which the total amount of drug in the body would be required to be dissolved, to reflect the drug concentration attained in plasma. The volume of distribution (V_d) has no direct physiological meaning: it is not a 'real' volume and is usually referred to as the apparent volume of distribution. Some drugs may have limited tissue distribution, hence their V_d reflects total plasma volume, e.g. gentamicin $V_d = 15$ litres, whereas other drugs show intensive distribution, e.g. amiodarone $V_d = 2000$ litres.

HALF-LIFE

The time required to reduce the plasma concentration to one-half its initial value is defined as the half-life $(t_{1/2})$, i.e. $t_{1/2} = 0.693/k$. The time taken to reach steady-state serum concentrations, i.e. when the rate of administration is equal to the rate of elimination, is approximately equal to $5 \times t_{1/2}$. At steady state the changes in serum concentrations within a dosing interval are the same.

CLEARANCE

Drug clearance can be defined as the volume of plasma in the vascular compartment cleared of drug per unit of time by the processes of metabolism and excretion. Clearance is constant for all drugs that are eliminated by first-order kinetics. Drugs can be cleared by renal excretion or metabolism or both. With respect to the kidney and liver, clearances, are additive, i.e.

$$Cl_{(total)} = Cl_{renal} + Cl_{non-renal}$$

Mathematically, clearance is the product of the first-order elimination rate constant (k) and the apparent volume of distribution (V_d). Thus:

$$Cl_{(total)} = k \times V_d$$

Relationship with half-life $(t_{1/2})$:

$$(t_{1/2}) = 0.693 \times V_d/Cl$$

NON-LINEAR PHARMACOKINETICS: BASIC PARAMETERS

Drugs such as phenytoin will show non-linear drug handing. The processes of metabolism are non-linear. The rate of metabolism shows zero order. In practice, Michaelis–Menten pharmacokinetics are applied, and the equations are summarised below.

If a patient receives different doses of phenytoin, e.g. 200 mg/day, 250 mg/day, 300 mg/day or 400 mg/day, the steady-state plasma concentration varies exponentially with time, i.e. a small change in the total daily dose of phenytoin shows a disproportionate increase in the steady-state concentration (Cp_{ss}) (Fig. 26.1).

Daily dose

If the rate of metabolism of phenytoin is considered, given different dosages, Figure 26.2 describes the profile. As the dose of phenytoin increases, the rate of elimination increases until it reaches a plateau where the rate of elimination is constant despite increases in the total daily dose of phenytoin (Fig. 26.2).

The profile can be described as follows.

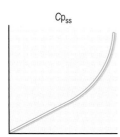

Fig. 26.1 Plasma concentration at steady state (Cp_{ss}) following different doses of phenytoin.

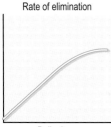

Fig. 26.2 Profile of elimination following phenytoin administration.

Rate of elimination

$$\frac{-dX}{dt} = \frac{V_m \times Cp_{ss}}{K_m \times Cp_{ss}}$$

Hence, the model that appears to fit the pattern for the metabolic elimination of phenytoin is not linear and is the one proposed by Michaelis and Menten. The velocity (V) or rate at which an enzyme can metabolise a substrate (S) can be described by the following equation:

$$V = \frac{V_m \times S}{K_m \times S}$$

where V is the rate of metabolism, V_m (sometimes referred to as V_{max}) is the maximum rate of metabolism and K_m is the substrate concentration (S) at which V will be half V_m, i.e. when half the total enzyme is complexed with the substrate (Fig. 26.3).

At steady state we know that the rate of administration is equal to the rate of elimination; hence, in the clinical situation, the daily dose R (or D) is substituted for velocity V, and the steady-state phenytoin concentration (Cp_{ss}) is substituted for substrate concentration S. Further equations can be described for steady-state concentrations.

Following the rate of elimination described in Figure 26.2, at steady state the rate of administration is equal to the rate of elimination. Rate of administration can be stated as SFD/τ where D/τ can equal R. Hence:

$$RSF = \frac{V_m \times Cp_{ss}}{K_m \times Cp_{ss}}$$

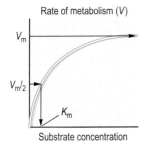

Fig. 26.3 Rate of metabolism following phenytoin administration.

where V_m is the maximum metabolic capacity, i.e. the total amount of drug that can be eliminated at saturation and K_m is the Michaelis constant – this by definition is the concentration at which the metabolism is operating at half the maximum capacity.

All drugs will show non-linear handling if they are administered in high enough doses. However, only a small number of drugs show non-linear handling in doses used clinically.

To assess whether a drug will show linear or non-linear drug handling in therapeutic doses depends on the drug's Michaelis constant, K_m.

For example:

If a drug has a K_m that is much greater than Cp_{ss}, i.e. plasma levels seen with normal therapeutic doses of the drug, the rate of elimination can be described as:

$$\frac{-dX}{dt} = \frac{V_m \times Cp_{ss}}{K_m \times Cp_{ss}}$$

Since K_m is $>>>$ Cp_{ss}, the equation simplifies to:

$$\frac{-dX}{dt} = \frac{V_m \times Cp_{ss}}{K_m}$$

Since V_m and K_m are constants, this is now showing a first-order process.

In another simulation a drug has a K_m which is much smaller than Cp_{ss}, i.e. plasma levels seen with normal therapeutic doses of the drug.

$$\frac{-dX}{dt} = \frac{V_m \times Cp_{ss}}{K_m \times Cp_{ss}}$$

Since K_m is $<<<$ Cp_{ss}, the equation simplifies to

$$\frac{-dX}{dt} = \frac{V_m}{K_m} \tag{1}$$

Since V_m and K_m are constants, this is now showing a zero-order process.

Hence the relationship between the Michaelis constant (K_m) of the drug and the plasma levels of the drug normally achieved with therapeutic dosage will determine whether the drug will show linear first-order or zero saturation pharmacokinetics.

Practical clinical use of non-linear equations

The above equation can be used to calculate predicted Cp_{ss} from a given dosage regimen, to estimate the patient's V_m using population K_m.

To describe the relationship between the total daily dose (R[mg/day]) and the steady-state serum concentration:

$$R \times F \times S = \frac{V_m \times Cp_{ss}}{K_m \times Cp_{ss}} \qquad (2)$$

$$Cp_{ss} = \frac{K_m \times (R \times F \times S)}{V_m - (R \times F \times S)} \qquad (3)$$

$$R \times F \times S = \frac{(V_m - K_m) \times R}{Cp_{ss}} \qquad (4)$$

$$Cp_{ss} = \frac{(V_m)(Cp_{ss}) - K_m}{(R \times F \times S)} \qquad (5)$$

Or:

$$Cp_{ss} = \frac{(D_{max})(Cp_{ss}) - K_m}{D} \qquad (6)$$

NB: The last three equations are linear relationships.

Clearance (Cl) is the parameter that relates the rate of elimination to the plasma concentration.

Since:

$$Cl = R/Cp_{ss}$$

Then

$$Cl = \frac{V_m}{K_m + Cp_{ss}} \qquad (7)$$

Since

$$\text{Apparent } t_{1/2} = (0.693 \times V_d)/Cl$$

Then

$$t_{1/2} = \{0.93 \times Vd(K_m + Cp_{ss})\}/ V_m \qquad (8)$$

From the above equations, it can be noted that the clearance and half-life will alter depending on the steady-state concentration. Thus it is V_m and K_m that should be used to describe the kinetics of phenytoin and not clearance and half-life.

TABLE 26.1 Basic pharmacokinetic equations

Pharmacokinetic equation	Comments on the clinical use of the equations
Single intravenous bolus injection $Cp_t = Cp° \, e^{-kt}$	This equation describes the serum concentration at time (t) after a single intravenous dose. This equation can be used to calculate monoexponential decay. If you have a toxic serum concentration use this equation to estimate the time for decay of a toxic level to a desired serum concentration (see below)
e^{-kt}	Fraction of a dose remaining
$1 - e^{-kt}$	Fraction of a dose eliminated
$Cp° = \dfrac{SFD}{V_d}$	Loading dose. Let $Cp°$ equal the desired serum concentration
$t_{1/2} = \dfrac{0.693}{k}$	The half-life can be estimated using this equation. Times to reach steady-state serum concentrations are 4–5 times the half-life
$Cl = kV_d$	The total body clearance can be calculated using this equation
Single oral dose $Cp_t = Cp° \dfrac{k_a}{k_a - k}\left(e^{-kt} - e^{-k_a t}\right)$	This equation is used to calculate the serum concentration at any time (t) after a single oral dose
Multiple intravenous bolus injections (a) $Cp_{ss_t} = Cp° \dfrac{\left(e^{-kt}\right)}{\left(1 - e^{-k\tau}\right)}$	This equation is used to calculate the serum concentration at any time (t) within a dosing interval at steady state following multiple bolus intravenous dosing
(b) $Cp_{ss_{max}} = Cp° \dfrac{1}{\left(1 - e^{-k\tau}\right)}$	This equation is used to calculate the maximum serum concentration at state, i.e. $t = 0$. To estimate the peak serum concentration then (t) must be selected, e.g. for gentamicin t peak = 1 hour
(c) $Cp_{ss_{min}} = Cp° \dfrac{e^{-k\tau}}{\left(1 - e^{-k\tau}\right)}$	This equation is used to calculate the minimum

TABLE 26.1 Basic pharmacokinetic equations – cont'd

Pharmacokinetic equation	Comments on the clinical use of the equations
	concentration at steady state following multiple intravenous bolus dosing
Intravenous infusion prior to steady state $$Cp_t = \frac{DS}{\tau Cl}(1 - e^{-kt})$$	This equation can be used to calculate a serum concentration at any time (t) after starting an intravenous infusion
Intravenous infusion at steady state $$Cp_{ss} = \frac{DS}{\tau Cl}$$	This equation can be used to calculate the steady-state serum concentration during an intravenous infusion
Multiple oral dosing at steady state $$Cp_{ss} = \frac{Cp^\circ k_a}{(k_a - k)}\left[\frac{e^{-kt}}{(1-e^{-k\tau})} - \frac{e^{-k_a t}}{(1-e^{-k_a \tau})}\right]$$	This equation is used to calculate a concentration any time (t) within a dosing interval, at steady state following oral dosing
The maximum concentration is given by: $$Cp_{ss_{max}} = \frac{Cp^\circ k_a}{(k_a - k)}\left[\frac{e^{-kt_{ss_{max}}}}{(1-e^{-k\tau})} - \frac{e^{-k_a t_{ss_{max}}}}{(1-e^{-k_a \tau})}\right]$$	This equation calculates the peak concentration at steady state following oral dosing
The time at which the maximum concentration occurs: $$t_{ss_{max}} = \frac{1}{(k_a - k)}\ln\left[\frac{k_a(1-e^{-k\tau})}{k(1-e^{-k_a \tau})}\right]$$	This equation calculates the time to reach a peak concentration at steady state following oral dosing
The minimum concentration is given by: $$Cp_{ss_{min}} = \frac{Cp^\circ k_a}{(k_a - k)}\left[\frac{e^{-k\tau}}{(1-e^{-k\tau})} - \frac{e^{-k_a \tau}}{(1-e^{-k_a \tau})}\right]$$	The minimum or trough concentration at steady state, i.e. at the beginning of a dosage interval
Loading doses $$Ld = \frac{V_d Cp}{SF}$$ $$Ld = \frac{V_d(Cp_{desired} - Cp_{observed})}{SF}$$	This equation can be used to calculate loading doses following oral or intravenous administration. Select the target serum concentration usually in the middle of the therapeutic range
The average steady-state concentration (Cp_{ss}) $$Cp_{ss_{min}} = \frac{SF \text{ dose}}{Cl\tau}$$	This equation can be used to calculate maintenance doses (dose/) following oral or intravenous administration

TABLE 26.1 Basic pharmacokinetic equations – cont'd	
Pharmacokinetic equation	Comments on the clinical use of the equations
Time for decay $= \dfrac{\ln Cp_1 - \ln Cp_2}{k}$	Toxic level decay equation which assumes first-order elimination, complete absorption and distribution

Cp_t is serum drug concentration at any time (t); $Cp°$ is initial serum concentration at time 0h; k is first-order elimination rate concentration; k_a is first-order absorption rate constant; V_d is volume of distribution; Cl is total body clearance; S is salt factor; F is bioavailability; Cp_{ss_t} is steady-state serum concentration at any time (t); Cp_{ss} is average steady-state serum concentration; $Cp_{ss_{min}}$ is trough or minimum serum concentration at steady state; $Cp_{ss_{max}}$ is peak or maximum serum concentration at steady state; $t_{ss_{max}}$ is time of peak serum concentration at steady state; D is dose; Ld is loading dose; τ is dosing interval; ln is natural log.

PHENYTOIN TOXIC LEVEL DECAY

To decay a toxic plasma concentration Cp^1 to a desired plasma concentration Cp:

$$Cp^1_{t_{decay}} = \frac{[K_m \times \ln(Cp)] + (Cp^1 - Cp)}{V_m / V_d},$$

where t_{decay} = time (days) to allow Cp^1 to fall to Cp; ln = natural log.

PHENYTOIN SERUM LEVELS IN THE PRESENCE OF ALTERED PLASMA PROTEIN BINDING

To calculate a 'corrected' Cp_{ss} for a patient with a low serum albumin:

$$Cp_{adjusted} = \frac{Cp^*}{(1-\alpha)\left(\dfrac{P^1}{P}\right) + \alpha}$$

where $Cp_{adjusted}$ = plasma concentration that would be expected if the patient had a normal serum albumin; Cp^* = steady-state serum level observed; P^1 = serum albumin concentration observed; P = 'normal' serum albumin concentration, 40g/l; α = phenytoin free fraction (0.1).

To calculate a 'corrected' Cp_{ss} for a patient with both uraemia and hypoalbuminaemia:

$$Cp_{adjusted} = \frac{Cp^*}{(1-\alpha)\left(0.44\dfrac{P^1}{P}\right) + \alpha}$$

where 0.44 = empirical adjustment factor and $\alpha = 0.2$.

PHARMACOKINETIC APPLICATIONS

Table 26.1 summarises the basic pharmacokinetic equations that can be applied on the wards.

CHAPTER 27

Comparative doses of corticosteroids

Apart from the dose differences of corticosteroids there are qualitative differences in their actions. Consequently, side-effects may occur when one steroid is substituted for another. For further details see Table 27.1.

TABLE 27.1 Comparative doses of corticosteroids for systemic use based on glucocorticoid properties

Corticosteroid	Dose (mg)
Betamethasone	0.7
Cortisone	25
Dexamethasone	0.75
Hydrocortisone	20
Methylprednisolone	4
Prednisolone	5
Prednisone	5
Triamcinolone	4

CHAPTER 28

Calculating body surface area from weight and height

The nomogram shown in Figure 28.1 may be used to calculate the body surface area from the weight and height of the patient. Mark the patient's weight and height on the chart, and then draw a line between the two points. Read off the surface area from the point where this line crosses the middle line.

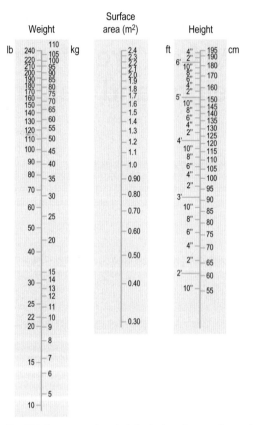

Fig. 28.1 A nomogram for calculating body surface area from weight and height.

CHAPTER 29

Abbreviations

A & E accident and emergency

ABG arterial blood gases

ACE angiotensin-converting enzyme

ACTH adrenocorticotrophic hormone

ADH antidiuretic hormone

AF atrial fibrillation

AIDS acquired immunodeficiency syndrome

ALL acute lymphoblastic leukaemia

AML acute myeloid leukaemia

ANF antinuclear factor

APTT activated partial thromboplastin time

ARDS adult respiratory distress syndrome

ARF acute renal failure

ASD atrial septal defect

ASO antistreptolysin O

AST aspartate transaminase

ATN acute tubular necrosis

AXR abdominal X-ray

BBB bundle branch block

BD bis diurnale (twice a day)

BMT bone marrow transplant

BNF *British National Formulary*

BP blood pressure

BTS blood transfusion service

CABG coronary artery bypass graft

CAH chronic active hepatitis

CAPD chronic ambulatory peritoneal dialysis

CCF congestive cardiac failure

CCU coronary care unit

CLL chronic lymphatic leukaemia

CML chronic myeloid leukaemia

CMV cytomegalovirus

CNS central nervous system

COP colloid osmotic pressure

COPD chronic obstructive pulmonary disease

CSF cerebrospinal fluid

CSU catheter specimen of urine

CT computed tomography

CVA cerebrovascular accident

CVP central venous pressure

CVS cardiovascular system

CXR chest X-ray

DIC disseminated intravascular coagulation

DIP distal interphalangeal

DM diabetes mellitus

DVT deep venous thrombosis

EBV Epstein–Barr virus

ECF extracellular fluid

ECG electrocardiogram

EEG electroencephalogram

ELISA enzyme-linked immunosorbent assay

EMG electromyography

ERCP endoscopic retrograde cholangiopancreatography

ESR erythrocyte sedimentation rate

FBC full blood count

FEV_1 forced expiratory volume in 1 second

FFP fresh frozen plasma

FSH follicle-stimulating hormone

FVC forced vital capacity

GABA gamma-aminobutyric acid

GFR glomerular filtration rate

GGTP gamma-glutamyl transpeptidase

GH growth hormone

GI gastrointestinal

GIT gastrointestinal tract

GKI glucose/potassium/insulin

GN glomerulonephritis

GVH graft-versus-host disease

HBV hepatitis B virus

HIV human immunodeficiency virus

HLA human leukocyte antigen

HSV herpes simplex virus

IBD inflammatory bowel disease

IBW ideal body weight

ICF intracellular fluid

ICP intracranial pressure

IHD ischaemic heart disease

IM infectious mononucleosis

IMHP intramuscular high potency

INR international normalised ratio

ISQ idem status quo (i.e. unchanged)

ITP idiopathic thrombocyto-penic purpura

IVC inferior vena cava

IVHP intravenous high potency

IVU intravenous urography

JVP jugular venous pressure

KCCT kaolin cephalin clotting time

LA left atrium

LBBB left bundle branch block

LFTs liver function tests

LH luteinising hormone

LIF left iliac fossa

LV left ventricle

LVF left ventricular failure

MCHC mean corpuscular haemoglobin concentration

MCV mean corpuscular volume

MEN multiple endocrine neoplasia

MI myocardial infarction

MIBG meta-iodo benzyl guanidine

NSAID non-steroidal anti-inflammatory drugs

OGTT oral glucose tolerance test

OM olim mane (once daily in the morning)

PA pulmonary artery, pernicious anaemia

PCV packed cell volume

PDA patent ductus arteriosus

PE pulmonary embolism

PEEP positive end-expiratory pressure

PEFR peak expiratory flow rate

PFTs pulmonary function tests

PIP proximal interphalangeal

PR per rectum

PRN pro re nata (as required)

PRV polycythaemia rubra vera

PT prothrombin time

PTC percutaneous transhepatic cholangiogram

PTH parathyroid hormone

PTT partial thromboplastin time

PUO pyrexia of unknown origin

QDS quater diurnale summen-sum (four times a day)

RA rheumatoid arthritis

RAST radioallergosorbent test

RBBB right bundle branch block

RCC red cell count

RIF right iliac fossa

RVF right ventricular failure

SLE systemic lupus erythematosus

ST sinus tachycardia

SVC superior vena cava

SVT supraventricular tachycardia

TB tuberculosis

TBG thyroid-binding globulin

TDS ter diurnale summensum (three times a day)

TIA transient ischaemic attack

TIBC total iron-binding capacity

TIP terminal interphalangeal

TPN total parenteral nutrition

TRH thyrotrophin-releasing hormone

TSH thyroid-stimulating hormone

U&E urea and electrolytes

URTI upper respiratory tract infection

US ultrasound

UTI urinary tract infection

VF ventricular fibrillation

VSD ventricular septal defect

VT ventricular tachycardia

VWF von Willebrand factor

WBC white blood count

WPW Wolff–Parkinson–White

INDEX